# Clinical Decision Making™ Series

## Published

*Friedman:*
   Obstetrical Decision Making
*Friedman:*
   Gynecological Decision Making
*Holt, Mattox and Gates:*
   Decision Making in Otolaryngology

## Forthcoming

*Berman:*
   Pediatric Decision Making
*Don:*
   Decision Making in Critical Care
*Dubovsky, Feiger and Eiseman:*
   Decision Making in Psychiatry
*Goldstone:*
   Decision Making in Vascular Surgery
*Korones:*
   Neonatal Decision Making
*Montgomery:*
   Decision Making in Emergency Cardiology
*Resnick, Caldamone, and Spirnak:*
   Urological Decision Making
*Wheeler, Feinstein, Scott:*
   Decision Making in Radiology

*Consulting Editor:* Ben Eiseman, M.D.

# Orthopaedic Decision Making

## ROBERT W. BUCHOLZ, M.D.

*Associate Professor*
*Division of Orthopaedic Surgery*
*Southwestern Medical School*
*The University of Texas Health*
*Science Center at Dallas*
*Dallas, Texas*

## FREDERICK G. LIPPERT, III, M.D.

*Associate Professor*
*Department of Orthopaedics*
*University of Washington School of Medicine*

*Chief, Department of Orthopaedics*
*Seattle Veterans Administration Hospital*
*Seattle, Washington*

## DENNIS R. WENGER, M.D.

*Associate Professor*
*Division of Orthopaedic Surgery*
*Southwestern Medical School*
*The University of Texas Health*
*Science Center at Dallas*

*Assistant Chief of Staff*
*Texas Scottish Rite Hospital for Crippled Children*
*Dallas, Texas*

## MARYBETH EZAKI, M.D.

*Assistant Professor*
*Division of Orthopaedic Surgery*
*Southwestern Medical School*
*The University of Texas Health*
*Science Center at Dallas*
*Dallas, Texas*

1984

**B.C. Decker Inc.** • Philadelphia • Toronto
**The C.V. Mosby Company** • Saint Louis • Toronto • London

Publisher:      **B.C. Decker Inc.**
                3228 South Service Road
                Burlington, Ontario  L7N 3H8

                **B.C. Decker Inc.**
                Six Penn Center Plaza, Suite 305
                Philadelphia, Pennsylvania  19103

North American and worldwide sales and distribution:

                **The C.V. Mosby Company**
                11830 Westline Industrial Drive
                Saint Louis, Missouri  63141

In Canada:      **The C.V. Mosby Company, Ltd.**
                120 Melford Drive
                Toronto, Ontario  M1B 2X5

Orthopaedic Decision Making                              ISBN 0-941158-10-1

Library of Congress catalog card number:    82-83699

Last digit is print number:  10  9  8  7  6  5  4  3  2  1

# PREFACE

Orthopaedic practice demands repetitive, complex decision making. Confronted with a musculoskeletal problem, the orthopaedist draws upon his understanding of basic medical and surgical principles, his experience, and familiarity with the literature to formulate a reasonable plan for diagnosis and therapy. All decisions are necessarily influenced by nonscientific considerations such as limited facilities, patient noncompliance, and financial constraints as well as the current limitations of orthopaedic science. Despite these impediments, we all strive for purism in our decision making.

Basic orthopaedic decision making is often muddled by the constant deluge of new information, recent innovations, and unfortunately, faddish techniques. This book of decision trees or algorithms may be viewed as a return to basics. Each chapter covers an orthopaedic problem which is analyzed diagrammatically, stressing the critical variables in arriving at a diagnosis or therapy. Principles and rules, not specific techniques, are emphasized. The algorithmic approach forces the reader to think systematically; even if he disagrees with the fundamental preferences of the author, the book will have served its purpose. Indeed, this educational exercise will be most valuable if it stimulates the reader to construct his own decision trees based on his experience, capabilities, and practice setting.

Four orthopaedic specialty areas, reflecting the interests and expertise of the authors, are covered: trauma, adult reconstruction, pediatric orthopaedics, and the hand. Other topics such as sports medicine, musculoskeletal oncology, and rehabilitation receive proportionately less coverage. The authors have attempted to convey the accepted standard of care but naturally, the algorithms manifest their biases to a degree. References have been carefully selected to provide a comprehensive overview of the subject.

It is hoped that this text will assist all individuals who care for patients with extremity and spinal disorders. As educators involved in university training programs, we have consciously targeted the work for residents in orthopaedics. Other medical specialists, especially general surgeons, emergency room physicians, plastic surgeons, and pediatricians, as well as general practitioners, may find this systematic approach to orthopaedics useful. It may also serve as a basis for review prior to board certification and recertification in orthopaedics.

We wish to gratefully acknowledge Cynthia Turner for her medical illustrations; Lisa Sloan, Carol Foster, and Cynthia Buchanan for their assiduous handling of secretarial duties; and Brian Decker for his seemingly endless patience with us.

Robert W. Bucholz, M.D.
Frederick G. Lippert, III, M.D.
Dennis R. Wenger, M.D.
Marybeth Ezaki, M.D.

# CONTENTS

## ORTHOPAEDIC TRAUMA

### ROBERT W. BUCHOLZ, M.D.

# ADULT ORTHOPAEDICS

## FREDERICK G. LIPPERT, III, M.D.

## CHILDREN'S ORTHOPAEDICS

### DENNIS R. WENGER, M.D.

# HAND SURGERY

## MARYBETH EZAKI, M.D.

# INTRODUCTION

This text represents one of a series of books on surgical decision making. Medical educators are constantly searching for innovative and improved teaching techniques. Algorithms and decision trees, common tools employed in the business world, have been slow to appear in their application to medicine. This is an initial effort to portray diagrammatically current orthopaedic decision making. Future refinements, embellishments, and digressions will be required, as diagnostic and therapeutic modalities increase in sophistication and the science of orthopaedic surgery advances.

Each chapter is presented as an algorithm. The algorithmic heading may be a patient's symptom (the "sprained ankle", heel pain, febrile child with limb pain, altered sensation in the hand) or a musculoskeletal sign (knee instability, chronic knee effusion, toeing in and out in the child). The resultant algorithm cascades down through additional pertinent history, physical findings, and laboratory examinations to end in a differential diagnosis. Therapeutic algorithms, alternatively, commence with a given diagnosis (acromioclavicular dislocation, degenerative arthritis of the hip, slipped capital femoral epiphysis, bite wounds) and flow through variables which influence decisions on therapy. Most trauma algorithms, as would be expected, fall into this latter group, while the reconstructive, pediatric, and hand decision trees furnish a mix of diagnostic and therapeutic problems.

The algorithms are structured so that they may be used independently of the comments. The headings at each branch are self-explanatory with specific treatment recommendations enclosed in boxes. Tangential loops along branches are intended to remind the reader of common variants in a given decision. The comments clarify and expand the information in the algorithm. Distinctions, guidelines, and exceptions to rules, not to be viewed as hedging, are offered in the comments. The bibliography is selected to both substantiate critical branches in the decision tree and provide the reader with sources of the detailed information. Use of the listed references is strongly encouraged.

# PRINCIPLES OF FRACTURE MANAGEMENT

## COMMENTS

A.  All life-threatening injuries take precedence over any fracture or dislocation. Resuscitative measures aimed at monitoring and stabilizing vital signs should be performed on an emergency basis. Hemorrhage into fracture sites and surrounding soft tissues may exceed 2 units in closed femoral fractures, and 7 to 8 units after unstable pelvic fractures. Blood loss secondary to open fractures is unpredictable.

B.  The status of the soft tissues profoundly influences the ideal treatment of any fracture. The extremity must be inspected circumferentially to reveal any break in the skin. Distal neurovascular function should be carefully documented with any abnormalities appropriately evaluated. Occult injuries to the adjacent joints are best detected by physical examination. Splint the extremity in neutral position. Manipulative realignment of the limb prior to diagnostic radiographs is only warranted if there is severe neurovascular compromise from an angulated fracture.

C.  The key to accurate diagnosis is correlation of the radiographs with the physical findings. The treating physician, not the radiologist, is thus responsible for the definitive diagnosis. Special, nonstandard radiographic views such as obliques, stress views, and tomographs aid in clarifying equivocal cases. Stress fractures may be diagnosed early with scintigraphy.

D.  All open fractures should be treated aggressively. Broad spectrum antibiotics, generally a cephalosporin, should be administered as early as possible. Thorough debridement in the operating room is mandatory. The presence of gross contamination or major soft tissue defects may alter the ideal treatment of a given fracture.

E.  Controversy surrounds what constitutes the preferred treatment of many fractures. With the advent of new techniques and implants, fracture care is a rapidly evolving art.[1,2,3] Therefore, the algorithms which follow necessarily reflect the current preference of the author.

## REFERENCES

1.  Rockwood C, Green D. Fractures. Philadelphia: JB Lippincott, 1975.
2.  Muller M, Allgower M, Schneider R, Willenegger H. *Manual of Internal Fixation*. Berlin: Springer-Verlag, 2nd edition, 1979.
3.  Mears D. External Skeletal Fixation. Baltimore: Williams & Wilkins, 1983.

FRACTURE AND/OR DISLOCATION

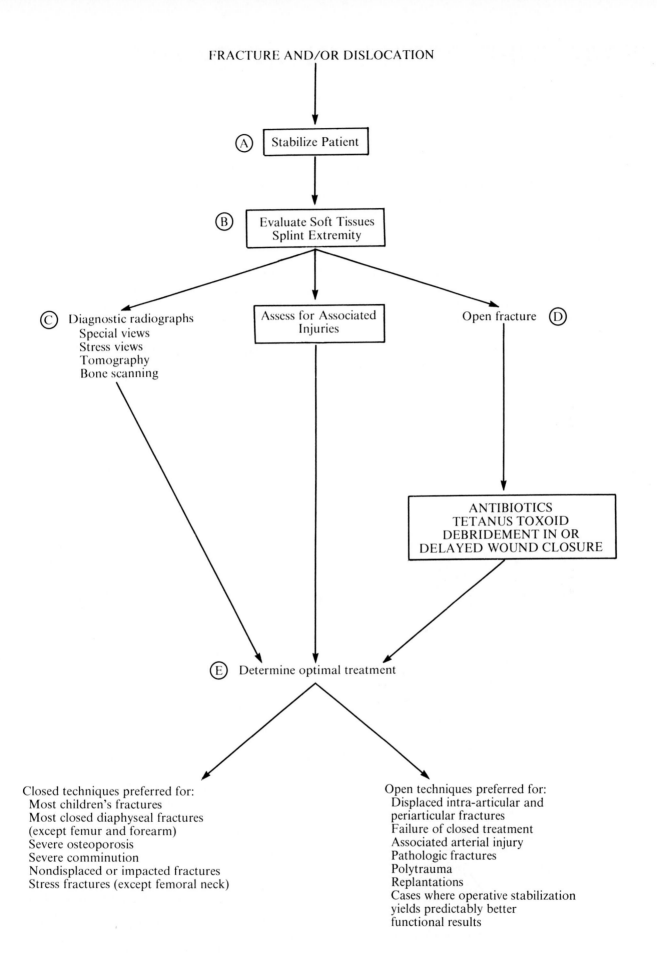

(A) Stabilize Patient

(B) Evaluate Soft Tissues
Splint Extremity

(C) Diagnostic radiographs
Special views
Stress views
Tomography
Bone scanning

Assess for Associated
Injuries

Open fracture (D)

ANTIBIOTICS
TETANUS TOXOID
DEBRIDEMENT IN OR
DELAYED WOUND CLOSURE

(E) Determine optimal treatment

Closed techniques preferred for:
Most children's fractures
Most closed diaphyseal fractures
(except femur and forearm)
Severe osteoporosis
Severe comminution
Nondisplaced or impacted fractures
Stress fractures (except femoral neck)

Open techniques preferred for:
Displaced intra-articular and
periarticular fractures
Failure of closed treatment
Associated arterial injury
Pathologic fractures
Polytrauma
Replantations
Cases where operative stabilization
yields predictably better
functional results

# FRACTURE OF THE ATLANTOAXIAL COMPLEX

## COMMENTS

A. The radiographic signs of atlantoaxial injuries are often subtle. The prevertebral soft tissue shadow on the lateral radiograph should be less than 5 mm wide at C2 and 10 mm wide in front of the ring of the atlas. Localized increases in the soft tissue shadow width may signify an occult fracture or subluxation.

B. Polytomography is rarely indicated in the routine evaluation of atlantoaxial injuries. Occasionally the detection and categorization of nondisplaced odontoid fractures necessitates its use.

C. CT scans are especially helpful in identifying and evaluating Jefferson fractures and atlantoaxial rotatory subluxation.

D. Spreading of the lateral masses of the atlas of greater than 7 mm on the open-mouth odontoid view indicates probable transverse ligament disruption.[1]

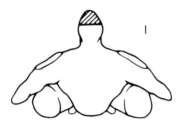

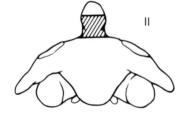

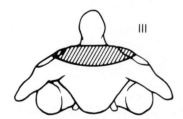

Anderson-D'Alonzo classification of odontoid fractures.

E. Healing of the various components of a Jefferson fracture can be evaluated by CT scanning. The status of the transverse ligament is determined by lateral flexion-extension radiographs.[2] Nonunion of either the anterior ring or posterior ring fractures associated with transverse ligament disruption may require special fusion constructs to restore upper cervical spine stability.[3]

F. The Anderson-D'Alonzo classification (see figure) of odontoid fractures is useful in predicting the likelihood of fracture union with nonoperative treatment.[4] Type III fractures extend into the cancellous bone of the axis and have an excellent prognosis with adequate external immobilization. Type II fractures through the body or base of the odontoid have an incidence of nonunion reported at between 30 and 60%.

G. Controversy surrounds the ideal treatment of type II odontoid fractures.[5] Such variables as patient age, fracture obliquity and displacement, associated injuries, and patient preference must be considered.

H. Bilateral pedicle fractures of the axis (hangman's fracture, traumatic spondylolisthesis of the axis) are usually associated with variable injury to the C2–C3 interspace anteriorly and the atlantoaxial membrane posteriorly. Interruption of the posterior longitudinal ligament allows significant horizontal translation of the cervicocranium on C3, resulting in neurologic damage.[6]

I. Absolute prerequisites for obtaining flexion-extension radiographs include: (1) absence of any demonstrable neurologic deficit, (2) absence of an altered state of consciousness, including intoxication, and (3) ability of the patient to actively flex and extend his neck without assistance. If adequate flexion-extension views are unobtainable, the fracture must be managed as a potentially unstable lesion.[7]

J. Only intermediate class orthoses (e.g., Yale brace, somi-brace, four-poster brace, or cervicothoracic orthosis) should be used. Soft cervical collars provide insufficient immobilization of the neck.[8]

## REFERENCES

1. Spence K, Decker S, Sell K. Bursting atlantal fracture associated with rupture of the transverse ligament. J Bone Joint Surg. 1970; 52A:543.
2. Fielding J, VanCochran G, Lawsing J, Hohl M. Tears of the transverse ligament of the atlas. J Bone Joint Surg. 1974; 56A:1683.

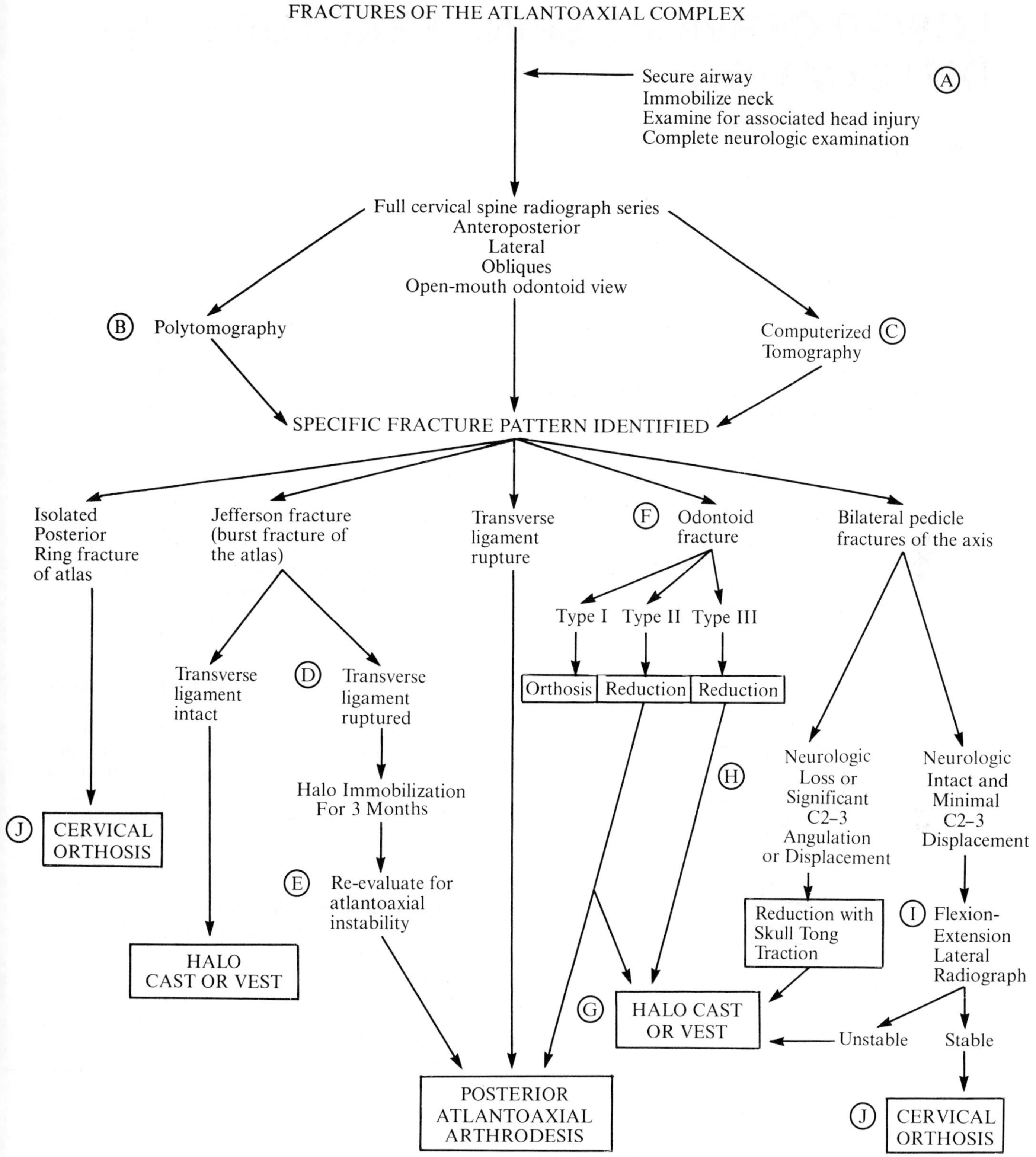

# FRACTURES OF THE ATLANTOAXIAL COMPLEX

(A)
Secure airway
Immobilize neck
Examine for associated head injury
Complete neurologic examination

↓

Full cervical spine radiograph series
Anteroposterior
Lateral
Obliques
Open-mouth odontoid view

(B) Polytomography
(C) Computerized Tomography

→ SPECIFIC FRACTURE PATTERN IDENTIFIED

- Isolated Posterior Ring fracture of atlas
- Jefferson fracture (burst fracture of the atlas)
- Transverse ligament rupture
- (F) Odontoid fracture
- Bilateral pedicle fractures of the axis

**Jefferson fracture:**
- Transverse ligament intact
- (D) Transverse ligament ruptured → Halo Immobilization For 3 Months → (E) Re-evaluate for atlantoaxial instability

**Odontoid fracture:** Type I, Type II, Type III
| Orthosis | Reduction | Reduction |

(H)

**Bilateral pedicle fractures of the axis:**
- Neurologic Loss or Significant C2–3 Angulation or Displacement → Reduction with Skull Tong Traction
- Neurologic Intact and Minimal C2–3 Displacement → (I) Flexion-Extension Lateral Radiograph → Unstable / Stable

(J) CERVICAL ORTHOSIS

HALO CAST OR VEST

(G) HALO CAST OR VEST

POSTERIOR ATLANTOAXIAL ARTHRODESIS

(J) CERVICAL ORTHOSIS

3. Schlike L, Callahan R. A rational approach to burst fractures of the atlas. Clin Orthop Rel Res. 1981; 154:18.
4. Anderson L, D'Alonzo R. Fractures of the odontoid process of the axis. J Bone Joint Surg. 1974; 56A:1663.
5. Southwick W. Management of fractures of the dens. J Bone Joint Surg. 1980; 62A:482.
6. Bucholz R. Unstable hangman's fractures. Clin Orthop Rel Res. 1981; 154:119.
7. Brashear H, Venters G, Preston E. Fractures of the neural arch of the axis. J Bone Joint Surg. 1975; 57A:879.
8. Johnson R, Hart D, Simmons E, Ramsby G, Southwick W. Cervical orthoses—study comparing their effectiveness in restricting cervical motion in normal subjects. J Bone Joint Surg. 1977; 59A:332.

# LOWER CERVICAL SPINE FRACTURE OR DISLOCATION

## COMMENTS

A. All polytrauma patients with altered states of consciousness and all patients with pain or point tenderness in the neck warrant a diagnosis of possible cervical spine fracture or dislocation. If the emergency cross-table lateral radiograph is normal or equivocal, a full cervical spine series is required. The entire cervical spine from the occiput to C7 must be adequately visualized on lateral radiographs, often necessitating a swimmers view of the cervicothoracic junction. Elective cervical tomography assists in detecting fractures of the pedicles, lamina, and facet joints. As in upper cervical spine injuries, the absolute prerequisites for flexion-extension radiographs include an unaltered mental status, the absence of any neurologic symptoms or signs, and the capability of the patient to flex and extend actively without any manipulation by the physician. Occult ligamentous injuries may be disclosed by flexion-extension views, which are mainly indicated in cases of presumptive stable fracture patterns.

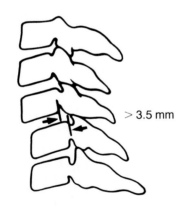

> 3.5 mm

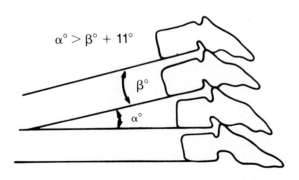

$\alpha° > \beta° + 11°$

$\beta°$

$\alpha°$

Criteria for lower cervical spine instability.

B. An unstable cervical spine injury is one in which there is sufficient osseous or ligamentous disruption so that under physiologic loads, displacement of the spinal elements results in nerve root or spinal cord damage. Quantitative measures of spine stability are imprecise. Generally, either a horizontal translation of greater than 3.5 mm of one vertebral body on an adjacent vertebra or an angulation between two vertebrae of 11° more than contiguous vertebra implies probable instability.[1] All cervical spine fractures should be presumed unstable until definitively proved otherwise.

C. Stable patterns include isolated compression fractures of the vertebral body, lateral mass fractures, spinous process fractures, and most fractures secondary to penetrating neck trauma. Cervical pain and muscular spasm may prevent adequate flexion and extension during diagnostic radiographs. Follow-up flexion-extension radiographs are thus required to rule out unsuspected ligamentous injuries.

D. With careful monitoring of neurologic symptoms and signs, closed reduction is attempted with skull tong traction, occasionally supplemented with manual manipulation under radiographic control. All cases with demonstrable neurologic loss or grossly unstable fracture patterns need emergency closed reduction. The required traction weight, ranging up to 35 lb for C7–T1 dislocations, varies with the fracture level.[2]

E. The inconsistent healing of posterior ligamentous tears gives rise to a high incidence of chronic spinal instability.

F. The posterior surgical approach is preferred in nearly all cases necessitating open reduction or fusion, or both. It permits reduction of jumped facets under direct visualization, provides a more rigid fusion construct, and minimizes further surgical compromise of the supporting spinal structures.

G. Major osseous injuries generally heal without the need for surgical fusion. Satisfactory alignment during healing can be achieved with traction or halo immobilization. Prolonged traction treatment is the less attractive alternative because of the complications of bed rest, the need for lengthy hospitalization, and the delays in commencing rehabilitation of the patient with spinal cord injury. If properly utilized, the halo device provides sufficient stabilization in most cases for early mobilization of the patient.[3]

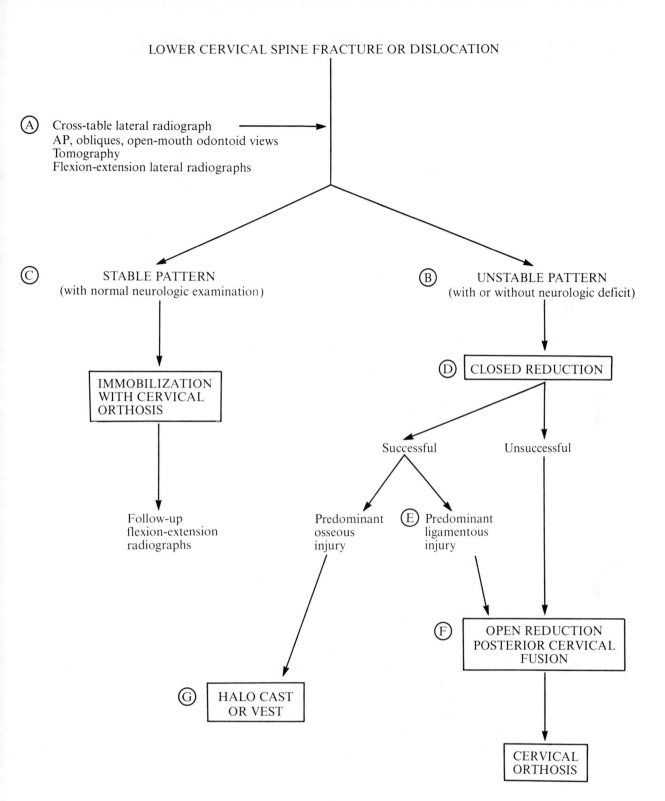

LOWER CERVICAL SPINE FRACTURE OR DISLOCATION

(A) Cross-table lateral radiograph
AP, obliques, open-mouth odontoid views
Tomography
Flexion-extension lateral radiographs

(C) STABLE PATTERN
(with normal neurologic examination)

(B) UNSTABLE PATTERN
(with or without neurologic deficit)

IMMOBILIZATION
WITH CERVICAL
ORTHOSIS

(D) CLOSED REDUCTION

Successful                    Unsuccessful

Follow-up
flexion-extension
radiographs

Predominant        (E) Predominant
osseous                 ligamentous
injury                     injury

(F) OPEN REDUCTION
POSTERIOR CERVICAL
FUSION

(G) HALO CAST
OR VEST

CERVICAL
ORTHOSIS

## REFERENCES

1. White A, Johnson R, Panjabi M, Southwick W. Biomechanical analysis of clinical stability in the cervical spine. Clin Orthop Rel Res. 1975; 109:85–96.
2. Johnson R, Southwick W. Surgical approaches to the spine. In *The Spine*. Rothman R, Simeone F, eds. Philadelphia, WB Saunders. 1975; 1:69–132.
3. Nickel V, Perry J, Garrett A, Heppenstall M. The halo-A spinal skeletal traction device. J Bone Joint Surg. 1968; 50A:1400.

# THORACOLUMBAR FRACTURE AND DISLOCATION

## COMMENTS

A. Hyperflexion forces cause most thoracolumbar injuries, approximately half of which occur at the thoracolumbar junction. All resuscitative and diagnostic measures performed prior to and during radiography of the spine must be done with the patient immobilized in a supine position. Plain AP and lateral radiographs are often of poor quality and fail to visualize adequately all spinal elements. CT scanning has replaced polytomography as the best adjunctive test for defining spinal pathology.

B. Nearly all major thoracolumbar injuries result in a vertebral body fracture. The concomitant posterior element injury is usually trivial, often merely a ligamentous sprain. If there is sufficient posterior osseous or ligamentous disruption to permit significant spinal displacement with real or potential neurologic compromise, the injury is defined as unstable.[1] Unless there is gross spinal angulation or translation on the diagnostic radiographs or a presenting neurologic deficit, instability may be difficult to verify. CT scanning helps, but no quantitative guidelines for stability are universally accepted. Most classification schemes are based on mechanisms of injury.[2] Stable injuries generally include isolated compression and wedge fractures of the vertebral body, rare hyperextension injuries such as traumatic spondylolisthesis, and transverse or spinous process fractures secondary to direct trauma or muscular contractions. Major flexion-distraction, flexion-rotation, burst (axial load), and shear forces lead to unstable fracture patterns.

C. No conventional orthoses provide firm immobilization of the thoracolumbar spine. After a short period of bed rest, symptomatic relief of pain from stable fractures can however be achieved with corsets or spinal braces e.g., Knight-Taylor or Jewett.

D. Flexion-distraction forces to the spine, often experienced by persons wearing lap seat belts during a traffic accident, can cause transverse fractures through both anterior and posterior spinal elements (Chance fracture). Due to the broad cancellous fracture surfaces, these fractures, which commonly occur in the upper or midlumbar region, heal readily and are not prone to late instability.

E. Spinal cord injury with unstable thoracolumbar fracture-dislocations can result from cord compression (burst fractures), cord crushing (flexion-rotation and shear fractures), or cord traction (flexion-distraction dislocations). Decompression of the neural elements is best accomplished by realignment and stabilization of the spine. Open reduction and internal fixation with Harrington instrumentation are preferred to closed techniques, since improved fracture reduction, early patient mobilization and rehabilitation, and decreased hospitalization are usually realized.[3] Laminectomy should be limited to those rare cases with a well-documented progressive neurologic loss. Reduction or extraction of retropulsed posterior body fragments from the neural canal commonly seen in burst fractures can be done through either an anterior or posterolateral approach, depending upon the experience of the surgeon.

The timing of operative treatment and the role of routine spinal arthrodesis remain controversial. In general, unstable patterns with a partial neurologic deficit should be reduced and stabilized immediately, whereas those with no neural deficit or a complete lesion can be surgically stabilized on an elective basis. Bone grafting and fusion are mainly indicated in paraplegic patients and patients with pure ligamentous injuries.

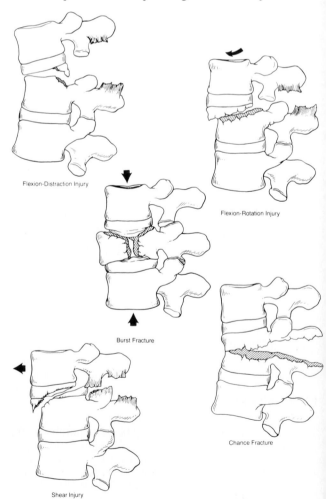

Flexion-Distraction Injury

Flexion-Rotation Injury

Burst Fracture

Chance Fracture

Shear Injury

THORACOLUMBAR INJURY

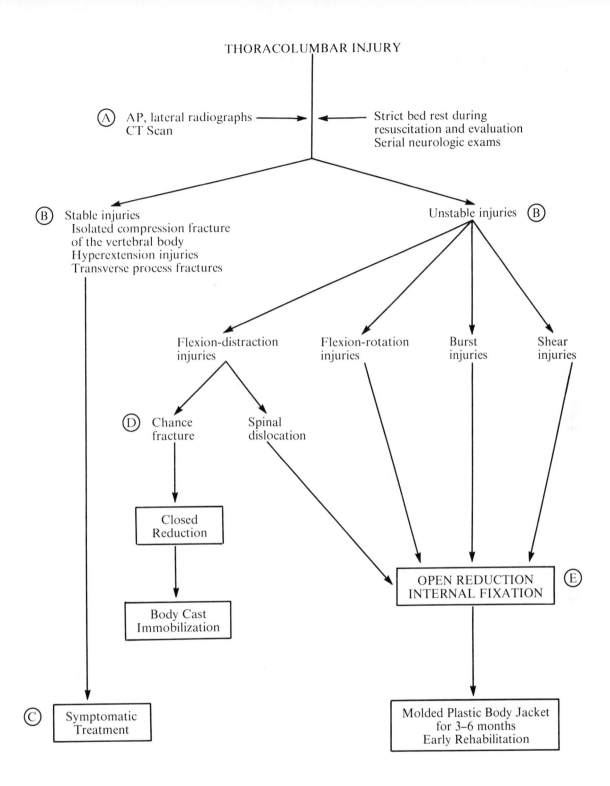

**REFERENCES**

1. Kelly R, Whitesides T. Treatment of lumbodorsal fracture-dislocations. Ann Surg. 1968; 167:705.
2. Holdsworth F. Fractures, dislocations and fracture-dislocations of the spine. J Bone Joint Surg. 1970; 52A:1534.
3. Dickson J, Harrington P, Erwin W. Results of reduction and stabilization of the severely fractured thoracic and lumbar spine. J Bone Joint Surg. 1978; 60A:799.

# FRACTURE OF THE CLAVICLE

## COMMENTS

A. Associated neurovascular injuries can be detected by careful physical examination of the upper extremities.

B. More than 99% of all adult clavicle fractures involve the medial and middle third portions and are managed by closed reduction. Neurovascular complications are rare.

C. Vertically displaced butterfly fragments can occasionally tent the overlying skin to the point of delayed opening of the fracture site. Often these fragments can be gently manipulated to relieve the skin pressure, but in some cases surgical reduction or extraction of the offending fragment is necessary. Rarely, displaced fragments are approached operatively to improve the cosmetic appearance in young females.

D. Neurovascular compromise is usually secondary to narrowing of the space between the clavicle and the first rib by displaced fracture fragments. The vascular injury may involve direct compression of the subclavian artery or vein, thrombosis of the vessels, traumatic aneurysms of the subclavian artery, or, rarely, the development of a subclavian arteriovenous fistula.[1] Brachial plexus injuries may be caused by a traction mechanism or direct compression by an inferiorly displaced distal fragment. Treatment varies depending upon the nature of the neurovascular injury.[1]

E. Anteroposterior radiographic stress views of both shoulders with 10- to 15-lb weights in both hands will document the status of the coracoclavicular ligaments. If the ligaments are lacerated, the proximal fragment will be superiorly displaced by muscle forces and the distal fragment inferiorly displaced by the weight of the arm.

F. With complete coracoclavicular ligament disruption (see figure), there is poor bony apposition and, thus, a propensity to delayed union or nonunion. Open reduction and fixation with a coracoid screw or transacromial pin (similar to the techniques for acromioclavicular separations) will improve the chances for successful union and full return of function.[2]

G. The risks of open reduction and internal fixation of midshaft clavicle fractures are great. All series report high incidences of implant failure, nonunion, and infection. The most common techniques used for stabilization include plates[3] and intramedullary devices.[4]

H. Nearly all adult midshaft clavicle fractures are unstable. Although reduction can frequently be achieved by external manipulation, the maintainence of reduction is impossible by external support alone. However, healed displaced clavicle fractures are compatible with normal shoulder and arm function. The role of external supports is therefore mainly patient comfort. A variety of supports, including figure-of-8 straps, Velpeau dressings, sling and swathes, modified shoulder spicas, and so forth, have been described.[4]

## REFERENCES

1. Howard F, Shafer S. Injuries to the clavicle with neurovascular complications. J Bone Joint Surg. 1965; 47A:1335.
2. Neer C. Fractures of the distal third of the clavicle. Clin Orthop Rel Res. 1968; 58:43.
3. Muller M, Allgower M, Schneider R, Willenegger H. (ed). *Manual of Internal Fixation*. Berlin: Springer-Verlag. 1979; 166–67.
4. Rowe C. An atlas of anatomy and treatment of midclavicular fractures. Clin Orthop Rel Res. 1968; 58:29.

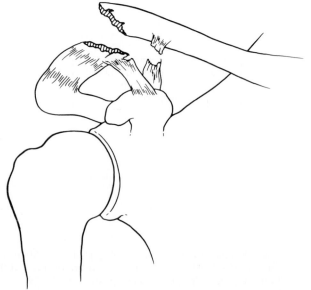

Distal clavicle fracture with disruption of the coracoclavicular ligaments.

# FRACTURE OF THE CLAVICLE

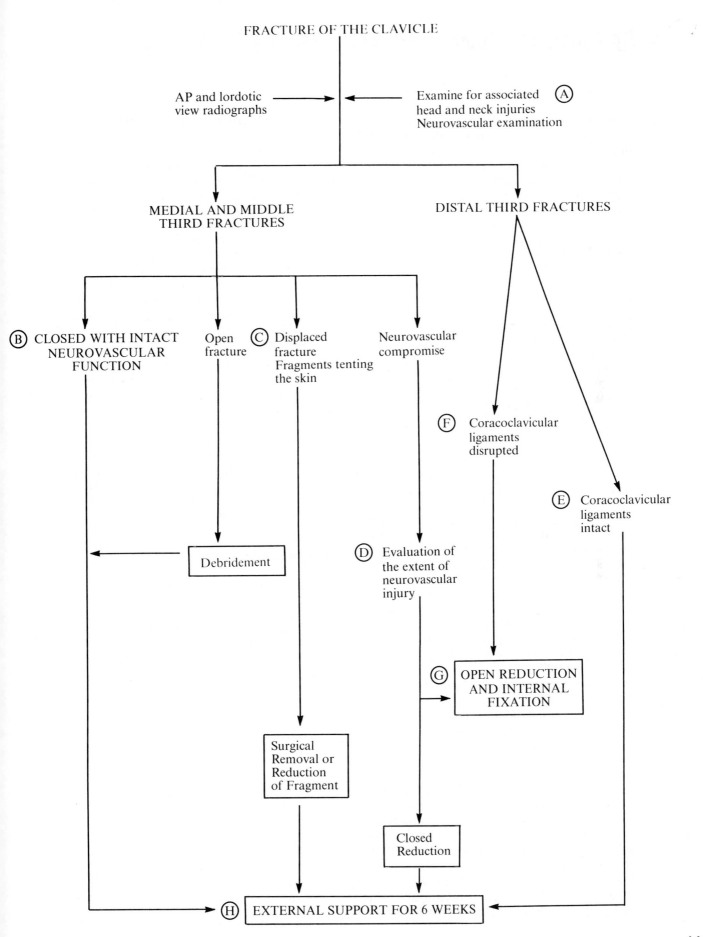

AP and lordotic view radiographs → ← Examine for associated head and neck injuries Neurovascular examination (A)

**MEDIAL AND MIDDLE THIRD FRACTURES**

**DISTAL THIRD FRACTURES**

(B) **CLOSED WITH INTACT NEUROVASCULAR FUNCTION**

Open fracture

(C) Displaced fracture Fragments tenting the skin

Neurovascular compromise

(F) Coracoclavicular ligaments disrupted

(E) Coracoclavicular ligaments intact

Debridement

(D) Evaluation of the extent of neurovascular injury

(G) → **OPEN REDUCTION AND INTERNAL FIXATION**

Surgical Removal or Reduction of Fragment

Closed Reduction

(H) **EXTERNAL SUPPORT FOR 6 WEEKS**

**11**

# STERNOCLAVICULAR DISLOCATION

## COMMENTS

A. The stability of the sternoclavicular joint depends on the supporting ligaments, including the costo-clavicular ligament, the anterior and posterior capsular ligaments, the intra-articular discal ligament, and the interclavicular ligament. Lateral compression forces transmitted through the clavicle may cause anterior or posterior displacement of the medial end of the clavicle, the former being much more common. Lesser trauma results in ligamentous sprains without disruption of the articulation. These mild injuries are easily managed by temporary immobilization of the shoulder. Although the clinical signs of complete anterior or posterior dislocations are usually obvious, their radiographic diagnosis is difficult owing to overlying bony shadows on the AP and lateral views. A 40° cephalic tilt view with the beam aimed at the manubrium demonstrates the joint with minimal superimposition of other thoracic structures.[1] Standard chest radiographs should be routinely ordered to detect associated pulmonary injuries.

B. The vital vascular structures situated behind the joint include the aorta, the superior vena cava, and the right pulmonary artery. Posterior dislocations may compress not only these vessels, but also the lungs, trachea, or esophagus. Nearly one-fourth of patients with posterior sternoclavicular dislocations have a complaint from vessel, esophageal, or pulmonary injury.[2] Physical signs of dyspnea, tachypnea, venous congestion in the neck, and diminished pulses in the ipsilateral arm may be apparent. These symptoms and signs will readily resolve with prompt reduction of the posterior sternoclavicular dislocation. More severe visceral injuries, such as pneumothorax, obviously take precedence over the joint disruption.

C. Reduction may be effected with the patient supine or in a seated position. With counterpressure of a pad between the scapulae, longitudinal traction is applied to the abducted arm. The medial end of the clavicle may be manipulated with direct digital pressure in anterior dislocations or with pulling in posterior dislocations.

The medial clavicular growth plate closes around the age of 25. In children and young adults, types I and II epiphyseal separations may masquerade as sternoclavicular dislocations. Closed reduction of these physeal injuries is occasionally necessary.

D. Anterior dislocations are easy to reduce, but often are unstable. Many operative repairs using combinations of Steinmann pins, muscle releases, and tendinous and ligamentous reconstructions have been described.[1] Because of the major forces acting on the destabilized joint, internal fixation with pins is imperative to hold the corrected position. Owing to serious intraoperative and postoperative complications, including death from migration of Steinmann pins, it is advisable to abstain from placing pins across the sternoclavicular joint.[1] Redisplaced unstable anterior dislocations are thus best treated with only short-term immobilization for pain.

E. Posterior dislocations are stable after closed reduction. In the unusual case necessitating open reduction, internal fixation is not needed and, indeed, should be avoided.

F. Rigid external immobilization of the sternoclavicular joint is impossible. Partial immobilization and pain relief can be achieved with the use of a figure-of-8 harness, a sling, or a clavicular strap.

G. Both reduced and unreduced dislocations may lead infrequently to chronic sternoclavicular degeneration and pain. In the incapacitating case, resection of the end of the clavicle medial to the attachments of the costoclavicular ligaments is preferable to any operative attempt at joint reconstruction.

## REFERENCES

1. Rockwood C. Dislocation of the sternoclavicular joint. In *Fractures*. Edited by Rockwood C and Green D. Philadelphia: JB Lippincott. 1975; 756–787.
2. Worman L, Leagus C. Intrathoracic injury following retrosternal dislocation of the clavicle. J Trauma 1967; 7:416.

STERNOCLAVICULAR DISLOCATION

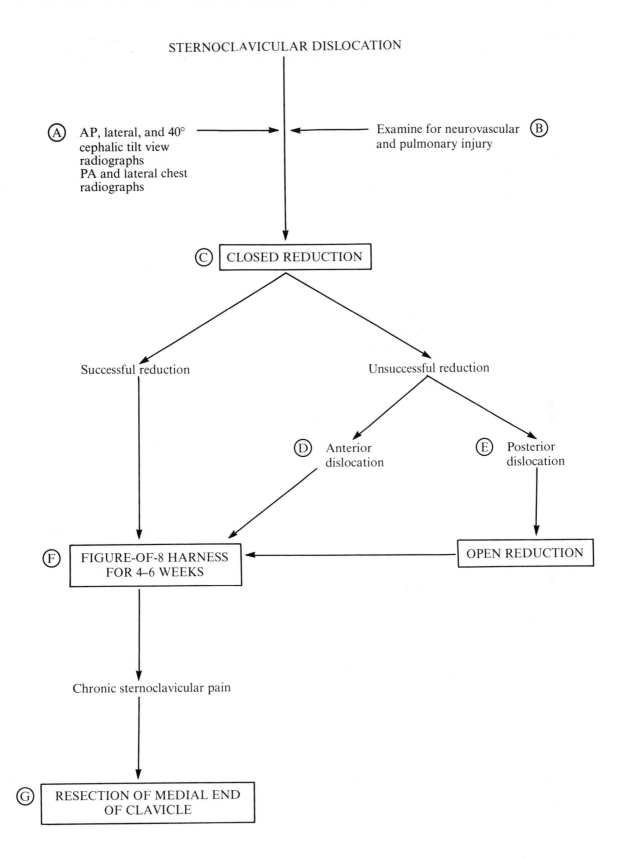

(A) AP, lateral, and 40°
cephalic tilt view
radiographs
PA and lateral chest
radiographs

Examine for neurovascular
and pulmonary injury (B)

(C) CLOSED REDUCTION

Successful reduction

Unsuccessful reduction

(D) Anterior
dislocation

(E) Posterior
dislocation

(F) FIGURE-OF-8 HARNESS
FOR 4–6 WEEKS

OPEN REDUCTION

Chronic sternoclavicular pain

(G) RESECTION OF MEDIAL END
OF CLAVICLE

# ACROMIOCLAVICULAR DISLOCATION

## COMMENTS

A. Classification of acromioclavicular (AC) injuries is based on the degree of disruption of the acromioclavicular and coracoclavicular (CC) ligaments.[1] Tearing of the AC ligaments with sparing of the CC ligaments defines a grade I sprain, with no radiographically apparent joint subluxation. Grade II injuries involve a greater disruption of the joint, with partial tearing of the CC ligaments leading to slight vertical displacement of the distal calvicle. Further complete interruption of the continuity of the CC ligaments permits total AC dislocation (grade III). Radiographic distinction between grade I–II and grade III injuries is essential for appropriate therapeutic decisions. The AC joints are best visualized when the x-ray beam is directed cephalad 10–15° on the AP view. In addition to a resting AP view of both joints, a stress radiograph with 5–10 lb of weight suspended from both wrists should be obtained routinely. Grade III injuries demonstrate vertical displacement of the distal clavicle above the entire height of the joint and an increase in the distance (10–12 mm) between the coracoid process and the inferior border of the clavicle of 5 mm or more.[2]

B. Grade I sprains and grade II subluxations can be managed by sling immobilization for several days, followed by range of motion exercises. Strenuous athletic activity and heavy lifting should be avoided for 3–6 months following grade II separations.

C. Many nonoperative and operative methods have been recommended for grade III AC dislocations. Most techniques devised to maintain reduction by external means have been discarded owing to the risks of skin sloughs. Temporary immobilization of an unreduced dislocation in a sling followed by early motion and rehabilitation results in satisfactory functional recovery in many patients.[3] The prominent end of the distal clavicle is rarely of greater cosmetic concern than the disfiguring scar that follows operative repairs. Complete joint reduction is probably necessary for full functional return, especially in young physically active patients. Surgical reduction and fixation is therefore advisable in all patients under 50 years of age and in older patients with high functional demands. Major soft tissue injury over the anticipated operative site may preclude surgical repair.

D. Numerous operative techniques using combinations of ligament repairs or reconstructions; fixation with pins, cancellous screws, or sutures; and excision of the distal clavicle have been described. All procedures yield comparable long-term results, and thus the more complex operations generally are not warranted. Attention should be focused on debridement of damaged joint tissues, accurate reduction of the AC joint, and rigid internal fixation.[4] Poor operative results usually arise from inadequate fixation leading to postoperative redisplacement of the joint. Although most patients compensate for the loss of normal clavicular rotation, any internal fixation that stabilizes the AC joint can restrict full shoulder abduction and elevation. Routine extraction of all pins and screws is therefore indicated at 6–12 weeks.

E. Chronic AC pain after nonoperative or operative treatment of grade II and III injuries is caused by impingement and degeneration of the joint surfaces. If incapacitating symptoms persist for more than a year, elective excision of the distal 1–2 cm of the clavicle should be considered.

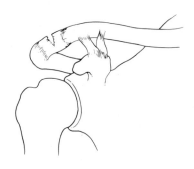

GRADE 1

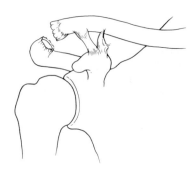

GRADE 2

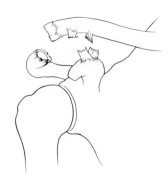

GRADE 3

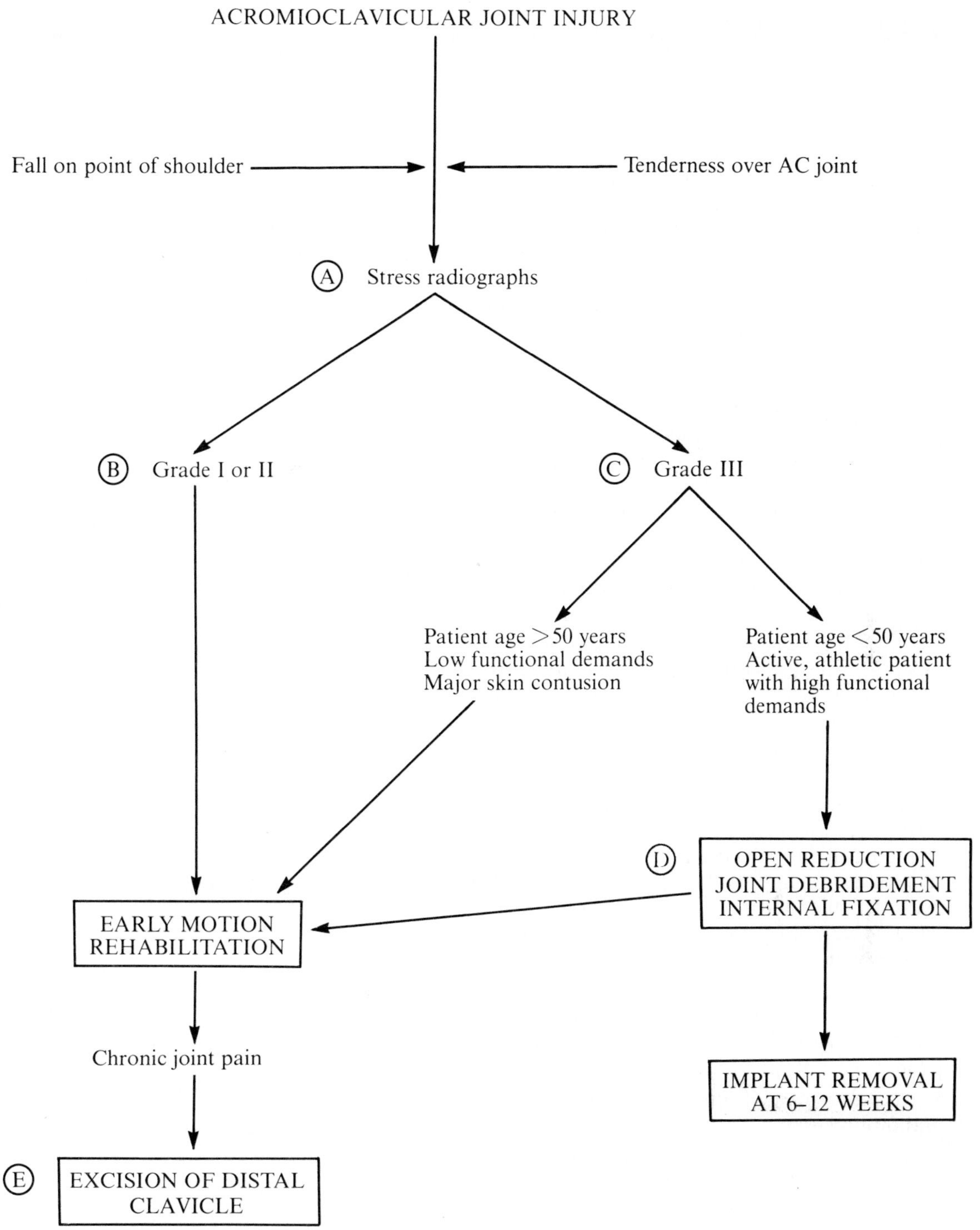

ACROMIOCLAVICULAR JOINT INJURY

Fall on point of shoulder ──────→ ←────── Tenderness over AC joint

(A) Stress radiographs

(B) Grade I or II                    (C) Grade III

                    Patient age > 50 years          Patient age < 50 years
                    Low functional demands          Active, athletic patient
                    Major skin contusion            with high functional
                                                    demands

                                                    (D) OPEN REDUCTION
                                                        JOINT DEBRIDEMENT
                                                        INTERNAL FIXATION

EARLY MOTION
REHABILITATION

Chronic joint pain                                  IMPLANT REMOVAL
                                                    AT 6–12 WEEKS

(E) EXCISION OF DISTAL
    CLAVICLE

**REFERENCES**

1. Tossy J, Mead N, Sigmond H. Acromioclavicular separations: useful and practical classification for treatment. Clin Orthop Rel Res. 1963; 28:111.
2. Rockwood C. Acromioclavicular injuries. In *Fractures*. Edited by Rockwood C, Green D. Philadelphia: J B Lippincott. 1975; 721–756.
3. Imatani R, Hanlon J, Cady G. Acute complete acromioclavicular separation. J Bone Joint Surg. 1975; 57A:328.
4. Weitzman G. Treatment of acute acromioclavicular joint dislocation by a modified Bosworth method. J Bone Joint Surg. 1967; 49A:1167.

# FRACTURE OF THE SCAPULA

## COMMENTS

A. Scapular fractures are generally high-energy injuries sustained in automobile or motorcycle accidents. Common associated injuries to the head, spine, and viscera deserve more immediate attention than the fracture itself. Imatani noted a high incidence of rib fractures (27%), clavicle fractures (23%), pulmonary injuries (23%), and brachial plexus injuries (8%) in his large series of scapular fractures.[1] Every effort, including routine chest radiographs, should be made to detect these serious associated injuries.

B. Scapular body and acromial fractures are well visualized on anteroposterior and tangential radiographic views. Coracoid and glenoid fractures require an axillary view; scapular neck fractures frequently necessitate oblique views for proper delineation of the fracture pattern and displacement.

C. Scapular body and spine fractures are secondary to direct trauma to the posterior aspect of the trunk. Because of a thick muscular envelope, scapular fractures rarely fail to unite; reduction is unnecessary. Healing proceeds rapidly, permitting early mobilization of the shoulder.

D. Two-thirds of all scapular fractures in Imatani's series were localized to the scapular neck. They are generally impacted and thus have a prognosis similar to that of humeral neck fractures. The extra-articular location of the fracture must be documented radiographically to ensure that the glenoid articular surface has remained intact.

E. Isolated coracoid and acromial fractures result from direct trauma. Nonunion and persistent symptoms from such injuries rarely occur.[2]

F. Early range of motion exercises can be instituted after 2–3 weeks of sling or sling-and-swathe immobilization.

G. Displaced acromial fractures impinging on the rotator cuff or the glenohumeral joint should be anatomically reduced and fixed with a screw or Steinmann pin.

H. Anterior or posterior rim fractures of the glenoid frequently accompany shoulder dislocations. These minor avulsion fractures may be ignored during the treatment of the shoulder dislocation. Distinct major articular fractures of the glenoid are secondary to lateral blows to the adducted shoulder.[3] If such a pattern is evident on the axillary radiograph, the shoulder should be reduced and then tested for stability. Persistent displacement of the glenoid fragment or recurrent subluxation of the joint with gentle ranging necessitate open reduction and internal fixation.[4] With adequate restoration and fixation of the glenoid, no further imbrication of the capsule or surrounding musculature is needed to prevent recurrent dislocation of the shoulder.

## REFERENCES

1. Imatani R. Fractures of the scapula: a review of 53 fractures. J Trauma. 1975; 15:473–478.
2. Benton J, Nelson C. Avulsion of the coracoid process in an athlete. J Bone Joint Surg. 1971; 53A:356–358.
3. Aston J, Gregory C. Dislocation of the shoulder with significant fracture of the glenoid. J Bone Joint Surg. 1973; 55A:1531–1533.
4. Muller M, Allgower M, Schneider R, Willenegger H. *Manual of Internal Fixation*. 2nd ed. Berlin: Springer-Verlag. 1979, pp. 164–165.

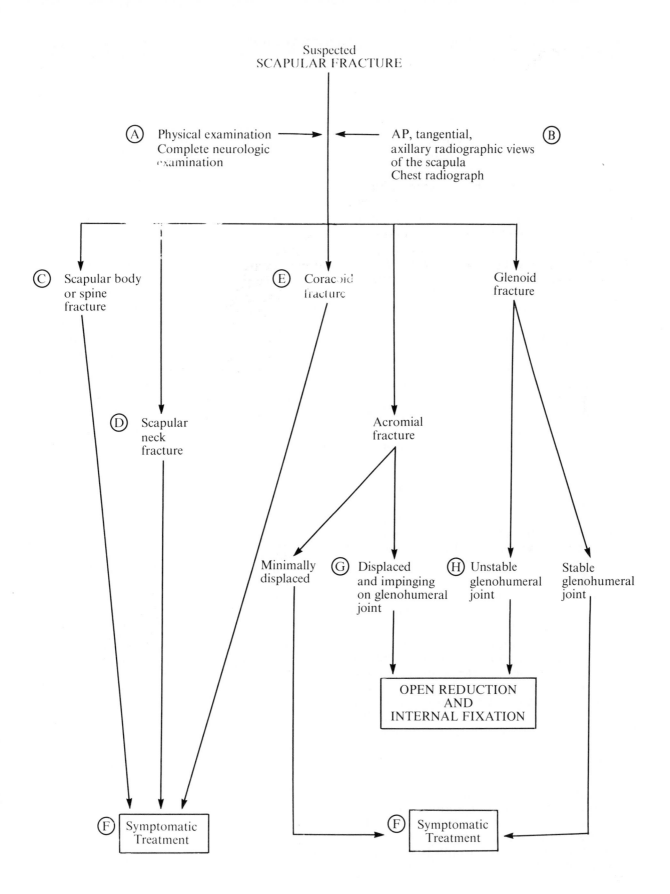

Suspected
SCAPULAR FRACTURE

(A) Physical examination
Complete neurologic
examination

(B) AP, tangential,
axillary radiographic views
of the scapula
Chest radiograph

(C) Scapular body
or spine
fracture

(E) Coracoid
fracture

Glenoid
fracture

(D) Scapular
neck
fracture

Acromial
fracture

Minimally
displaced

(G) Displaced
and impinging
on glenohumeral
joint

(H) Unstable
glenohumeral
joint

Stable
glenohumeral
joint

OPEN REDUCTION
AND
INTERNAL FIXATION

(F) Symptomatic
Treatment

(F) Symptomatic
Treatment

# FRACTURE OF THE PROXIMAL HUMERUS

## COMMENTS

A. Complete assessment of fracture displacement and associated humeral head subluxation or dislocation necessitates biplane radiographs taken at a right angle to one another. Axillary views are especially helpful in evaluating posterior glenohumeral dislocations.

B. Approximately 80 to 90% of all proximal humeral fractures are minimally displaced. In these generally older patients, the surrounding periosteum, capsule, and ligaments maintain the fracture fragments in satisfactory position during the healing phase.

C. Restoration of shoulder function and avoidance of joint adhesions are the primary goals of treatment. Several weeks of immobilization with a sling, collar and cuff, or Velpeau dressing followed by active and passive range of motion exercises can be expected to yield a full recovery of function.

D. Neer classified displaced proximal humeral fractures according to the number of fractures of its four major anatomic components—the humeral head, the greater tuberosity, the lesser tuberosity, and the proximal humeral shaft. Significant displacement is defined as greater than one centimeter translation or 45° angulation of one fragment in relation to another fragment. This four part classification scheme aids in the interpretation and therapeutic decision making in these complex fracture patterns.[1]

E. Following closed or, if necessary, open reduction of the shoulder dislocation, associated proximal humeral fractures should be re-evaluated for displacement and angulation.

F. Severely angulated surgical neck fractures may result in significant loss of functional motion, especially abduction and elevation. If manipulative reduction fails to restore satisfactory alignment, traction or a hanging arm cast may be successful.[2] Open reduction with internal fixation, however, offers the best opportunity in the young patient for early return of shoulder function.

G. Fractures of the greater tuberosity displaced more than one centimeter are resistant to closed reduction because of the deforming muscle forces. Associated rotator cuff tears should be repaired at the time of open reduction. Isolated fractures of the lesser tuberosity rarely occur and should alert the physician to a possible occult posterior shoulder dislocation.

H. The most frequent three-part fracture pattern is with one tuberosity intact with the humeral head and the other tuberosity displaced along with shaft displacement. Because of the incorrectable displacement, open reduction and fixation are preferred.[3]

I. Various techniques of internal fixation have been recommended.[3,4] All operative methods are demanding, especially in comminuted fractures. Elderly, osteoporotic patients with comminuted displaced fractures achieve better functional results with closed treatment and early motion.

J. Humeral head articular injuries may involve impaction fractures (usually associated with posterior dislocations) or head-splitting fractures. With greater than 50% of the articular surface damaged, chronic symptoms of instability and pain are likely. Complete fractures through the anatomic neck may also lead to avascular necrosis of the humeral head. If possible, primary prosthetic replacement of the humeral head should be limited to the elderly patient with minimal functional demands.

## REFERENCES

1. Neer C. Displaced proximal humeral fractures. Part I: Classification and evaluation. J Bone Joint Surg. 1970; 52A:1077–1089.
2. Connolly J. (Ed.). *DePalma's, The Management of Fractures and Dislocations*. 3rd ed. Philadelphia: WB Saunders, 1981; pp. 686–718.
3. Neer C. Displaced proximal humeral fractures, Part II: Treatment of three-part and four-part displacement. J Bone Joint Surg. 1970; 52A:1090–1103.
4. Muller M, Algower M, Schneider R, Willenegger H. *Manual of Internal Fixation*. 2nd ed. Berlin: Springer-Verlag, 1979; pp. 125–126.

INJURY TO THE PROXIMAL HUMERUS

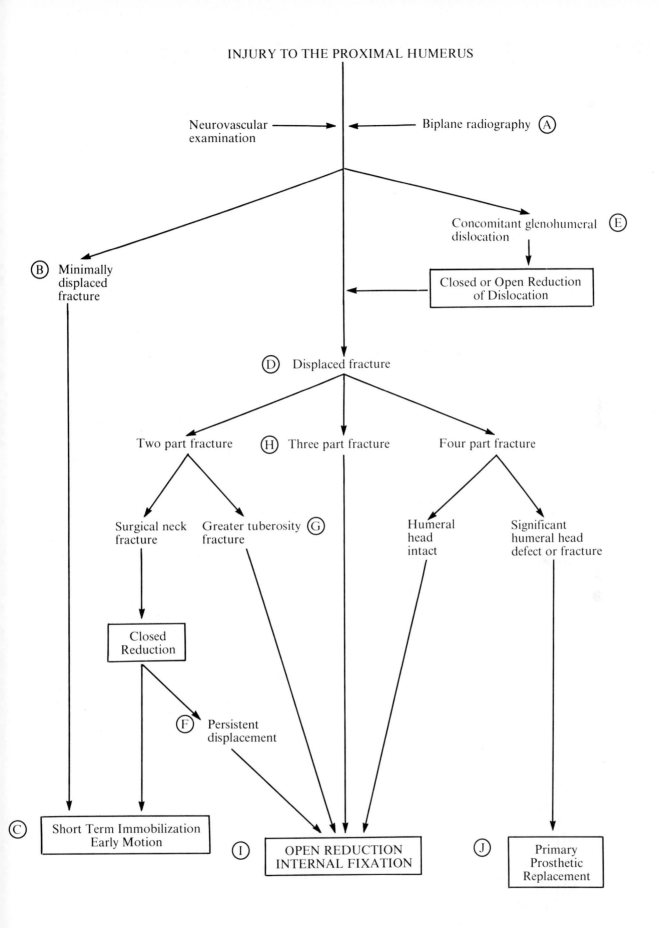

# FRACTURE OF THE HUMERAL SHAFT

## COMMENTS

A. With the patient in a sitting position, gravity and the weight of the arm usually suffice in achieving a satisfactory reduction. The limits of acceptability of a reduction vary with the patient's age, sex, and body habitus, the fracture pattern, and the degree of fracture comminution. Moderate overriding and angulation generally are consistent with a satisfactory functional and cosmetic result. Fracture distraction may lead to delayed or nonunion, and must be avoided.

B. Radial nerve injury may occur with any pattern of humeral shaft fracture. The nerve contacts directly the bone at the junction of the midshaft and distal one-third of the humerus. Holstein described a spiral fracture at this level, in which the distal bone fragment is displaced proximally and angulated radially, as having a high incidence of associated radial palsy[1] (see figure). If radial nerve function is present prior to reduction and then lost during the reduction maneuvers, it must be assumed that the nerve is trapped in the fracture site. Open reduction with freeing of the nerve and compression plating of the fracture are indicated. Routine surgery on all humeral fractures with absent radial nerve function at the time of initial evaluation is not warranted. Spontaneous recovery of neural function is likely in most cases.

C. Fracture splinting can be accomplished with coaptation splints, a hanging arm cast, Velpeau casting, an ordinary collar and hand sling,[2] an adjustable humeral orthosis, a shoulder spica cast, or a variety of other devices. Any technique that assures good osseous apposition and alignment is acceptable. Care must be taken not to distract transverse fractures, especially when using a hanging arm cast. Early elbow and shoulder function within several weeks of injury are desirable.

D. Humeral shaft fractures associated with concomitant displaced periarticular fractures and "floating elbow" injuries often are best managed with rigid internal stabilization of all fractures.

E. Dynamic compression plates are ideal for most humeral fractures.[3] Never should lag screws alone be utilized.

F. The upper humeral shaft is cylindrical in shape while the shaft flattens distally in the anteroposterior plane. The humerus therefore is not well suited anatomically for intramedullary rodding. Commonly employed devices include Rush, Ender, and Kuntscher rods. Their use should be limited to displaced, irreducible segmental fractures, pathologic fractures, and other rare clinical settings. When inserted through the greater tuberosity, intramedullary rods may be complicated by shoulder stiffness and contractures.

G. Humeral shaft fractures associated with massive soft tissue injuries can be stabilized with external fixation, employing widely spaced, preloaded half pins and a unilateral bar. Once the soft tissue injury has healed, definitive fracture care should be switched to some form of internal or external fixation. Humeral fracture distraction and subsequent nonunion are common with prolonged use of external fixators.

## REFERENCES

1. Holstein A, Lewis G. Fractures of the humerus with radial nerve paralysis. J Bone Joint Surg. 1963; 45A:1382–1388.
2. Spak I. Humeral shaft fractures–treatment with a simple hand sling. Acta Orthop. Scand. 1978; 49:234–239.
3. Muller M, Allgower M, Schneider R, Willenegger H. *Manual of Internal Fixation*. Berlin: Springer-Verlag, 1979; pp. 174–175.

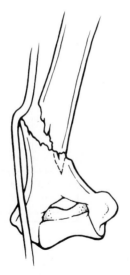

Holstein Fracture

# FRACTURE OF THE HUMERAL SHAFT

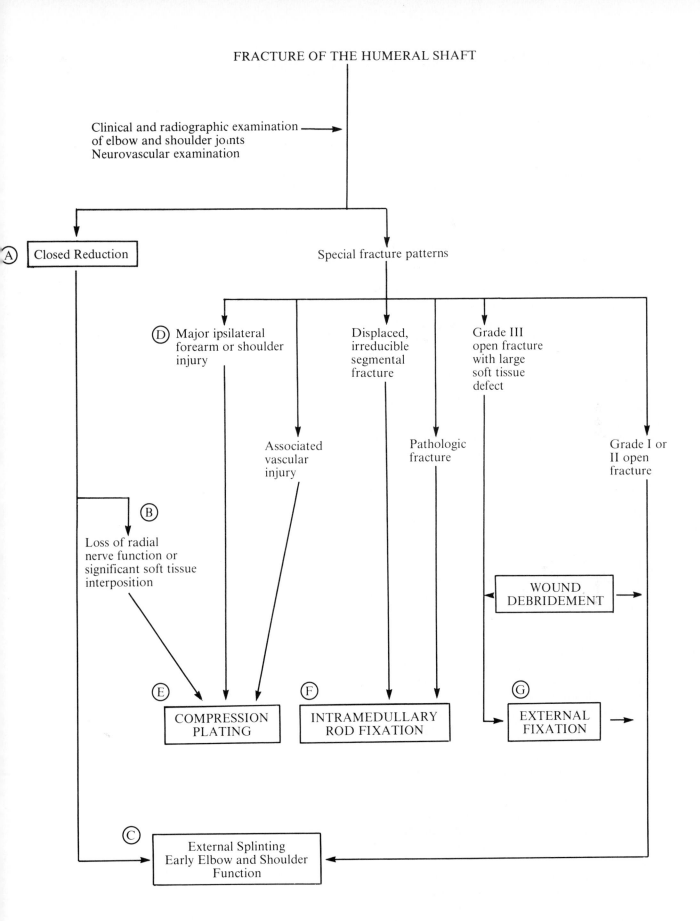

Clinical and radiographic examination of elbow and shoulder joints
Neurovascular examination

Ⓐ Closed Reduction

Special fracture patterns

Ⓓ Major ipsilateral forearm or shoulder injury

Displaced, irreducible segmental fracture

Grade III open fracture with large soft tissue defect

Associated vascular injury

Pathologic fracture

Grade I or II open fracture

Ⓑ Loss of radial nerve function or significant soft tissue interposition

WOUND DEBRIDEMENT

Ⓔ COMPRESSION PLATING

Ⓕ INTRAMEDULLARY ROD FIXATION

Ⓖ EXTERNAL FIXATION

Ⓒ External Splinting
Early Elbow and Shoulder Function

21

# DISLOCATION OF THE ELBOW

## COMMENTS

A. Over 90% of all elbow dislocations occur posteriorly. Rarer patterns include lateral, medial, anterior, and divergent dislocations as well as isolated dislocations of the radial head or olecranon. Posterior dislocations result from axial force on the outstretched hand with the elbow hyperextended. Associated neural damage, especially neuropraxic injury to the ulnar nerve, may be sustained in dislocations secondary to severe trauma.[1] The neurovascular status of the limb must be examined carefully prior to any attempt to reduce the dislocation.

B. Closed reduction can be obtained routinely with the patent under general anesthesia, heavy sedation, or regional block. Numerous reduction techniques have been described.[2]

C. The postreduction anteroposterior and lateral radiographs must be closely inspected for any joint widening, joint irregularity, or osseous malalignment signaling an incongruous reduction. Radiographs of the contralateral elbow may help in interpreting subtle abnormalities of the injured elbow.

D. Reduced posterior dislocations are generally stable with the elbow flexed greater than 90°. Redislocation or subluxation at 30° or more of elbow flexion defines an unstable reduction. Fluoroscopic examination is useful in evaluating potential instability.

E. Unstable elbow dislocations without concomitant fractures or with only minor ligamentous avulsion fractures should be immoblilzed in their most stable position, usually hyperflexion for posterior dislocations. Radial head and neck fractures may be reduced closed or open, but should not be excised, since further compromise of elbow stability may result. External support is maintained for 3 to 4 weeks.

F. Displaced fractures of the medial epicondyle, coronoid process or olecranon may predispose the elbow to recurrent dislocations. Medial epicondyle fragments can also be entrapped in the joint, especially in adolescent patients.[1] Coronoid process fractures with severe proximal displacement are also biomechanically significant. Anatomical reduction and internal fixation of these fractures in unstable dislocations restore the osseous and ligamentous stability of the joint.

G. Short-term immobilization (7 to 10 days) and early active range of motion exercises minimize the frequency and severity of late complications including myositis ossificans and loss of elbow extension. Prolonged immobilization over 4 weeks will invariably lead to some degree of elbow contracture.

## REFERENCES

1. Linscheid R, Wheeler D. Elbow dislocations. JAMA. 1965; 194:1171–1176.
2. Eppright R, Wilkins K. Fractures and dislocations of the elbow. In *Fractures*. Edited by Rockwood and Green. Philadelphia: JB Lippincott. 1975; 1:487–563.

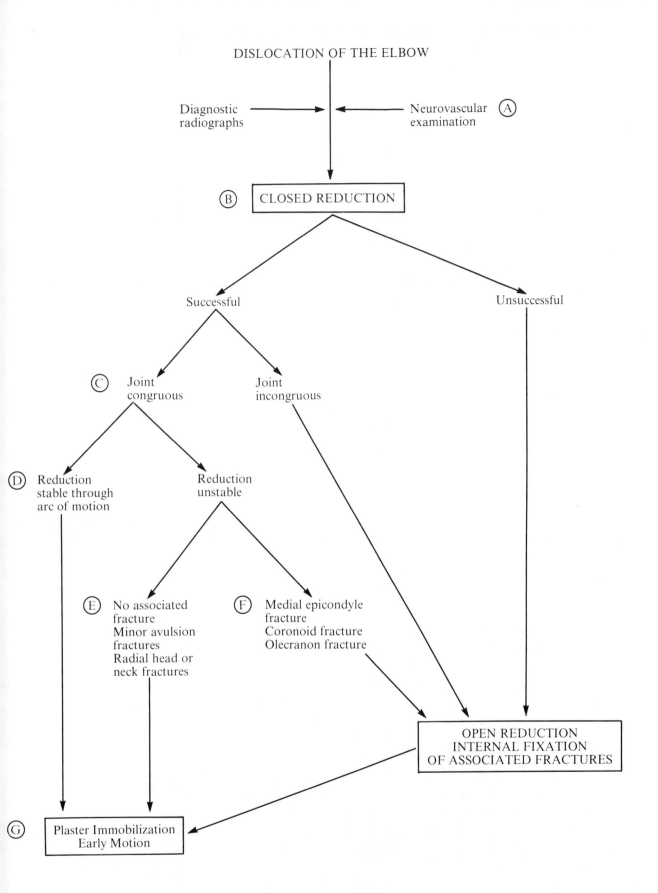

DISLOCATION OF THE ELBOW

Diagnostic radiographs → ← Neurovascular examination (A)

(B) CLOSED REDUCTION

Successful

Unsuccessful

(C) Joint congruous

Joint incongruous

(D) Reduction stable through arc of motion

Reduction unstable

(E) No associated fracture
Minor avulsion fractures
Radial head or neck fractures

(F) Medial epicondyle fracture
Coronoid fracture
Olecranon fracture

OPEN REDUCTION INTERNAL FIXATION OF ASSOCIATED FRACTURES

(G) Plaster Immobilization Early Motion

# FRACTURE OF THE FOREARM

## COMMENTS

A. Routine wrist and elbow examinations and radiographs are indicated in all forearm fractures to ascertain whether associated joint subluxation or dislocation has occurred. The index of suspicion should be high in cases with only an apparent isolated fracture of the radius or ulna.

B. Posterior interosseous nerve palsy, signalled by loss of active finger extension, is usually sustained in either anterior Monteggia fracture-dislocations or proximal radial shaft/neck fractures. Standard distal neurovascular examination will disclose the rarer associated nerve and vessel injuries.

C. Galeazzi fracture-dislocation, a fracture of the distal radius shaft with subluxation of the distal radioulnar joint, cannot be managed satisfactorily by closed techniques in adults. Following open reduction and rigid compression plating of the radial fracture, the dorsally subluxed or dislocated ulna is manipulated. The joint may be unstable even in the ideal fully supinated position, thus necessitating adjunctive percutaneous Steinmann pin fixation of the joint in the reduced position.[1]

D. Isolated ulnar or radial shaft fractures may result from direct blows (e.g., nightstick ulnar fractures) or penetrating injuries (e.g., low velocity gunshot wounds). Closed reduction and long arm cast immobilization suffice for most fractures. Indications for open reduction and internal fixation include loss of the normal lateral bow of the radius, angulation in any plane of greater than 10°, and cortical apposition of 50% or less.

E. Adult forearm fractures almost invariably are displaced. Full functional recovery requires restoration of the length and normal rotatory and axial alignments of both bones. Closed techniques yield poor anatomical and functional results.

F. Intramedullary devices, such as the Sage nail, Rush rod, Steinmann pin, and Kuntscher nail, have been largely discarded due to problems with their operative insertion and inadequate fixation of the fracture fragments. Compression plates provide rigid stabilization, leading to primary bone healing. Success of the technique hinges on precise reduction, plate selection and application, and rigid interfragmental fixation.[2] Complications, including nonunion (2 to 3% incidence), infection (3%), refracture (3%), and synostosis (1.2%), are usually attributable to technical errors.[3] Open forearm fractures may be managed by one of two means. Following immediate extensive debridement and cleansing of a grade I or II injury, primary plating may be performed. Alternatively, debridement may be followed by delayed closure, and subsequent plating at 10 to 14 days. Grade III injuries demand individualized care with osseous stabilization by external fixation or plating.

G. Fractures of the proximal one-third of the ulna associated with dislocations of the radial head constitute the Monteggia lesion. The Bado classification is based on the plane of displacement.[4] The type I pattern, characterized by anterior dislocation of the radial head and anterior angulations of the ulnar diaphyseal fracture (classic Monteggia fracture-dislocation), represents 60% of all Monteggia injuries. Types II to IV involve posterior or lateral radial head dislocation with or without concomitant radial shaft fracture.

H. Unlike Monteggia fractures in children, the injury in adults demands operative stabilization. Manipulative reduction of the radial head displacement is accomplished easily after plate fixation of the ulnar fracture. Failure of reduction usually implies buttonholing of the radial head through the joint capsule. Open reduction need not be followed by reconstruction of the annular ligament, which is intact in most cases.[5] Joint alignment is maintained by plaster immobilization in the stable position (elbow flexion and forearm supination for the type I injuries).

I. Most poor results after Galeazzi and Monteggia fracture-dislocations are secondary to redisplacement of the joint subluxations or dislocations. Check radiographs at 7 to 10 days confirming the maintenance of the reduction are therefore essential.

## REFERENCES

1. Mikic Z. Galeazzi fracture-dislocations. J Bone Joint Surg. 1975; 57A:1071.
2. Muller M, Allgower M, Schneideer R, Willenegger H. *Manual of Internal Fixation*. 2nd ed., New York: Springer-Verlag, 1979; pp. 182–193.
3. Anderson L, Sisk T, Tooms R, Park W. Compression-plate fixation in acute diaphyseal fractures of the radius and ulna. J Bone Joint Surg. 1975; 57A:287.
4. Bado J. The Monteggia lesion. Clin Orth Rel Res. 1967; 50:71.
5. Reckling F. Unstable fracture-dislocations of the forearm (Monteggia and Galeazzi lesions). J Bone Joint Surg. 1982; 64A:857.

Suspected
FRACTURE OF THE FOREARM

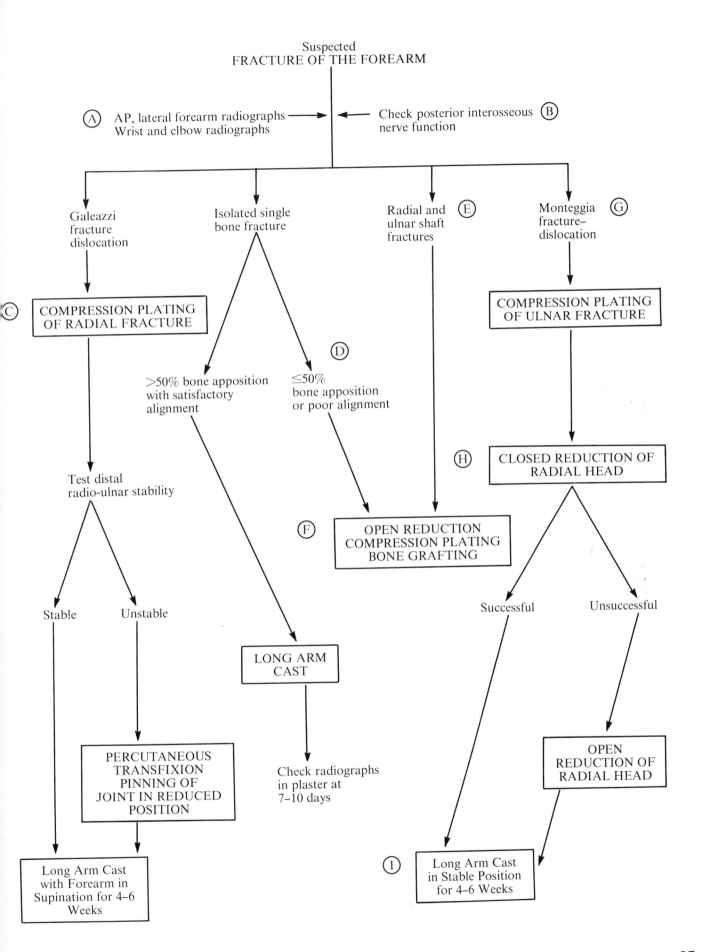

(A) AP, lateral forearm radiographs
Wrist and elbow radiographs

(B) Check posterior interosseous
nerve function

Galeazzi
fracture
dislocation

Isolated single
bone fracture

(E) Radial and
ulnar shaft
fractures

(G) Monteggia
fracture–
dislocation

(C) COMPRESSION PLATING
OF RADIAL FRACTURE

COMPRESSION PLATING
OF ULNAR FRACTURE

>50% bone apposition
with satisfactory
alignment

(D) ≤50%
bone apposition
or poor alignment

(H) CLOSED REDUCTION OF
RADIAL HEAD

Test distal
radio-ulnar stability

(F) OPEN REDUCTION
COMPRESSION PLATING
BONE GRAFTING

Stable

Unstable

Successful

Unsuccessful

LONG ARM
CAST

PERCUTANEOUS
TRANSFIXION
PINNING OF
JOINT IN REDUCED
POSITION

Check radiographs
in plaster at
7–10 days

OPEN
REDUCTION OF
RADIAL HEAD

Long Arm Cast
with Forearm in
Supination for 4–6
Weeks

(I) Long Arm Cast
in Stable Position
for 4–6 Weeks

**25**

# FRACTURE OF THE DISTAL RADIUS

## COMMENTS

A. Median nerve dysfunction may arise from stretching or compression of the nerve by fracture fragments or from immobilization of the wrist in excessive volar flexion following fracture manipulation. Carpal tunnel release and neural decompression should be performed when sensory or motor signs of neural compromise appear and are unrelieved by change in wrist position.

B. Once the specific fracture pattern and planes of displacement are identified, correct manipulative maneuvers can be undertaken.[1] The ideal position of immobilization depends upon the fracture type, with the most common dorsally angulated (Colles') pattern best casted in ulnar deviation, slight volar flexion, and neutral rotation. Extremes of flexion and pronation should be avoided. Alternative bracing techniques and positions of immobilization have been reported.[2]

C. The criteria for a satisfactory reduction vary with the age of the patient, his functional demands, and the fracture pattern. Postreduction radiographs are inspected carefully to verify the restoration of normal radial length, radial tilt, and volar tilt (see figure). With Colles' fractures, the dorsal tilt is least important from a functional standpoint. Many authors have noted a direct correlation between anatomic and functional results.[3]

D. Dorsal comminution of the typical Colles' fracture frequently permits settling and reangulation of a reduced fracture, even when it is held in a well-molded cast. Serial check radiographs are thus mandatory to detect redisplacement of the fracture.

E. Fractures often necessitating open reduction and internal fixation include displaced dorsal or volar rim fracture-dislocations (Barton and reverse Barton fractures) and high-energy comminuted intra-articular fractures in young adults.[4,5] Severely comminuted intra-articular fractures not amenable to anatomic open reduction can be managed with the pins and plaster or external fixation techniques.

## REFERENCES

1. Osterman A, and Bora F. Injuries of the wrist. In *Fracture Treatment and Healing*. Edited by B Heppenstall. Philadelphia: WB Saunders, 1980; 504–558.
2. Sarmiento A, Pratt G, Berry N, Sinclair W. Colles' fractures—functional bracing in supination. J Bone Joint Surg. 1975; 57A:311.
3. Green D. Pins and plaster treatment of comminuted fractures of the distal end of the radius. J Bone Joint Surg. 1975; 57A:304.
4. Ellis J. Smith's and Barton's fractures: A method of treatment. J Bone Joint Surg. 1965; 47B:724.
5. Muller M, Allgower M, Schneider R, Willenegger H. *Manual of Internal Fixation*. 2nd ed. New York: Springer-Verlag, 1979; 196–197.

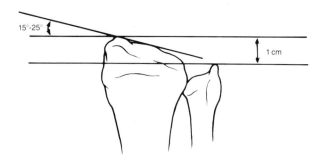

Normal Radial Length and Tilt

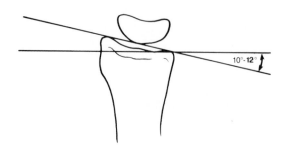

Normal Volar Tilt

DISTAL RADIUS FRACTURE

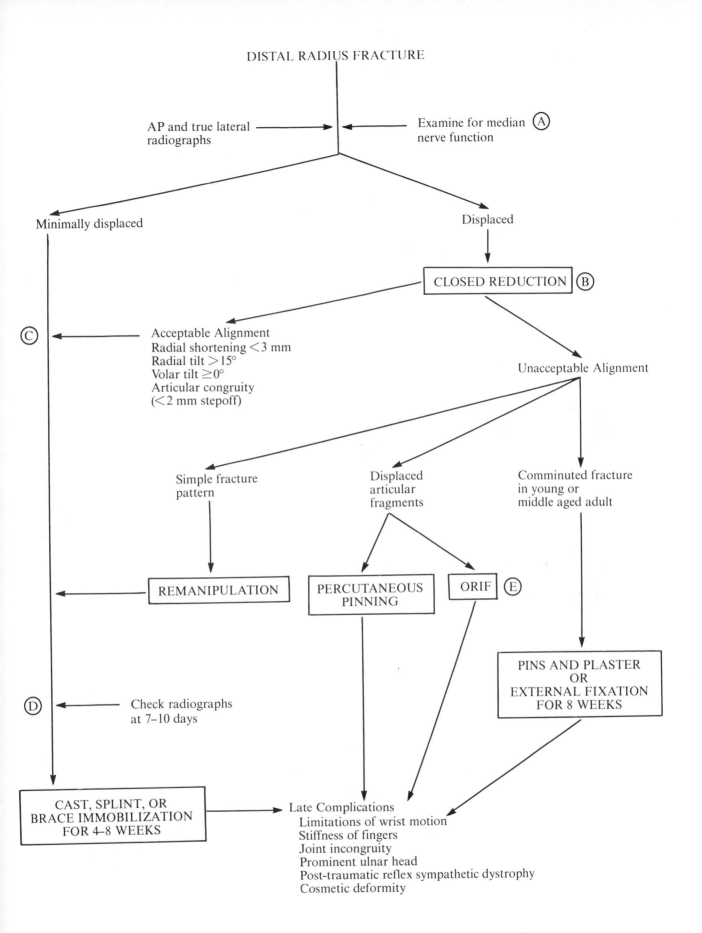

AP and true lateral radiographs → ← Examine for median (A) nerve function

Minimally displaced

Displaced

CLOSED REDUCTION (B)

(C) ← Acceptable Alignment
Radial shortening <3 mm
Radial tilt >15°
Volar tilt ≥0°
Articular congruity
(<2 mm stepoff)

Unacceptable Alignment

Simple fracture pattern

Displaced articular fragments

Comminuted fracture in young or middle aged adult

REMANIPULATION

PERCUTANEOUS PINNING

ORIF (E)

PINS AND PLASTER
OR
EXTERNAL FIXATION
FOR 8 WEEKS

(D) ← Check radiographs at 7–10 days

CAST, SPLINT, OR
BRACE IMMOBILIZATION
FOR 4–8 WEEKS

Late Complications
Limitations of wrist motion
Stiffness of fingers
Joint incongruity
Prominent ulnar head
Post-traumatic reflex sympathetic dystrophy
Cosmetic deformity

# FRACTURE OF THE PELVIC RING

## COMMENTS

A.  Associated abdominal and thoracic injuries take precedence over the pelvic fracture. Conolly and Hedberg have outlined an excellent emergency management protocol for pelvic fractures and their frequent concomitant visceral injuries.[1] See pp. 30 and 31 for the management of severe pelvic hemorrhage accompanying these fractures.

B.  Plain radiographs as well as special tilt and rotation views can fail to show occult posterior ring fractures and subluxation.[2,3] Computerized tomography aids especially in the evaluation of triplane displacement in unstable Malgaigne fractures.

C.  Minor fracture patterns and stable hemipelvis fractures retain sufficient posterior stability through the weight bearing portion of the pelvis that only symptomatic treatment is necessary. Bed rest, with or without pelvic slings and traction, usually suffices. The uniformly good results arise from the potential for early mobilization of the patient within several days of injury and the low incidence of late disability.

D.  The distinction between stable and unstable hemipelvis injuries is based on the degree of posterior ring disruption.[3,4] Stable patterns, such as anteroposterior compression (open book injury) and lateral compression injuries,[4] have only partial posterior disruption of the hemipelvis. Unstable injuries (vertical shear injuries in the Pennal classification) result in a free-floating hemipelvis (see figure). The hemipelvis is usually externally rotated with cephalad and posterior displacement.

E.  Indications for external fixation of stable Malgaigne fractures include severe pelvic hemorrhage and the need for early patient mobilization, especially in cases of polytrauma. Many fixation frame configurations are described.[5,6]

F.  An anatomic closed reduction of a displaced hemipelvis fracture is impossible to achieve. Most of the cephalad and posterior displacement can be corrected by proper positioning and manipulation of the pelvis. However, maintenance of the reduction by external means (traction, spica cast, or external fixation) is difficult. The choice between various external and internal modalities of stabilization depends on the patient's age, associated injuries, the fracture pattern, and experience of the treating physician. External fixation will not stabilize vertical shear fractures, though it may serve to minimize pelvic hemorrhage and lessen pelvic pain. Traction requires prolonged bed rest and constant attention. Combined anterior and posterior internal fixation is optimal treatment for unstable fractures, but the risk of such surgery is high. Surgery should be undertaken only when the benefits of anatomic reduction and rigid fixation outweigh the potential problems of hemorrhage, difficult exposure, and postoperative infection.

G.  Late complications occur almost exclusively with unstable hemipelvis fracture-dislocations. The high frequency of late sequelae can be decreased by careful reduction and meticulous management of the injury.[7]

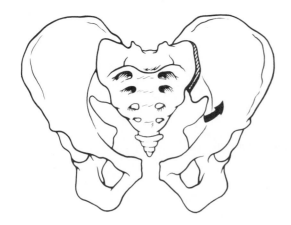

STABLE
Open Book Injury

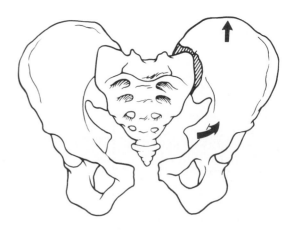

UNSTABLE
Vertical Shear Injury

# FRACTURE OF THE PELVIC RING

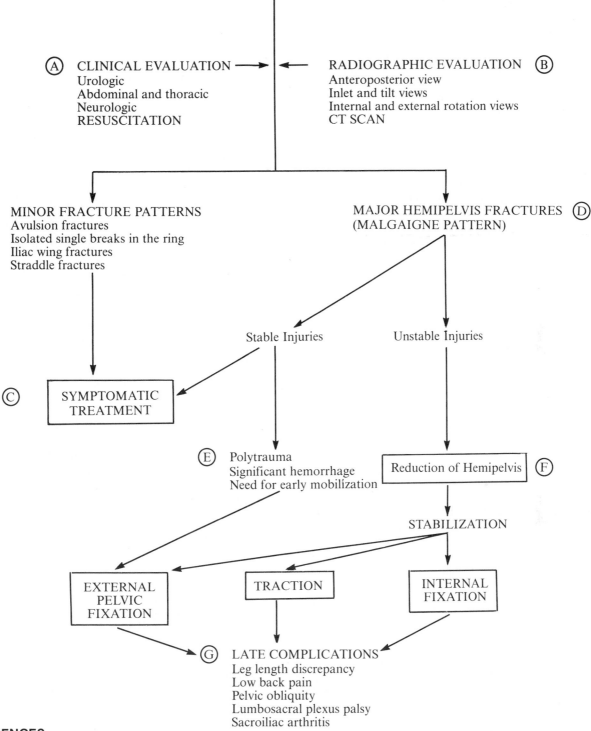

(A) CLINICAL EVALUATION ⟶ ⟵ RADIOGRAPHIC EVALUATION (B)
Urologic
Abdominal and thoracic
Neurologic
RESUSCITATION

Anteroposterior view
Inlet and tilt views
Internal and external rotation views
CT SCAN

MINOR FRACTURE PATTERNS
Avulsion fractures
Isolated single breaks in the ring
Iliac wing fractures
Straddle fractures

MAJOR HEMIPELVIS FRACTURES (D)
(MALGAIGNE PATTERN)

Stable Injuries     Unstable Injuries

(C) SYMPTOMATIC TREATMENT

(E) Polytrauma
Significant hemorrhage
Need for early mobilization

Reduction of Hemipelvis (F)

STABILIZATION

EXTERNAL PELVIC FIXATION     TRACTION     INTERNAL FIXATION

(G) LATE COMPLICATIONS
Leg length discrepancy
Low back pain
Pelvic obliquity
Lumbosacral plexus palsy
Sacroiliac arthritis

## REFERENCES

1. Conolly W, Hedberg E. Observations on fractures of the pelvis. J Trauma 1969; 9:104.
2. Gertzbein S, Chenowith D. Occult injuries of the pelvic ring. Clin Orth Rel Res. 1977; 128:202.
3. Bucholz R. The pathological anatomy of fracture-dislocations of the pelvis. J Bone Joint Surg. 1981; 63A:400.
4. Pennal G, Tile M, Waddell T, Garside H. Pelvic disruption: assessment and classification. Clin Orth Rel. Res. 1980; 151:1221.
5. Haraharju E, Slatis P. External fixation of double vertical pelvic fractures with a trapezoidal compression frame. Injury 1978; 10:142.
6. Brooker A, Edwards C (eds). External Fixation—The Current State of the Art. Baltimore: Williams and Wilkins, 1979; p. 123.
7. Slatis P, Huittinen V. Double vertical fractures of the pelvis. Acta Chir Scand. 1972; 138:799.

# HEMORRHAGE FROM PELVIC FRACTURE

## COMMENTS

A. The treatment of hemorrhagic shock is the first priority in pelvic fractures. Bleeding originates from the raw cancellous fracture surfaces as well as ruptured pelvic and lumbar retroperitoneal vessels. Patient movement and manipulation promote further bleeding and therefore should be permitted only when necessary.

B. It is often clinically difficult to localize the major sources of bleeding in the polytraumatized patient, especially attempting to differentiate continued pelvic hemorrhage from bleeding at other injury sites. Although brisk retroperitoneal bleeding is possible without any external manifestation of hemorrhage, an expanding gluteal, scrotal, or perineal hematoma suggests active bleeding at a pelvic fracture.

C. The keystone to treatment is the early institution and continuation of effective blood replacement. The appearance of shock is usually slow to develop, thereby allowing ample time for typing and cross-matching blood. Approximately one-half of all patients with pelvic fractures require transfusions. The average number of transfusions for Malgaigne fracture-dislocations is 7.4 units per patient.[1] Patients with all other fracture patterns necessitate an average of only 1.0 unit of blood.

D. Large pelvic vessel injuries occur in only 2% of all pelvic fractures. Physical signs of large vessel injury include diminished or absent distal pulses, a pulsatile hematoma, and an audible pelvic bruit. Massive uncontrollable bleeding may signal a large vessel injury or a concomitant intra-abdominal injury. It is advisable to proceed directly with peritoneal lavage or possible arteriography in such situations.

E. Undesirable motion of pelvic fracture fragments may be neutralized by the application of an external fixation device or, alternatively, an external counterpressure suit. The former requires an operative procedure, but has the added advantage of maintaining any fracture reduction and obliterating the potential pelvic dead space created by fracture displacement. Counterpressure or pneumatic trousers (G-suit, MAST trousers) are easily applied to the patient, but do not allow for controlled reduction of the fracture.[2] The increased systemic blood pressure recorded after inflation of the trousers is conjectured to be secondary to either an autotransfusion of blood from the legs and pelvis to the upper half of the body or an increase in peripheral vascular resistance. Whatever their mechanism of action, the trousers must be cautiously deflated once their use is no longer indicated. Contraindications to pneumatic trousers include impaired pulmonary function, cerebral edema, and injuries to the lower extremities which have a high probability of causing a compartment syndrome.

F. There is no absolute point at which either arteriography or surgical exploration is mandatory. Each case must be individualized on the basis of the patient's condition as well as the facilities and expertise at the treatment center. Selective transcatheter arterial embolization is feasible when the bleeding sites are well localized. A variety of different agents, such as autologous clot, Gelfoam, and intra-arterial steel coils, have been utilized for vessel occlusion.[3]

G. Surgical exploration to attempt direct control of pelvic hemorrhage is rarely indicated. Techniques for halting continued bleeding involve combinations of suture ligation, hypogastric artery ligation, aortic cross clamping, and compressive packing[4]. Massive intraoperative hemorrhage should be anticipated.[5] Due to the high operative mortality rate, all alternative methods of controlling hemorrhage should be exhausted prior to resorting to surgical exploration unless there is a well-documented associated intra-abdominal or large vessel injury. During laparotomies for intra-abdominal trauma, the retroperitoneal hematoma of a pelvic fracture should not be disturbed.

## REFERENCES

1. Hauser C, Perry J. Massive hemorrhage from pelvic fractures. Minn Med. 1966; 49:285.
2. Flint L, et al. Definitive control of bleeding from severe pelvic fractures. Ann Surg. 1979; 189:709.
3. Ben-Menachem Y, et al. Therapeutic arterial embolization in trauma. J Trauma. 1979; 19:944.
4. Hawkins L, Pomerantz M, and Eiseman B. Laparotomy at the time of pelvic fracture. J Trauma. 1970; 10:619.
5. Riska E, et al. Operative control of massive hemorrhages in comminuted pelvic fractures. Acta Orthop Scand. 1979; 50:362.

UNSTABLE PELVIC FRACTURE

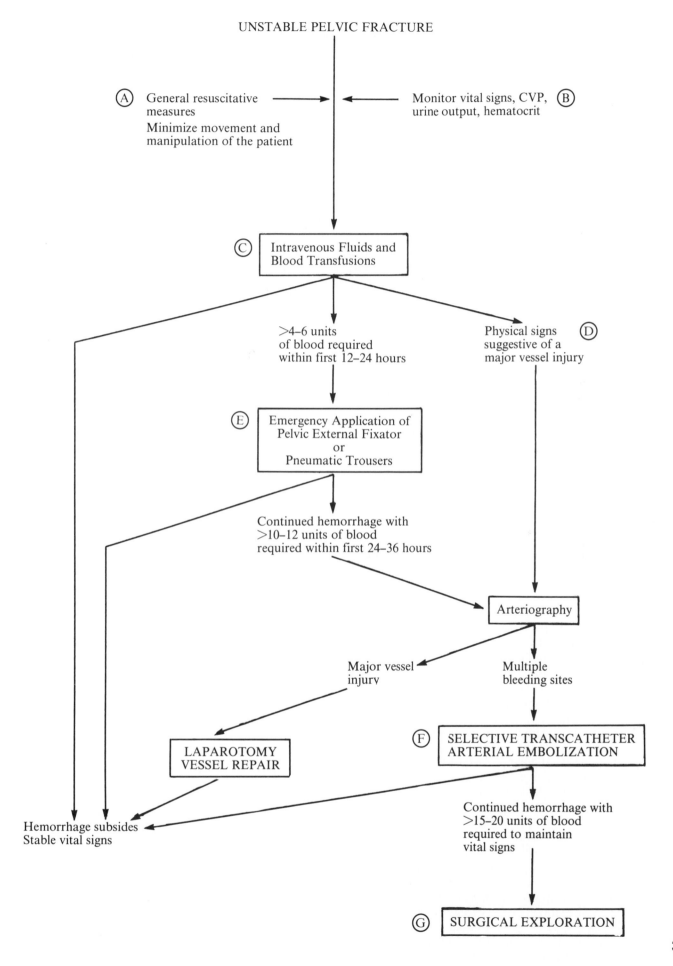

(A) General resuscitative measures
Minimize movement and manipulation of the patient

(B) Monitor vital signs, CVP, urine output, hematocrit

(C) Intravenous Fluids and Blood Transfusions

>4–6 units of blood required within first 12–24 hours

(D) Physical signs suggestive of a major vessel injury

(E) Emergency Application of Pelvic External Fixator or Pneumatic Trousers

Continued hemorrhage with >10–12 units of blood required within first 24–36 hours

Arteriography

Major vessel injury

Multiple bleeding sites

LAPAROTOMY VESSEL REPAIR

(F) SELECTIVE TRANSCATHETER ARTERIAL EMBOLIZATION

Hemorrhage subsides Stable vital signs

Continued hemorrhage with >15–20 units of blood required to maintain vital signs

(G) SURGICAL EXPLORATION

# CENTRAL ACETABULAR FRACTURE

## COMMENTS

A.  The proper treatment of central acetabular fractures, with or without femoral head subluxation, depends on an accurate determination of the fracture pattern. The status of the anterior and posterior acetabular columns as well as the dome of the acetabulum can be defined by careful scrutiny of the AP and both oblique (Judet) pelvic radiographs.[1]

B.  Hairline acetabular fractures in reliable patients may be managed with early motion and non-weight bearing crutch ambulation for 3 months. However, nondisplaced fractures with fracture lines extending through the acetabular dome may displace secondarily and should be treated with bed rest and gentle traction.

C.  A central acetabular fracture-subluxation, as with any intra-articular fracture of a weight bearing joint, demands anatomic restoration. Owing to the difficulty of surgical approaches, the frequently discouraging degree of comminution, and the recent development of a predictably good salvage procedure in total hip replacement, surgeons often have compromised their orthopedic principles in the handling of these injuries. Following closed reduction under general anesthesia, the decision to proceed with surgery is based on the congruence of the reduction and the status of the acetabular dome.

D.  If the femoral head articulates well with an intact acetabular dome, displaced medial acetabular wall fragments may be ignored. Longitudinal skeletal traction, supplemented with lateral traction through trochanteric pins, is standardly required for 8–12 weeks.[2] Extension of the fracture lines up to the dome, with a resulting small dome fragment, makes traction management less likely to succeed.

E.  If technically possible, surgical restoration of the acetabular anatomy optimizes the opportunity for a good functional result. Surgical treatment of inadequately reduced fractures is especially indicated in young patients, in polytrauma patients requiring early mobilization, and in cases where the experience of the surgeon with such major pelvic operations is extensive. The surgical approach depends on the preoperative assessment of acetabular columns, the dome, and associated pelvic injuries. Detailed recommendations on approaches and techniques have been offered by Tile[3] and Letournel.[4,5]

F.  Long-term complications of central acetabular fracture-subluxations are usually secondary to either unrecognized trauma to the joint cartilage or joint incongruity. Avascular necrosis of the femoral head is an infrequent sequela of this injury in comparison to its incidence in posterior fracture-dislocations of the hip.

## REFERENCES

1.  Judet R, Judet J, Letournel E. Fractures of the acetabulum: classification and surgical approaches for open reduction. J Bone Joint Surg. 1964; 46A:1615.
2.  Tipton W, D'Ambrosia R, Ryle G. Non-operative management of central fracture dislocations of the hip. J Bone Joint Surg. 1975; 57A:888.
3.  Tile M. Fractures of the acetabulum. Orth Clin N Am. 1980; 11:481.
4.  Letournel E. Acetabulum fracture—classification and management. Clin Orth Rel Res. 1980; 151:81.
5.  Letournel, E., Judet, R. Fractures of the Acetabulum. New York: Springer-Verlag, 1981.

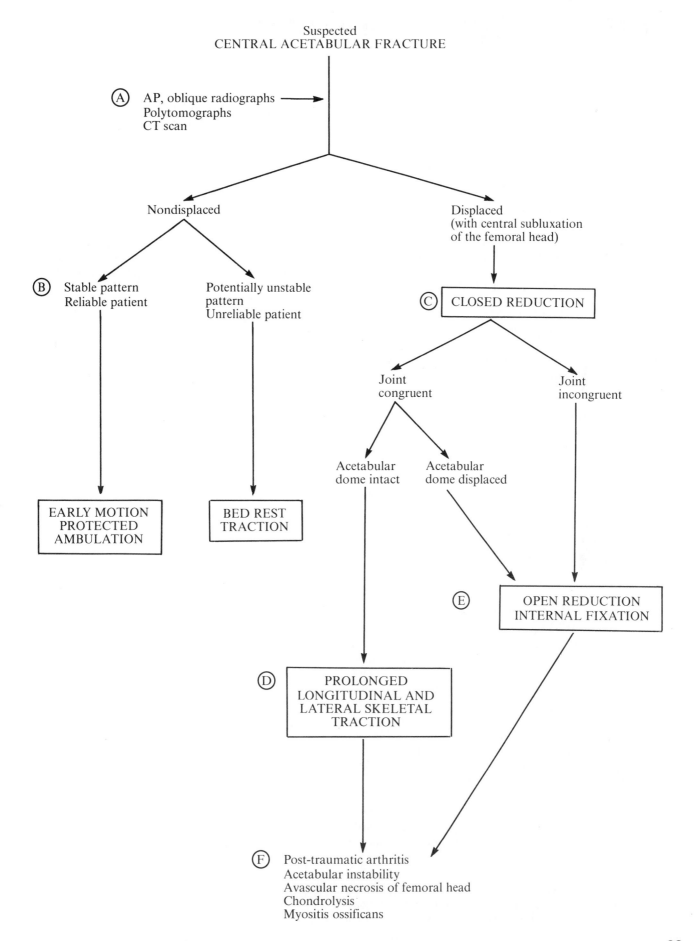

Suspected
CENTRAL ACETABULAR FRACTURE

Ⓐ AP, oblique radiographs
Polytomographs
CT scan

Nondisplaced

Displaced
(with central subluxation
of the femoral head)

Ⓑ Stable pattern
Reliable patient

Potentially unstable
pattern
Unreliable patient

Ⓒ CLOSED REDUCTION

EARLY MOTION
PROTECTED
AMBULATION

BED REST
TRACTION

Joint
congruent

Joint
incongruent

Acetabular
dome intact

Acetabular
dome displaced

Ⓔ OPEN REDUCTION
INTERNAL FIXATION

Ⓓ PROLONGED
LONGITUDINAL AND
LATERAL SKELETAL
TRACTION

Ⓕ Post-traumatic arthritis
Acetabular instability
Avascular necrosis of femoral head
Chondrolysis
Myositis ossificans

# DISLOCATION OF THE HIP

## COMMENTS

A. Sciatic nerve injury occurs in approximately 10% of all posterior fracture-dislocations of the hip. Spontaneous neural recovery can be expected in a majority of cases if appropriate treatment of the dislocation is instituted.

B. Anterior and Judet (oblique) radiographic views are sufficient to evaluate the dislocation and concomitant posterior or anterior acetabular rim fractures. The Epstein classification scheme of posterior hip dislocations is useful in treatment planning.[1] The five injury patterns include:

Type I: pure posterior dislocation without fracture
Type II: single large posterior acetabular rim fragment
Type III: acetabular rim comminution
Type IV: rim comminution and acetabular floor fracture
Type V: femoral head fracture

Anterior hip dislocations may be divided into pubic (superior) and obturator (inferior) types.

C. Anterior dislocations result from forced hip abduction, whereas posterior dislocations are usually secondary to a force applied to the flexed knee with the hip in flexion. The specific injury pattern dictates the proper manipulative maneuver for reduction.[1] Closed reduction should be performed on an emergency basis. Patient relaxation can be achieved with intravenous medications in the emergency room or, ideally, with general anesthesia in the operating room. A maximum of two or three attempts at closed reduction should be tried prior to resorting to operative reduction.

D. If closed reduction is attained the hip is gently flexed to 90°. If the hip subluxes or dislocates it should be relocated, and the surgeon should proceed with operative stabilization.

E. Widening of the joint space on postreduction radiographs signifies interposition of bone, cartilage, labrum, or capsule between the femoral head and acetabulum. Polytomography or computed tomography may be useful in detecting interposed osteochondral fragments in cases with questionable widening on plain radiographs.

F. Bed rest, with or without traction, is discontinued as soon as the patient is comfortable. Early weight bearing does not increase the frequency of late complications.[1]

G. Posterior dislocations are approached posteriorly, whereas anterior dislocations necessitate an anterior exposure. Following careful redislocation of the hip, the joint is debrided of all displaced osseous and soft tissues. Associated femoral head and neck fractures must be reduced and fixed, except for small inferior head fragments, which can be discarded. Interfragmental screw fixation is used for acetabular rim fractures. Posterior column buttress plates are needed occasionally for comminuted rim fractures.

H. Avascular necrosis of the femoral head becomes manifest radiographically at an average of 18 months after injury. The incidence of avascular necrosis is 15% for posterior dislocations and 4% for anterior dislocations.[1] Delays in initial treatment increase the frequency of this complication. The incidence of post-traumatic degenerative arthritis is similar for anterior and posterior dislocations.

## REFERENCE

1. Epstein H. *Traumatic Dislocation of the Hip*. Baltimore: Williams & Wilkins, 1980.

HIP DISLOCATION

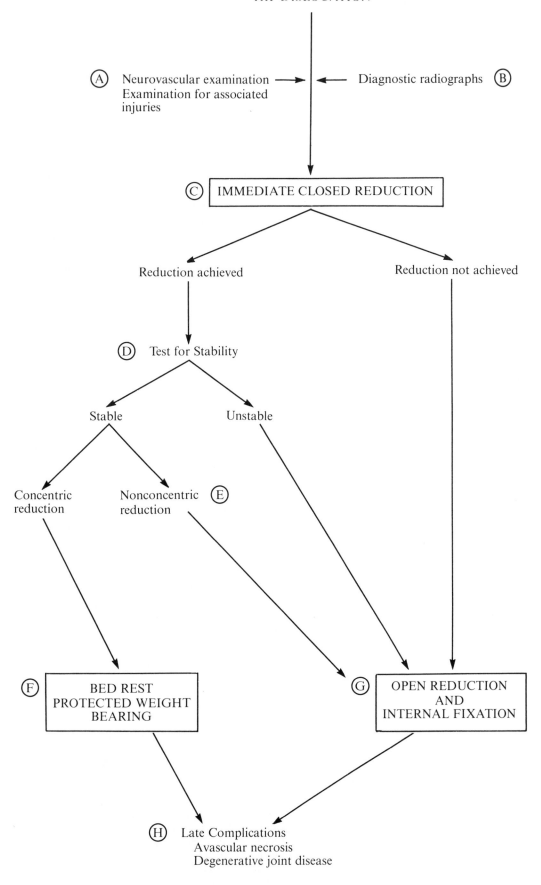

# FEMORAL NECK FRACTURE

## COMMENTS

A. Tomography of the hip is useful in detecting occasional nondisplaced and stress fractures of the femoral neck.

B. The Garden classification (see figure) stage I and II fractures do not require preoperative manipulation prior to in situ pinning.[1] Attempts to disimpact stage I fractures and improve their reduction should not be made. The incidence of complications in undisturbed stage I and II fractures that have been adequately stabilized is low. Approximately 10–15% of impacted femoral neck fractures will displace with nonoperative treatment.[2]

C. The principles in the management of displaced femoral neck fractures include early anatomic reduction, fracture impaction, and rigid fixation. Treatment is aimed at restoring the osseous anatomy and stability of the proximal femur.

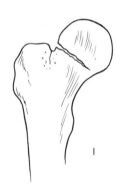

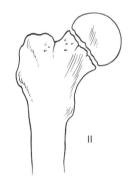

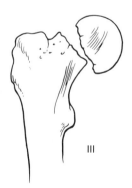

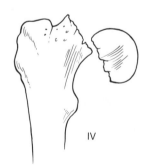

Garden classification of femoral neck fractures.

D. Various techniques of closed reduction on a fracture table have been described.[1] It is preferable to perform a closed reduction as soon after injury as possible, though controversy persists over the frequency of complications when reduction is delayed. Impaction of the fracture fragments is essential, since there is no periosteum along the femoral neck that can produce new bone to span a defect. Only an anatomic or slight valgus reduction should be accepted prior to proceeding with internal fixation.

E. A posterior muscle pedicle graft augments fracture stabilization and reduces the incidence of avascular necrosis with late segmental collapse.[3] Its use is indicated in young adults with displaced subcapital or transcervical fractures, and in older adults with fractures necessitating open reduction.

F. Primary femoral head replacement should be reserved for elderly patients with a limited life expectancy. Physiologic age is a better criterion than chronologic age in deciding to resort to hemiarthroplasty. Many patients over 65 years of age and without significant medical problems should be treated by closed reduction and pinning.

G. Either multiple pins (Knowles, Deyerle, Hagie, Steinmann, cancellous screws) or a sliding nail or screw device can be used. Which implant is selected is of less importance than the adequacy of the reduction and the proper placement of the device across the fracture site. Intraoperative impaction of the fracture is imperative.

H. Avascular necrosis with segmental collapse and fracture nonunion occur most frequently in stage III and IV displaced fractures that are incompletely reduced and inadequately stabilized. Specific variables associated with various late complications of femoral neck fractures have been well defined.[4]

## REFERENCES

1. Garden RS. Reduction and fixation of subcapital fractures of the femur. Ortho Clin N Am. 1974; 5:683–712.
2. Bentley G. The case for internal fixation of impacted femoral neck fractures. Ortho Clin N Am. 1974; 5:729–742.
3. Meyers M, Moore T, Harvey J. Displaced fracture of the femoral neck treated with a muscle pedicle graft with emphasis on the treatment of those fractures in young adults. J Bone Joint Surg. 1975; 57A:718–720.
4. Barnes R, Brown J, Garden R, Nicoll E. Subcapital fractures of the femur—a prospective review. J Bone Joint Surg. 1976; 58B:2–24.

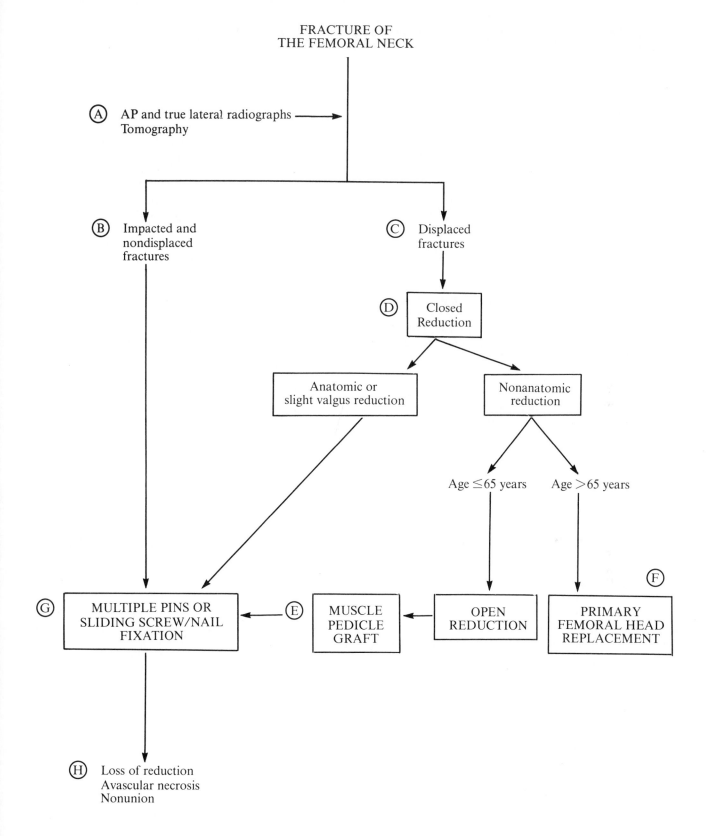

FRACTURE OF
THE FEMORAL NECK

Ⓐ AP and true lateral radiographs
   Tomography

Ⓑ Impacted and
   nondisplaced
   fractures

Ⓒ Displaced
   fractures

Ⓓ Closed
   Reduction

Anatomic or
slight valgus reduction

Nonanatomic
reduction

Age ≤65 years    Age >65 years

Ⓕ

Ⓖ MULTIPLE PINS OR
   SLIDING SCREW/NAIL
   FIXATION

Ⓔ MUSCLE
   PEDICLE
   GRAFT

OPEN
REDUCTION

PRIMARY
FEMORAL HEAD
REPLACEMENT

Ⓗ Loss of reduction
   Avascular necrosis
   Nonunion

# INTERTROCHANTERIC FRACTURE OF THE FEMUR

## COMMENTS

A. Intertrochanteric fracture, an injury of the elderly, has a high mortality rate. Rapid patient mobilization following surgical stabilization of the fracture lessens the frequency of life-threatening complications such as cardiopulmonary failure and thromboembolic disease. It also minimizes the incidence of decubitus ulcers and limb contractures. Most intertrochanteric fractures are four-part injuries, with secondary comminution of the greater and lesser trochanters. The presence of a large posteromedial fragment defines an unstable pattern (see figure). Restoration of bony apposition and stability by closed reduction on a fracture table is not possible in such cases with medial comminution.

B. Successful reduction restores the osseous stability by achieving medial cortical abutment or impaction of the major fracture fragments in a normal or slight valgus alignment. A sliding nail- or screw-plate device is preferred, since it permits controlled intraoperative compression of the fracture and telescopes postoperatively allowing the fracture to settle in a stable position and preventing nail protrusion through the femoral head. The device should act as an internal splint.[1] Complications arise when the surgical construct is inadequate to withstand the major forces to which the proximal femur is subjected. They include varus settling of the fracture, cutting out or protrusion of the nail or screw, and fatigue failure of the implant. Relative contraindications to surgery are a contaminated wound at the operative site, septicemia, and a delay in treatment of more than 3 weeks.

C. Reconstitution of the medial buttress of unstable fractures by interfragmental compression screws decreases the likelihood of limb shortening and abductor insufficiency. Most patients under 65 years of age and active patients over 65 years of age benefit from this additional surgery. Severe medial comminution or advanced osteoporosis may preclude successful interfragmental fixation.

D. Cancellous bone grafting of medial cortical defects is occasionally necessary in young patients with unstable fractures.

E. Elderly osteoporotic patients with unstable fractures may be managed by one of two techniques. First, the major head-neck and shaft fragments may be aligned on the fracture table so that femoral length is restored without concern for the trochanteric fractures. A sliding nail- or screw-plate implant allows postoperative settling and stabilization of the fracture as necessary. Alternatively, intraoperative medial bony contact and stability can be achieved by medial displacement of the shaft fragment or valgus osteotomy.[2,3] Although these procedures do obviate the need for "anatomically" nailed fractures to migrate into a stable position, they do shorten the limb and the abductor mechanism. The versatile compression hip screw is the most popular device for both stable and unstable intertrochanteric fractures.

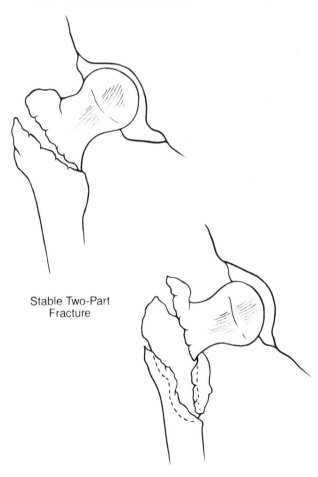

Stable Two-Part Fracture

Unstable Comminuted Fracture

## REFERENCES

1. Kyle R, Wright T, Burstein A. Biomechanical analysis of the sliding characteristics of compression hip screws. J Bone Joint Surg. 1980; 62A:1308
2. Dimon J, Hughston J. Unstable intertrochanteric fractures of the hip. J Bone Joint Surg. 1967; 49A:440.
3. Sarmiento A, Williams E. The unstable intertrochanteric fracture; treatment with a valgus osteotomy and I-beam nail plate. J Bone Joint Surg. 1970; 52A:1309.

INTERTROCHANTERIC FRACTURE

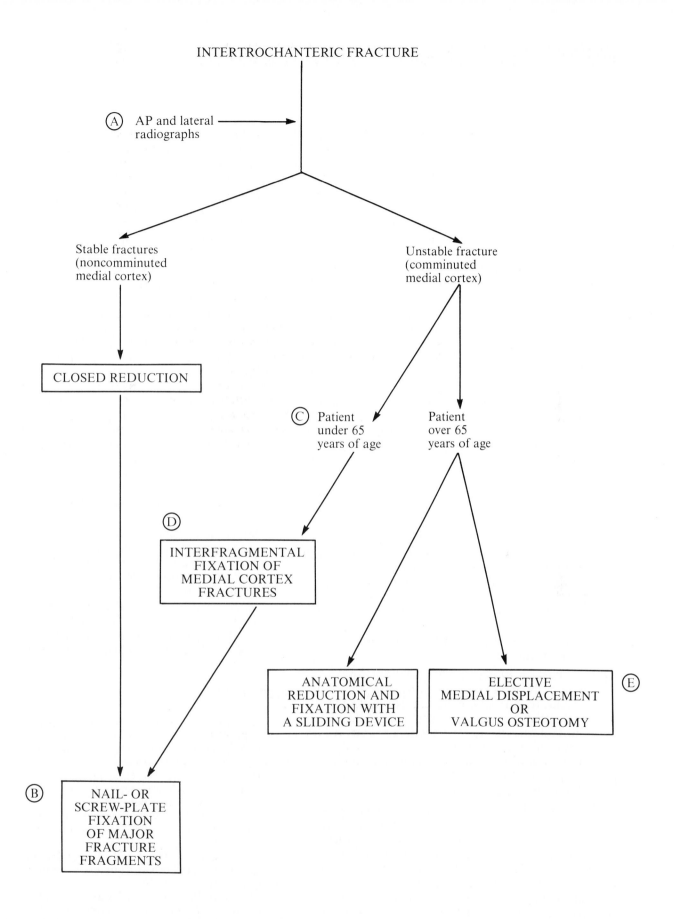

(A) AP and lateral radiographs

Stable fractures (noncomminuted medial cortex)

Unstable fracture (comminuted medial cortex)

CLOSED REDUCTION

(C) Patient under 65 years of age

Patient over 65 years of age

(D)

INTERFRAGMENTAL FIXATION OF MEDIAL CORTEX FRACTURES

ANATOMICAL REDUCTION AND FIXATION WITH A SLIDING DEVICE

ELECTIVE MEDIAL DISPLACEMENT OR VALGUS OSTEOTOMY (E)

(B) NAIL- OR SCREW-PLATE FIXATION OF MAJOR FRACTURE FRAGMENTS

# FEMORAL SHAFT FRACTURE

## COMMENTS

A. Femoral shaft fractures in adults are ideally treated by a rigid intramedullary nail, preferably inserted by the closed technique.[1,2,3] Available implants, including the Kuntscher, AO, Schneider, Hansen-Street and fluted nails, allow early mobilization and functional use of the injured extremity with maintenance of satisfactory length and alignment of the fracture. Therapeutic decision making centers on the feasibility of closed nailing, the potential for operative and postoperative complications, and the need for adjunctive stabilization.

B. Preoperative femur radiographs are evaluated for fracture location, anatomy, and comminution. Radiographic evidence for nondisplaced longitudinal cortical splits should be sought. When major fissures are discovered, they may require open cerclage prior to nailing of the fracture. A routine AP pelvis radiograph will detect concomitant hip fractures or dislocations. The presence of an ipsilateral hip injury may necessitate the selection of an alternative form of fixation, such as a compression plate, for the femoral shaft fracture.

C. Most femoral shaft fractures are high-energy injuries and thus are often associated with major abdominal, pelvic, or thoracic visceral injuries and significant bleeding into the thigh. The shaft fracture should be immobilized with skeletal traction during the emergency evaluation of blood loss and possible life-threatening injuries. If nailing is delayed for more than several days, radiographically documented distraction of the fracture is imperative. Longitudinal traction with 25–40 lb of weight will usually ensure adequate distraction.

D. The best fracture pattern for closed nailing is the minimally comminuted, transverse or short oblique fracture of the proximal or middle third of the shaft. Owing to the widening of the distal third of the shaft, intramedullary rods serve merely as internal splints for infraisthmal fractures. However, nailing remains the preferred treatment as long as the fracture is not excessively comminuted or spiral in configuration.

E. The essential requisite of a successful nailing of a femoral shaft fracture is the creation of a stable surgical construct. There should be sufficient cortical contact (usually a minimum of 50% of the circumference of the bone) of the proximal and distal fragments to prevent postoperative shortening of the fracture around the nail. The nail additionally must secure enough purchase of both fragments to ensure rotatory and varus/valgus stability. If the fracture is assessed preoperatively as being too proximal, too distal, or too comminuted to guarantee rigid stabilization by simple closed nailing, alternative treatments or supplemental internal fixation with cerclage wires or interlocking bolts must be considered.

F. The management of comminuted fractures, especially in the distal third of the shaft, must be individualized based on the facilities and experience of the surgeon. Balanced suspension skeletal traction demands constant vigilance by the staff to avoid malalignment of the fracture.[4] Roller traction, a recent modification of traditional skeletal traction, permits early mobilization of the patient and improved function of the knee.[5] Cast bracing maintains fracture alignment by the hydraulic effect of the thigh muscles encased in a well-molded plaster. Depending on the characteristics of the fracture, the application of the cast brace is performed by standard methods 2 to 8 weeks following injury. Union is achieved readily, but shortening and angulation are frequent complications.[6] External fixation has very limited usefulness in the care of femur fractures except in the presence of grade III soft tissue injuries.[7] Frequent problems with its use include pin tract infections, quadriceps entrapment, and loss of reduction. Most complications of femoral plating arise from failure to achieve sufficient skeletal stability at surgery, leading to intolerable stress on the implant. Refracture following successful plating is also common due to excessive fixation, with too much stress shielding at the fracture. Plating is best reserved for shaft fractures associated with femoral neck fractures that require operative fixation. Cancellous bone grafting should routinely be performed, especially in cases with medial cortical defects.

## REFERENCES

1. Kuntscher G. *Practice of Intramedullary Nailing.* Springfield IL: Charles C Thomas, 1967.
2. Bohler J. Closed intramedullary nailing of the femur. Clin Orthop. 1968; 60:51.
3. Hansen S, Winquist R. Closed intramedullary nailing of the femur—Kuntscher technique with reaming. Clin Orthop. 1979; 138:56.
4. Charnley J. *The Closed Treatment of Common Fractures.* 3rd ed. Edinburgh, Churchill-Livingstone, 1972, p. 166.
5. Montgomery S, Mooney V. Femur fractures: treatment with roller traction and early ambulation. Clin Orthop. 1981; 165:196.
6. Meggitt B, Juett D, Smith J. Cast-bracing for fractures of the femoral shaft. J Bone Joint Surg. 1981; 63B:12.
7. Fischer D. The Hoffman external fixation: technique of application. In *External Fixation—The Current State of the Art.* Edited by Brooker and Edwards. Baltimore: Williams & Wilkins, 1979, pp. 393–419.

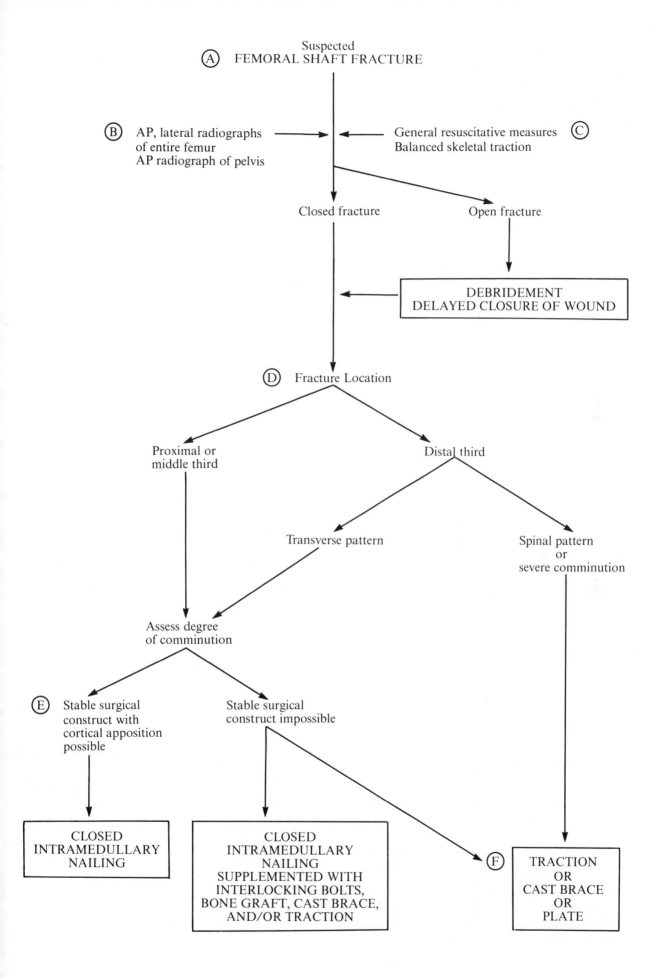

Suspected
Ⓐ FEMORAL SHAFT FRACTURE

Ⓑ AP, lateral radiographs of entire femur
AP radiograph of pelvis

Ⓒ General resuscitative measures
Balanced skeletal traction

Closed fracture

Open fracture

DEBRIDEMENT
DELAYED CLOSURE OF WOUND

Ⓓ Fracture Location

Proximal or middle third

Distal third

Transverse pattern

Spinal pattern
or
severe comminution

Assess degree of comminution

Ⓔ Stable surgical construct with cortical apposition possible

Stable surgical construct impossible

CLOSED
INTRAMEDULLARY
NAILING

CLOSED
INTRAMEDULLARY
NAILING
SUPPLEMENTED WITH
INTERLOCKING BOLTS,
BONE GRAFT, CAST BRACE,
AND/OR TRACTION

Ⓕ TRACTION
OR
CAST BRACE
OR
PLATE

# CLOSED INTRAMEDULLARY NAILING OF THE FEMUR

## COMMENTS

A. Preoperative distraction of the fracture, using skeletal traction of 25 to 40 pounds, facilitates the fracture reduction on the operative table. If the nailing is delayed for more than 2 or 3 days, a lateral radiograph of the femur demonstrating satisfactory fracture distraction should be obtained. If a complete stock of nails of variable length and width is not available, preoperative measurement of femoral length and anticipated nail length and width is necessary. This can be accomplished by clinical measurement of the contralateral femur from the trochanter to the knee joint, radiographic determination of femoral length by taping a known length nail to the thigh of the opposite leg, or the use of the Kuntscher ossimeter. The probable width of the nail to be used is 2 mm greater than the isthmal medullary width measured on the anteroposterior radiograph.

B. In the full lateral position on a Maquet or comparable fracture table, the patient's hip is placed in slight adduction and moderate flexion. Traction is applied through the tibial or femoral Steinmann pin, thus permitting flexion of the knee. Internal rotation of the leg of 10 to 15° usually guarantees correct rotatory alignment of the fracture fragments. Satisfactory reduction of the fracture must be achieved in both AP and lateral planes prior to the preparation and draping of the leg. The proximal fragment is usually flexed and adducted in relation to the distal fragment. Adduction can be corrected by lowering the leg or supporting the proximal fragment with a crutch under the thigh. Flexion is easily overcome by gentle external pressure over the anterior proximal aspect of the thigh. If near anatomic reduction in both planes is not accomplished, manipulation of the leg out of traction may be necessary.

C. The ideal location for the trochanteric entrance hole is the trochanteric fossa, located just medial to the tip of the trochanter and slightly posterior to the midline of the trochanter. Eccentric reaming and medial comminution of the proximal fragment are complications that occur frequently when an entrance hole is made too far laterally.

D. Any standard medullary instrumentation with flexible reamers can be utilized. A straight bulb-tipped guide rod is passed across the fracture into the distal fragment down to the distal femoral subchondral bone. If minor residual translatory displacement of the fracture makes its passage difficult, certain maneuvers may be used. These include bending the end of the guide rod; external pressure on the thigh with crutches, lead-gloved hands, or retractors; and the insertion of a narrow 9- or 10-mm nail into the proximal fragment to serve as a lever for fracture reduction.

E. Reaming is commenced with a 9-mm end cutting flexible reamer and then proceeds at 0.5-mm increments. In proximal and midshaft fractures, cortical contact of the nail of at least 2 to 3 cm on either side of the fracture is desirable. Over-reaming of the proximal fragment to 0.5 mm greater than the width of nail to be used is recommended to avoid nail incarceration and operative comminution of the fracture. The variable degree of anterior bow of the proximal fragment makes routine over-reaming of one full millimeter advisable in all distal shaft fractures.

F. Intraoperative measurement of the guide rod in the femur yields a precise optimal length for the nail. The selected prebent nail is then driven over a nail guide rod. When the tip of the nail reaches the fracture site, anatomic reduction must again be achieved by external pressure on the thigh. Following complete insertion of the nail and wound closure, plain radiographs of both the proximal and distal extents of the nail as well as the fracture site are obtained.

G. The postoperative management depends on the reliability of the patient and the stability of the fixation. If a stable surgical construct is achieved, progressive weight bearings as tolerated is begun. Quadriceps strengthening exercises are started within several weeks, and active range of motion exercises encouraged.

## REFERENCES

1. Kuntscher F. *Practice of Intramedullary Nailing. Springfield, Charles C Thomas, 1967.*
2. Hansen J, Winquist R. Closed intramedullary nailing of fracture of the femoral shaft—technical considerations. In *Instructional Course Lectures of the AAOS,* 1978.
3. Bucholz R, Mooney V. Fractures of the femoral shaft. In *Surgery of the Musculoskeletal System.* Edited by M Evarts. New York: Churchill-Livingstone, 1983.

# FEMORAL SHAFT FRACTURE

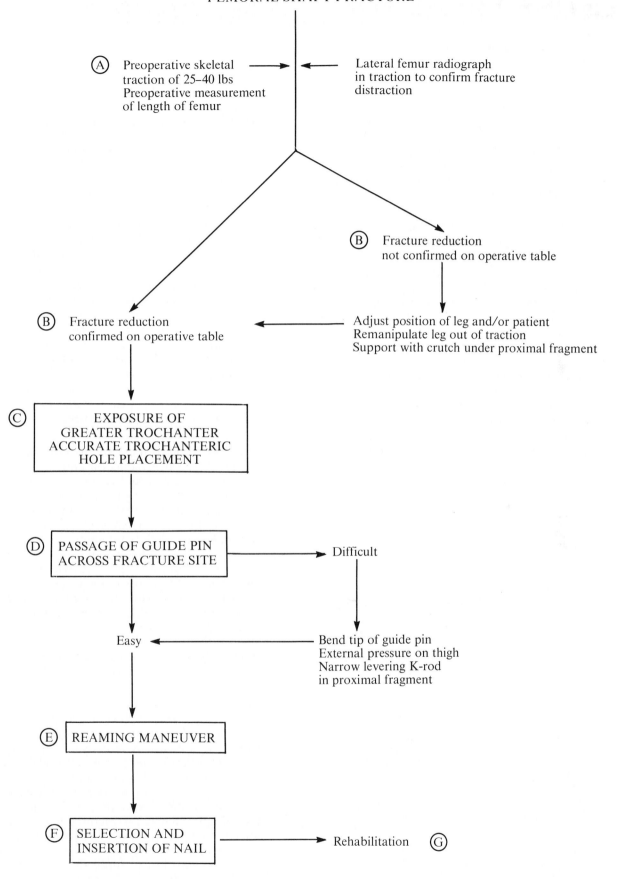

(A) Preoperative skeletal traction of 25–40 lbs
Preoperative measurement of length of femur

Lateral femur radiograph in traction to confirm fracture distraction

(B) Fracture reduction not confirmed on operative table

(B) Fracture reduction confirmed on operative table

Adjust position of leg and/or patient
Remanipulate leg out of traction
Support with crutch under proximal fragment

(C) EXPOSURE OF GREATER TROCHANTER ACCURATE TROCHANTERIC HOLE PLACEMENT

(D) PASSAGE OF GUIDE PIN ACROSS FRACTURE SITE

Difficult

Easy

Bend tip of guide pin
External pressure on thigh
Narrow levering K-rod in proximal fragment

(E) REAMING MANEUVER

(F) SELECTION AND INSERTION OF NAIL

Rehabilitation (G)

# FRACTURE OF THE DISTAL FEMUR

## COMMENTS

A. Most classification schemes for distal femur fractures are based on the distinction between simple and comminuted fractures, with or without intra-articular extension in one or more planes (see figure). Accurate radiographic assessment is essential in the selection of the ideal treatment, the preoperative planning of any surgical procedures, and the prediction of long-term complications. The tunnel view of the intercondylar notch is helpful in judging the extent of displacement of vertical fractures into the joint.

B. The rare nondisplaced and impacted supracondylar fractures usually occur in elderly patients. A well-molded long leg cast for 6 to 8 weeks, followed by cast bracing for an additional 4 to 6 weeks, is sufficient treatment in most cases. If check radiographs disclose an unacceptable loss of alignment, fracture manipulation and/or traction may be required. Although the criteria for acceptable alignment vary somewhat with the age of the adult patient, varus, valgus, and rotational alignment within 5° of normal, anterior and posterior alignment within 10 to 15° of normal, and shortening of one centimeter or less are consistent with good functional recovery.

C. The routine simple or comminuted transverse/short oblique supracondylar fracture may be managed by either surgical stabilization or skeletal traction. There are no absolute indications for open reduction and internal fixation, but surgery definitely yields superior results in certain fracture patterns. These included Y- or T-shaped fractures with displaced intra-articular extension, fractures irreducible by traction and manipulation, fractures with associated neurovascular injuries, "floating knee" injuries, and isolated medial or lateral femoral condylar fractures.

D. Complex distal femur fractures are among the most technically challenging fractures that confront the orthopedist. Without a full stock of implants, complete instrumentation, and most importantly, extensive experience in planning and performing such cases, anatomic reduction and rigid internal fixation may not be achieved.[1] Traction and cast brace treatment are preferable under these circumstances. The surgical risks are also magnified in cases with grade III soft tissue injury, active thigh infection, or severe osteoporosis.

E. Uniform good results are not automatically obtained by open reduction and internal fixation. The potential surgical benefit of improved function must be weighed in each case against the likelihood of achieving an anatomic reduction, absolutely rigid fixation, and early rehabilitation. Intramedullary implants (e.g., Rush rods or the Zickel supracondylar device) maintain alignment, but often allow excessive fracture shortening. Their use should be limited to elderly patients with advanced osteoporosis. The application of interfragmental screws, angled blade plates, and buttress plates demands strict adherence to the surgical principles of internal fixation.[1] Autogenous cancellous bone grafting is usually advisable, especially in the presence of a medial cortical defect.

F. Skeletal traction and cast brace treatment also necessitates close attention to details.[2,3,4] Initial traction of 15 to 20 pounds through a proximal tibial pin is routinely employed. The frequent problem of varus-internal rotation malalignment can be avoided by oblique placement of the tibial traction pin, proper positioning of the leg in the balanced suspension splint, and serial check radiographs. Knee contractures may be minimized by encouragement of active motion in the traction apparatus and early conversion at 4 to 8 weeks to a cast brace. Supplemental distal femoral pin traction is useful in correcting persistent flexion of the distal fragment.

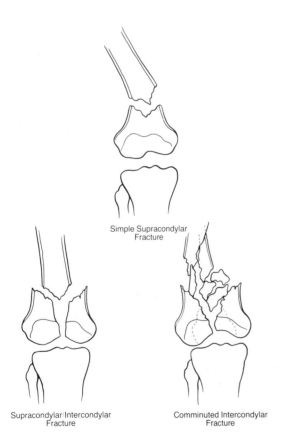

Simple Supracondylar
Fracture

Supracondylar/Intercondylar
Fracture

Comminuted Intercondylar
Fracture

# FRACTURE OF THE DISTAL FEMUR

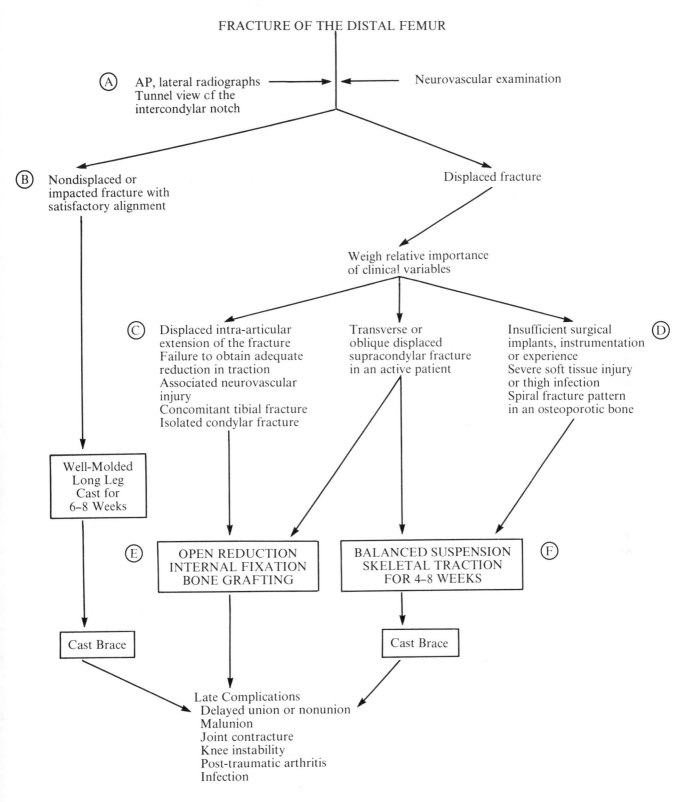

(A) AP, lateral radiographs
Tunnel view of the
intercondylar notch
→ ← Neurovascular examination

(B) Nondisplaced or
impacted fracture with
satisfactory alignment

Displaced fracture

Weigh relative importance
of clinical variables

(C) Displaced intra-articular
extension of the fracture
Failure to obtain adequate
reduction in traction
Associated neurovascular
injury
Concomitant tibial fracture
Isolated condylar fracture

Transverse or
oblique displaced
supracondylar fracture
in an active patient

Insufficient surgical
implants, instrumentation
or experience
Severe soft tissue injury
or thigh infection
Spiral fracture pattern
in an osteoporotic bone (D)

Well-Molded
Long Leg
Cast for
6–8 Weeks

(E) OPEN REDUCTION
INTERNAL FIXATION
BONE GRAFTING

BALANCED SUSPENSION
SKELETAL TRACTION
FOR 4–8 WEEKS (F)

Cast Brace

Cast Brace

Late Complications
Delayed union or nonunion
Malunion
Joint contracture
Knee instability
Post-traumatic arthritis
Infection

## REFERENCES

1.  Schatzker J, Lambert D. Supracondylar fractures of the femur. Clin Orth Rel Res. 1979; 138:77.
2.  Neer C, Grantham S, Shelton M. Supracondylar fracture of the adult femur. A study of one hundred and ten cases. J Bone Joint Surg. 1967; 49A:591.
3.  Charnley J. *The Closed Treatment of Common Fractures.* 3rd ed. Edinburgh: Churchill-Livingstone, 1972; p. 166.
4.  Mooney V, Nickel V, Harvey J, Snelson R. Cast-brace treatment for fractures of the distal part of the femur. J Bone Joint Surg. 1970; 52A:1563.

# EVALUATION OF THE ACUTELY INJURED KNEE

## COMMENTS

A.  This algorithm outlines the diagnostic evaluation of the acutely injured knee with normal radiographs. A spectrum of disabling soft tissue injuries involving disruptions of the extensor mechanism, ligamentous structures, menisci, and cartilaginous joint surfaces are possible. Prompt recognition of these diverse injuries is essential for their optimal treatment. The mechanism of injury influences the specific pattern of injury. Quadriceps or patellar tendon ruptures arise from sudden violent contraction of the extensor mechanism over a flexed knee, ligamentous tears from excessive forces in a varus/valgus or anterior/posterior direction, and meniscal lesions from twisting injuries. The ability of the patient to walk immediately following the trauma does not preclude a significant injury. Joint swelling appearing rapidly after an injury is indicative of a hemarthrosis from cruciate ligament disruption or chondral fracture. A gradual collection of joint fluid over 6 to 12 hours is more suggestive of a meniscal tear. A history of pre-existing knee problems or systemic illnesses should be sought. For example, patients with quadriceps or patellar tendon ruptures frequently provide a history of tendinitis, arthritis, disuse atrophy, collagen vascular disease, or previous steroid injections into the extensor mechanism.

B.  The sine qua non of any diagnostic work-up is a systematic physical examination. The detection of any localized signs of injury should be followed by detailed examinations (to be described).

C.  The presence of patellofemoral joint signs with a loss of active extension implies a probable rupture of the extensor mechanism. Disruption may occur at one of four levels—the quadriceps tendon, the patella, the patellar tendon, or the tibial tuberosity. Although radiographs are usually negative after soft tissue tears of the mechanism, a complete patellar tendon tear may present with a superiorly displaced patella on the lateral radiograph. A palpable gap at the site of rupture in either the quadriceps or patellar tendon may be evident in addition to localized tenderness, swelling, and ecchymosis. A partial rupture may result in loss of only the last few degrees of active extension and should not be confused with an internal derangement of the joint.

D.  Localized swelling and tenderness over the medial retinaculum of the patellofemoral joint may signify a spontaneously reduced patellar subluxation or dislocation. An apprehension (Fairbanks) test performed by gently pressing the patella laterally with the knee extended and observing the patient's reaction will confirm the diagnosis. A sunrise or tangential radiograph of the patellofemoral joint with the knee flexed 30 to 45° may disclose lateral tilting of the patella with widening of the joint space under the medial facet. Both the medial patellar facet and the lateral femoral condyle should be inspected closely for osteochondral or chondral fractures.

E.  The grading and testing of specific ligamentous injuries are discussed in a separate algorithm. Complete knee dislocations represent the most extreme form of such injuries. Approximately half of all knee dislocations have associated popliteal artery or common peroneal nerve injuries, thus making them true orthopaedic emergencies.[1] Anterior dislocations with the tibial plateau lying anterior to the femoral condyles are the most common pattern. Dislocations often are reduced in the field prior to emergency evaluation. Signs of vascular injury include diminished or absent distal pulses and an expanding hematoma in the popliteal space. If there is frank dislocation or subluxation of the joint at the time of evaluation, immediate closed reduction is mandatory to decompress the tented neurovascular structures. The ruptured ligaments may be repaired immediately, especially in open dislocations or cases necessitating vascular repair, or preferably, at 3 to 7 days after the injury.

F.  The combination of joint line tenderness and joint effusion after a twisting injury to the knee is highly suggestive of a meniscal tear. Displacement of a meniscal fragment between the tibial plateau and femoral condyles may cause loss of 5° or more of extension, locking of the joint in some degree of flexion or a positive McMurray test (a palpable clunk felt over the joint space as the knee is extended from a fully flexed and forcible internally or externally rotated position). Joint effusions and muscular spasm may produce many of these signs of meniscal tears. Aspiration of large effusions and instillation of local anesthetic into the joint followed by re-examination should therefore be performed in all questionable cases.

## REFERENCE

1.  Reckling F, Peltier L. Acute knee dislocations and their complications. J Trauma. 1969; 9:181.

ACUTELY INJURED KNEE

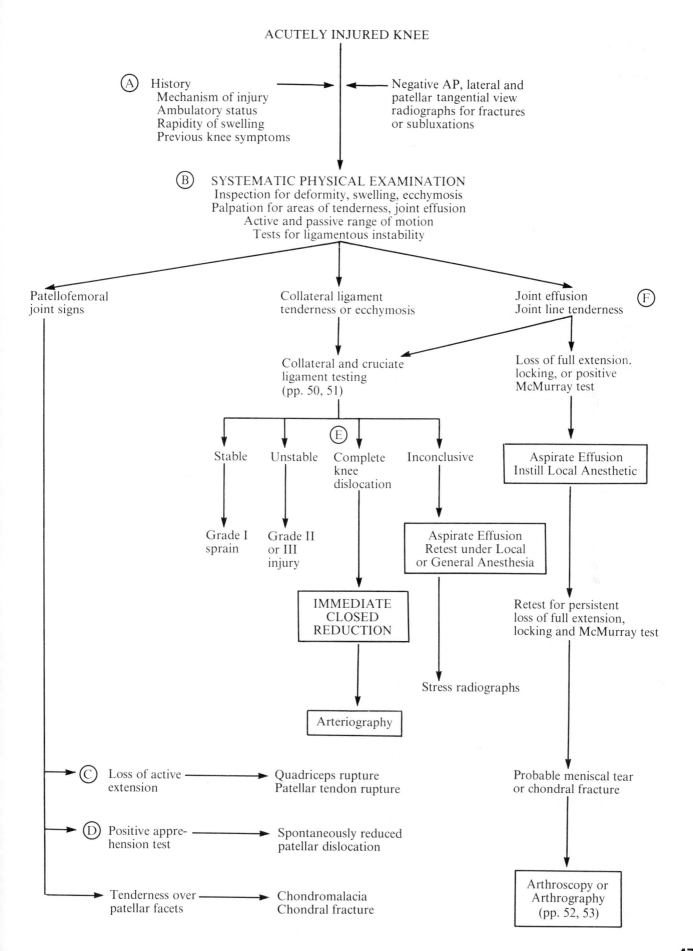

# FRACTURE OR DISLOCATION OF THE PATELLA

## COMMENTS

A. Fracture displacement and articular incongruity are evaluated best on the lateral radiograph while anteroposterior and sunrise (tangential) views aid in visualizing vertical fractures and osteochondral fragments. Bipartite patellas with the characteristic superolateral ossicles should not be mistakenly diagnosed as fractured.

B. The patella increases the mechanical advantage of the knee extensor mechanism (quadriceps tendon). The medial and lateral extensions of the vastus muscles around the patella constitute the extensor retinacula. Sparing of the retinacula during a complete fracture of the patella may permit some active knee extension. Retinacular disruption and total loss of active extension usually occur in fractures with greater than 3–4 mm displacement. If a transverse patellar fracture is allowed to heal in a displaced position, permanent extensor lag may be expected.

C. The prerequisites for cast treatment (a long leg or cylinder cast for 4 to 6 weeks) include an intact articular surface, minimal fracture displacement, and active knee extension. Chronic patellofemoral symptoms may result from direct cartilage trauma or from failure to reconstitute the articular congruity.

D. As with quadriceps and patellar tendon ruptures, the goal of surgery is to restore the extensor mechanism. Tension band wiring offers dynamic fixation of simple fractures.[1] Anchorage of the wire directly to the patella, using two vertical Steinmann pins, is probably necessary if early knee motion is anticipated.[2] Following visual confirmation of patellar articular reconstitution, the extensor retinacula should be repaired.

E. Partial patellectomy may be required in cases with severe comminution of either the proximal or distal poles. Extensive comminution necessitates total patellectomy. As much of the patella as possible should be saved to preserve its mechanical benefit.[3] Open fractures commonly are displaced and comminuted, thus requiring partial or total patellectomy during surgical debridement.

F. Lateral dislocations of the patella often reduce spontaneously. Tenderness over the medial aspect of the patella and a positive apprehension (Fairbanks) test should alert the physician to a probable reduced lateral dislocation. Following closed reduction by gentle extension of the knee, patellar dislocations must be evaluated radio-graphically to detect concomitant medial patellar facet fractures and lateral femoral condyle fractures. If these osteochondral fractures are displaced, arthrotomy with debridement or fixation of the fragments is necessary. Cast immobilization for 4 to 6 weeks is indicated for most acute patellar dislocations.

## REFERENCES

1. Muller M, Allgower M, Schneider R, Willenegger H. *Manual of Internal Fixation.* 2nd ed. New York: Springer-Verlag, 1979, pp. 248–253.
2. Weber M, Janecki C, McLeod P, Nelson C, Thompson J. Efficacy of various forms of fixation of transverse fractures of the patella. J Bone Joint Surg. 1980; 62A:215–220.
3. Kaufer J. Mechanical function of the patella. J Bone Joint Surg. 1971; 53A:1551–1560.

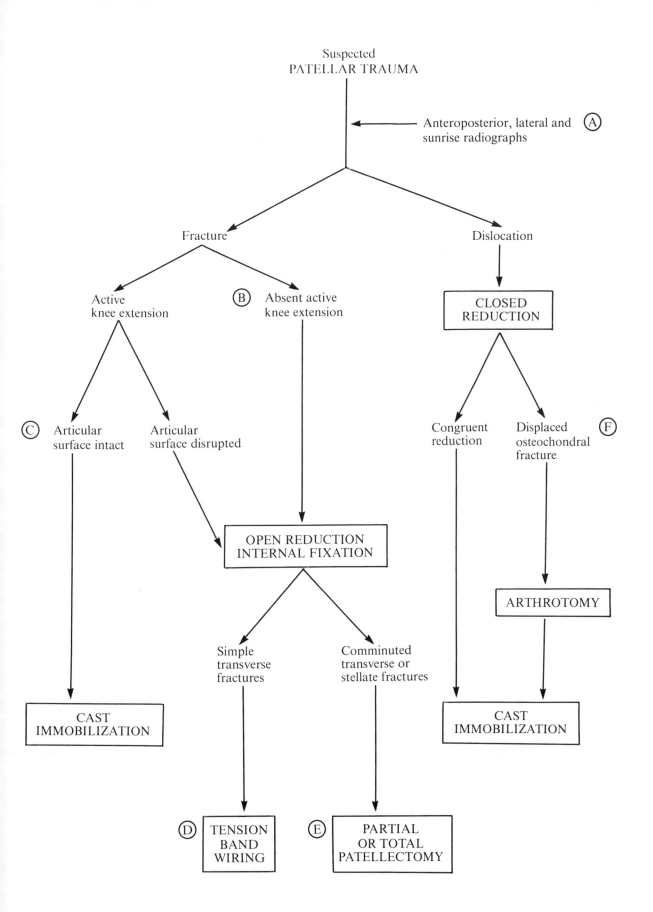

Suspected
PATELLAR TRAUMA

Anteroposterior, lateral and (A)
sunrise radiographs

Fracture

Dislocation

Active
knee extension

(B) Absent active
knee extension

CLOSED
REDUCTION

(C) Articular
surface intact

Articular
surface disrupted

Congruent
reduction

Displaced (F)
osteochondral
fracture

OPEN REDUCTION
INTERNAL FIXATION

ARTHROTOMY

Simple
transverse
fractures

Comminuted
transverse or
stellate fractures

CAST
IMMOBILIZATION

CAST
IMMOBILIZATION

(D) TENSION
BAND
WIRING

(E) PARTIAL
OR TOTAL
PATELLECTOMY

**49**

# KNEE LIGAMENT INJURY

## COMMENTS

A. Management of knee ligament injuries hinges on accurate clinical assessment of the extent of soft tissue disruption. Manual stress testing with the patient under local or general anesthesia should be used to localize systematically all significant ligamentous tears. Collateral ligament injuries may be graded as follows: Grade I: sprain with minimal laxity. Grade II: partial ligamentous tear with abnormal motion, but a firm resistant endpoint on stress testing. Grade III: complete tear with no solid endpoint on testing. Cruciate ligament disruptions are less amenable to grading, but an increase in anterior or posterior laxity of 1 cm compared to the contralateral normal knee is suggestive of a complete cruciate tear.

B. Routine knee radiographs are usually negative. However, avulsed bony prominences may signal a major disruption of the joint. Stress radiographs are useful in differentiating occult traumatic growth plate separations from ligamentous injuries in adolescent patients. Varus or valgus stress radiographs in adults with equivocal injuries should be obtained with both knees flexed 20 to 30°. An opening of 5 mm or more between the plateau and femoral condylar margins in excess of the contralateral knee suggests a probable collateral ligament rupture. If the measured distance is 12 mm greater than the normal knee, a concomitant cruciate ligament injury is likely.[1] Arthroscopy may be indicated to confirm a cruciate ligament injury or to rule out associated intra-articular pathology.

C. Stress to the knee in a given plane results in failure of the supporting structures in a predictable sequential order. Marshall and others have advanced the concept of lines of defense or prime stabilizers of the knee.[2] The application of this concept using experimental data from cadaveric studies has yielded the anatomic interpretations of various stress tests in this algorithm.[2] The anatomic structures are listed in order of their relative importance in preventing instability. A positive stress test implies definite injury to the prime stabilizers (labelled #1) and also may signify in more severe cases injury to other supplemental stabilizers (numbered 2 and 4 in order of their incidence of injury following the applied stress). Although controversy surrounds many of these tests and their interpretations, this outline does provide useful guidelines for predicting specific ligamentous tears. An alternative classification of knee ligament injuries distinguishes between single plane, rotatory, and combined instabilities.[3]

D. Valgus instability secondary to medial ligamentous tears should be checked with the knee in 30° flexion and full extension. Although grade III instability in 30° flexion can occur with isolated medial collateral ligament injury, comparable instability in full extension requires additional tears in the anterior cruciate ligament and posterior capsule.

E. Subluxation of 1 cm greater than the opposite knee on the anterior drawer test is a positive sign. Muscular spasm, tense joint effusion, or intact posterolateral cruciate band may occasionally cause a false-negative anterior drawer sign. Some authors therefore recommend testing anterior tibial subluxation with the knee extended (Lachman's test).

F. The posterior drawer test requires positioning of the leg similar to that in the anterior drawer maneuver, but with a posterior thrust applied to the proximal tibia. If marked swelling obscures the distinction between a positive anterior subluxation versus a postive posterior subluxation, stress radiographs may be helpful. The contours of both knees resting in 90° flexion should be inspected. Unilateral posterior sag of the tibia with loss of its tuberosity prominence anteriorly is also suggestive of a posterior cruciate tear.

G. A precise determination of ligamentous and capsular damage can consistently be achieved by the aforementioned medial-lateral and anterior-posterior stability tests. Rotatory tests stress multiple structures in a single maneuver, and thus merely confirm the results of the single plane tests.

H. When only the medial collateral ligament is ruptured, external rotation of the tibial plateau on the femoral condyles is possible if the flexed knee is externally rotated. Internal rotation of the foot tightens the intact posterolateral structures of the knee, thus blocking this rotatory subluxation.

I. The pivot shift, jerk, and Losee tests all detect anterior subluxation of the lateral tibial plateau on the femoral condyles (anterolateral instability or internal rotatory instability in extension). The pivot shift sign is elicited with the knee in extension and the foot held in forced internal rotation. The examiner exerts a valgus stress on the knee with his other hand and then flexes and extends the knee. As the knee is brought into 15 to 30° flexion, a sudden clunk from the reduction of the subluxed tibial plateau is felt. A similar clunk is sensed as the subluxation recurs. A positive test signifies an anterior cruciate tear. Lateral soft tissue lesions will accentuate the sign.

J. Most injuries involve multiplanar instability. Damage to the supporting knee structures can also lead to progressive instabilities as the remaining intact ligaments are stretched and attenuated by excessive abnormal forces. The

UNSTABLE KNEE

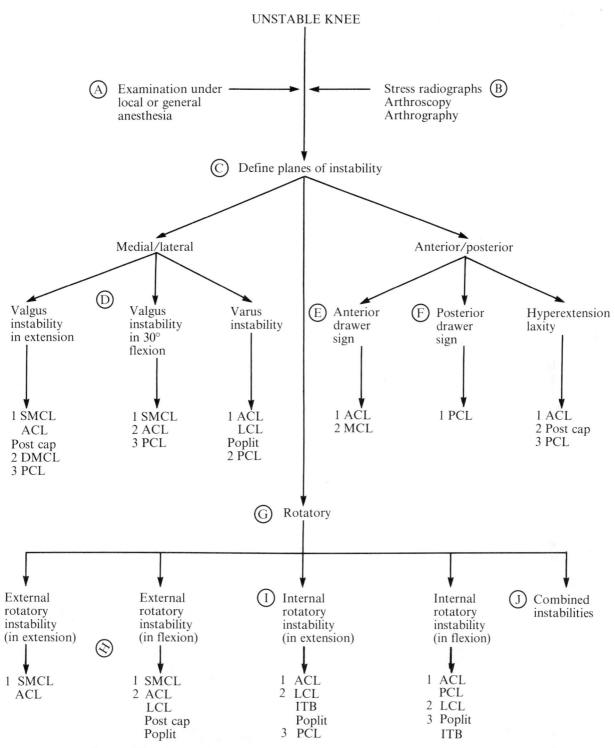

(A) Examination under
local or general
anesthesia

(B) Stress radiographs
Arthroscopy
Arthrography

(C) Define planes of instability

Medial/lateral

Anterior/posterior

(D) Valgus
instability
in extension

Valgus
instability
in 30°
flexion

Varus
instability

(E) Anterior
drawer
sign

(F) Posterior
drawer
sign

Hyperextension
laxity

1 SMCL
ACL
Post cap
2 DMCL
3 PCL

1 SMCL
2 ACL
3 PCL

1 ACL
LCL
Poplit
2 PCL

1 ACL
2 MCL

1 PCL

1 ACL
2 Post cap
3 PCL

(G) Rotatory

External
rotatory
instability
(in extension)

External
rotatory
instability
(in flexion)

(I) Internal
rotatory
instability
(in extension)

Internal
rotatory
instability
(in flexion)

(J) Combined
instabilities

(H)

1 SMCL
ACL

1 SMCL
2 ACL
LCL
Post cap
Poplit

1 ACL
2 LCL
ITB
Poplit
3 PCL

1 ACL
PCL
2 LCL
3 Poplit
ITB

treatment of specific ligamentous injuries remains controversial with many operative repairs recommended in the literature.[2,4]

knee joint instability. Clin Orthop. 1980; 147:15.

4. Hunter G, (Ed). Symposium on ligamentous injuries of the knee. Clin Orthop. 1980; 147:92.

## REFERENCES

1. Hastings D. The non-operative management of ligament injuries of the knee joint. Clin Orthop. 1980; 147:22.
2. Marshall J, Rubin R. Knee ligament injuries—a diagnostic and therapeutic approach. Orthop Clin N Amer. 1977; 8:641.
3. Fowler P. The classification and early diagnosis of

Abbreviations: ACL, anterior cruciate ligament. PCL, posterior cruciate ligament. MCL, medial collateral ligament. SMCL, superficial medial collateral ligament. DMCL, deep medial collateral ligament. Post cap, posterior capsule. Poplit, popliteus. LCL, lateral collateral ligament. ITB, iliotibial band.

# MENISCAL INJURY

## COMMENTS

A. As important stabilizers and load-sharing structures of the knee, the menisci serve a major role in normal joint function. Tears may occur either in the cartilagenous substance of a meniscus or along its fibrous attachments to the capsule. A history of a sudden twisting injury with a popping or catching sensation and subsequent locking of the joint is highly suggestive of a meniscal injury. Following an acute meniscal injury, a joint effusion gradually accumulates over a 6- to 12-hour period. Although the physical signs of joint-line tenderness, loss of full knee extension, and positive McMurray test (see section on The Acutely Injured Knee) strengthen one's clinical suspicion, a thorough history of the knee trauma and symptoms is essential for an accurate presumptive diagnosis of meniscal injury.

B. All patients with symptoms of meniscal injury that limit their normal activity should be evaluated by either arthroscopy or arthrography. Exploratory arthrotomy without preoperative documentation of a tear is not justified. The accuracy of arthrographic studies varies from 60 to 90%, depending on the technique and one's experience in their interpretation.[1,2] Arthroscopy is more accurate than arthrography in evaluating lateral meniscal tears as well as other intra-articular injury, such as cruciate ruptures and chondral fractures. Most orthopaedists now prefer diagnostic arthroscopy because the examination can be followed immediately with definitive endoscopic meniscectomy. Dandy has devised a detailed classification scheme of meniscal injuries for arthroscopic surgery.[3]

C. Meniscal tears may be grouped into several overlapping anatomic categories. Bucket-handle lesions arise from longitudinal tears near the posterior horn and propagate along the body of the meniscus. They may or may not be displaced into the intercondylar notch, thereby mechanically blocking knee extension. Arthroscopic excision of the bucket-handle fragment alone is indicated if the remaining rim of the meniscus is intact and stable.[4,5] Approximately 10% of cases require arthrotomy to complete the meniscectomy.[4]

D. Avulsion of an otherwise undamaged meniscus at its fibrous attachments to the capsule should be treated by suture repair rather than meniscectomy.

E. Meniscal flaps or tags may originate from partial bucket-handle injuries or horizontal fissures. They are frequently concealed above or below the posterior one-third of the meniscus. Limited horizontal cleavage, pedunculated or flap injuries to the meniscus, whether traumatic or degenerative in nature, should be managed by partial meniscectomy if there is a documented symptomatic tear and loss of knee extension. Guidelines for arthroscopic partial meniscectomy have been recommended by Dandy.[3] As wide a meniscal rim as possible should be preserved. Small meniscal fissures unrelated to the patient's complaints should not be excised.

F. Extensive tears with shredding of the meniscus necessitates total meniscectomy. The regenerated fibrous rim that often appears after complete meniscectomy serves little biomechanical function.

G. Endoscopic meniscectomy offers a shorter disability period and a more rapid rehabilitation than open surgery. Meniscectomy, however, is not a benign procedure. Long-term results are poorer in women and in cases with anterior cruciate insufficiency, coexisting degenerative disease, an extended delay in the diagnosis and treatment of the meniscal rupture, or a retained prolapsing posterior meniscal fragment.[6]

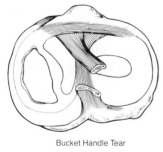

Bucket Handle Tear

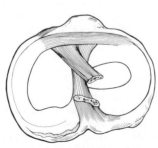

Peripheral Tear

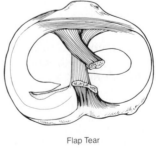

Flap Tear

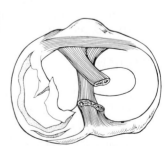

Extensive Complete Tear

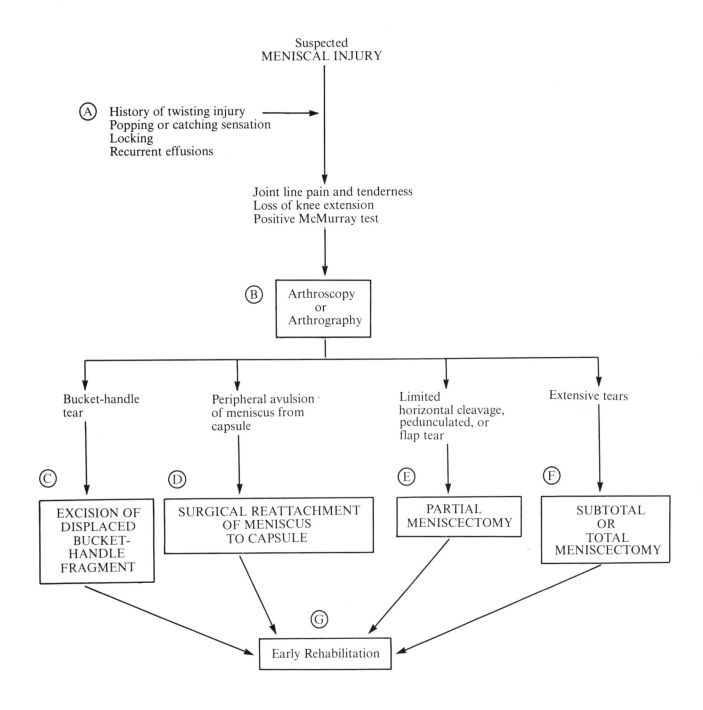

Suspected
MENISCAL INJURY

Ⓐ History of twisting injury
Popping or catching sensation
Locking
Recurrent effusions

Joint line pain and tenderness
Loss of knee extension
Positive McMurray test

Ⓑ Arthroscopy
or
Arthrography

Bucket-handle
tear

Peripheral avulsion
of meniscus from
capsule

Limited
horizontal cleavage,
pedunculated, or
flap tear

Extensive tears

Ⓒ EXCISION OF
DISPLACED
BUCKET-
HANDLE
FRAGMENT

Ⓓ SURGICAL REATTACHMENT
OF MENISCUS
TO CAPSULE

Ⓔ PARTIAL
MENISCECTOMY

Ⓕ SUBTOTAL
OR
TOTAL
MENISCECTOMY

Ⓖ Early Rehabilitation

## REFERENCES

1. Nicholas J, Freiberger R, Killoran P. Double-contrast arthrography of the knee—its valve in the management of two hundred and twenty-five knee derangements. J Bone Joint Surg. 1970; 52A:203.
2. Gillquist J, Hagberg G. Findings at arthroscopy and arthrography in knee injuries. Acta Orthop Scan. 1978; 49:398.
3. Dandy D. *Arthroscopic Surgery of the Knee*. Churchill-Livingstone: Edinburgh, 1981, pp. 70–110.
4. Gillquist J, Oretorp N. Arthroscopic partial meniscectomy—technique and long-term results. Clin Orthop. 1982; 167:29.
5. Northmore-Ball M, Dandy D. Long-term results of arthroscopic partial meniscectomy. Clin Orthop. 1982; 167:34.
6. Tapper E, Hoover N. Late results after meniscectomy. J Bone Joint Surg. 1969; 51A:517.

# TIBIAL PLATEAU FRACTURE

## COMMENTS

A. The tibial condylar surface slopes posteroinferiorly 10 to 15°. Accurate assessment of the amount of depression of articular fragments therefore necessitates an AP radiograph with the beam directed 10 to 15° inferiorly. Tomograms may be required in questionable cases. Since depression of the weight-bearing portion of the plateau may lead to varus or valgus instability, stress radiographs should be performed routinely in the evaluation of plateau fractures.

B. Under general or regional anesthesia, the integrity of the ligaments should be tested with the knee in full extension and in 15 to 30° flexion. Ligamentous disruptions may be suspected when there are radiographically evident avulsion fractures off the condylar edges, the tibial eminence, or the fibular head. The incidence of concomitant ligamentous injuries is highest in nondisplaced and split compression type plateau fractures, and lowest in isolated central compression fractures.[1] All grade III tears should be repaired, regardless of the treatment used for the plateau fracture.

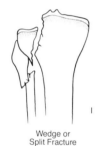

Wedge or
Split Fracture

I

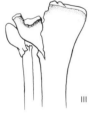

III

Split-Depression
Fracture

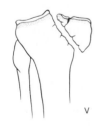

V

Total Condylar Fracture

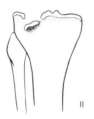

II

Central Depression
Fracture

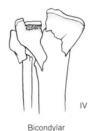

IV

Bicondylar
Fracture

C. The goal of any treatment is to restore knee motion, alignment, and stability. Dense intra-articular adhesions with resultant mechanical blockage of knee motion are a predictable consequence of prolonged immobilization.[2] Nondisplaced and stable central compression fractures therefore ought to be managed with early cast bracing.[3] Full weight bearing is commenced once early union is apparent, usually at 8 to 12 weeks.

D. The Hohl classification scheme provides a useful framework for therapeutic decisions.[2] Nondisplaced fractures, isolated central compression fractures, and split-compression fractures constitute over three-fourths of all plateau injuries. Split fractures (shear type condylar wedge fractures without articular depression), total condylar fractures (fracture lines extending up into the intercondylar eminence), and comminuted bicondylar fractures are common. Central depression of greater than 5 mm; medial, lateral, or inferior translation of more than 2 mm; or knee instability of 5° varus or valgus greater that the normal contralateral knee defines a displaced fracture. Owing to unsatisfactory closed reductions and loss of acceptable reductions in plaster, operative stabilization of displaced fractures is generally warranted.

E. Isolated central compression fractures, usually in the anterior aspect of the lateral condyle, that are less than 5 mm depressed and do not cause valgus instability can be treated by early motion in a cast brace.

F. Central compression fractures depressed greater than 5 mm are commonly associated with major varus/valgus instability, and should be elevated and stabilized. Autogenous cancellous bone graft fills the subarticular cavity under the raised osteocartilagenous fragment and prevents postoperative settling of the condylar surface.

G. Late complications of degenerative joint disease, knee contractures, and knee instability are minimized by accurate anatomical reduction and early active motion.[4] Open reduction and internal fixation of complex plateau fractures, however, may present formidable challenges to the surgeon. Surgical enthusiasm must be tempered by consideration of such variables as patient age, functional demands, soft tissue status, associated injuries, and operative experience of the surgeon. Specific indications for primary skeletal traction and/or case brace treatment include major skin loss and elderly patients with minimal functional demands.[3]

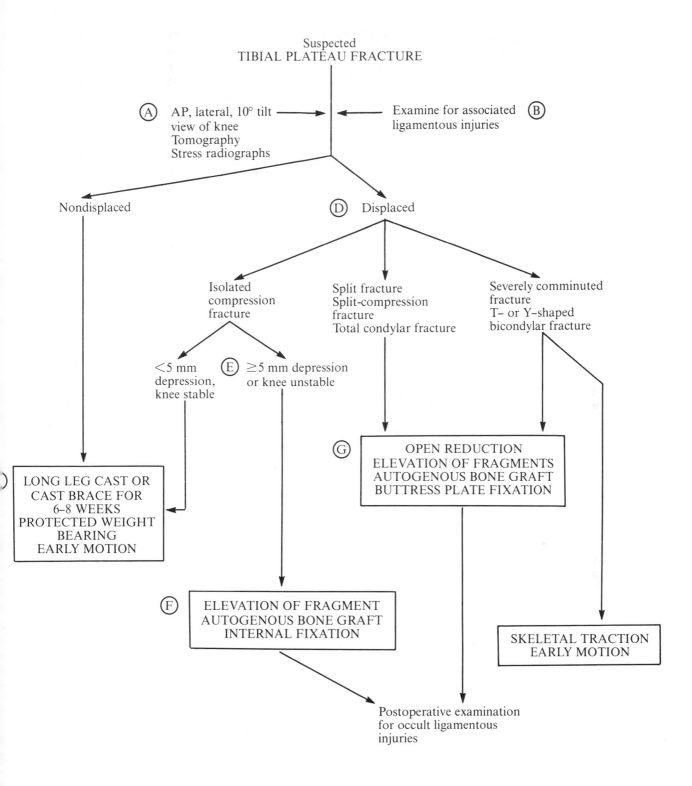

Suspected
**TIBIAL PLATEAU FRACTURE**

Ⓐ AP, lateral, 10° tilt → ← Examine for associated Ⓑ
view of knee                    ligamentous injuries
Tomography
Stress radiographs

Nondisplaced                    Ⓓ Displaced

Isolated              Split fracture          Severely comminuted
compression           Split-compression       fracture
fracture              fracture                T– or Y–shaped
                      Total condylar fracture bicondylar fracture

<5 mm          Ⓔ ≥5 mm depression
depression,       or knee unstable
knee stable

**LONG LEG CAST OR                    Ⓖ  OPEN REDUCTION
CAST BRACE FOR                            ELEVATION OF FRAGMENTS
6–8 WEEKS                                 AUTOGENOUS BONE GRAFT
PROTECTED WEIGHT                          BUTTRESS PLATE FIXATION
BEARING
EARLY MOTION**

Ⓕ  **ELEVATION OF FRAGMENT
AUTOGENOUS BONE GRAFT
INTERNAL FIXATION**

                                          **SKELETAL TRACTION
                                          EARLY MOTION**

Postoperative examination
for occult ligamentous
injuries

## REFERENCES

1. Moore T, Meyers M, Harvey J. Collateral ligament laxity of the knee—long-term comparison between plateau fractures and normal. J Bone Joint Surg. 1976; 58A:594.

2. Hohl M. Tibial condylar fractures. J Bone Joint Surg. 1967; 49A:1455.

3. Scotland T, Wardlaw D. The use of cast-bracing as treatment for fractures of the tibial plateau. J Bone Joint Surg. 1981; 63B:575.

4. Muller M, Allgower M, Schneider R, Willenegger H. *Manual of Internal Fixation*. Berlin: Springer-Verlag, 1979, pp. 256–263.

# TIBIAL SHAFT FRACTURE

## COMMENTS

A. The variables that most affect the outcome of tibial shaft fractures are the degree of initial displacement, the extent of fracture comminution, the severity of the soft tissue wounds, and the adequacy of the reduction. Acceptable reductions generally fall within 5° of varus or valgus, 5° of anterior or posterior angulation, and 5° of rotation compared to the normal contralateral tibia. While any fracture distraction must be avoided, shortening of up to 5 to 10 mm may be accepted, especially in comminuted, oblique fracture patterns. Translatory displacement of the major fragments is of less functional significance.

B. Reangulation and shortening of unstable fractures in plaster casts are common. Temporary non-weight bearing, cast wedgings, remanipulations, or, occasionally, reverting to external or internal fixation may be necessary to ensure healing in a satisfactory position. Serial check radiographs, using large casettes that permit visualization of the entire tibia and adjacent joints, provide the essential information for subsequent therapeutic decisions.

C. Early weight bearing appears to have a propitious effect on the healing process.[1] Besides improving muscle and joint function, the cyclic loading of the fracture with weight bearing accelerates the formation of callus. The frequent problems of shortening and reangulation demand close radiographic follow-up.[2] By 4 to 8 weeks, conversion to a total-contact below-knee cast is feasible for most fractures.[3]

D. Rigid internal fixation of both the femoral and tibial fractures in floating knee injuries optimizes the chance for full restoration of knee function. Similarly, internal fracture stabilization affords the best opportunity for aggressive management of concomitant vascular and knee ligament injuries.

E. As a load sharing device, the Lottes or Kuntscher intramedullary rod is preferred to plate fixation. The advantages are even greater if a closed technique with image intensification is utilized. Transverse or oblique mid-shaft fractures and segmental fractures in which satisfactory reduction cannot be achieved or maintained are ideal indications for an intramedullary rod. If the fracture extends beyond the middle third of the shaft, the rod acts solely as an internal splint. Fracture displacement or shortening around the rod may occur in such cases, thus making tibial plating a more reliable treatment alternative. Strict adherence to AFIF principles of plate fixation is mandatory.

F. Following thorough debridement and irrigation, fracture wounds should be dressed open, and subsequently closed at 4 to 7 days. A short course of antibiotic therapy is routine.[4] Most grade I and II injuries are amenable to standard cast treatment with minor modifications for the soft tissue wounds.

G. Extensive grade III injuries, with or without neurovascular compromise, often require several debridements of all necrotic tissue and multiple procedures to obtain soft tissue coverage. The soft tissue lesions take precedence over the osseous injury. External fixation allows easy access to the soft tissue and minimizes further tissue damage from fracture motion. It is imperative to avoid fracture distraction by the frame. Early substitution of cast immobilization or internal fixation for the external fixator once the wounds are healed is desirable in the majority of cases. Segmental osseous defects should be grafted early, preferable via a posterolateral approach.

## REFERENCES

1. Dehne E, Metz C, Deffer P. Nonoperative treatment of the fractured tibia by immediate weight bearing. J Trauma 1961; 1:514.
2. Brown P, Urban J. Early weight-bearing treatment of open fractures of the tibia. J Bone Joint Surg. 1969; 51A:59.
3. Sarmiento A. A functional below-the-knee cast for tibial fractures. J Bone Joint Surg. 1967; 49A:855.
4. Gustilo R, Anderson J. Prevention of infection in the treatment of one thousand and twenty-five open fractures of long bones. J Bone Joint Surg. 1976; 58A:453.

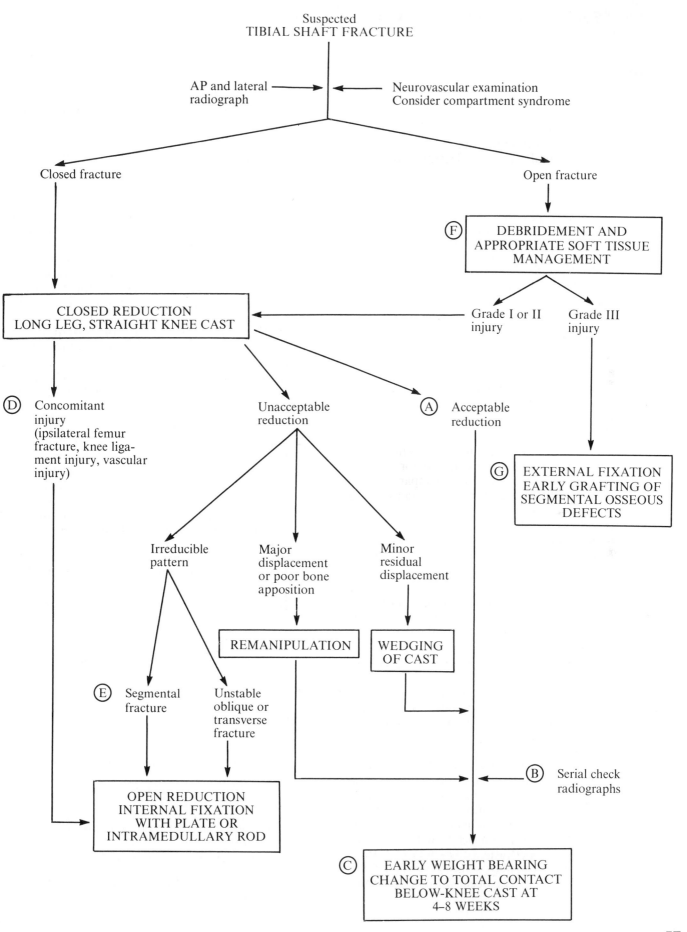

Suspected
TIBIAL SHAFT FRACTURE

AP and lateral
radiograph

Neurovascular examination
Consider compartment syndrome

Closed fracture

Open fracture

(F) DEBRIDEMENT AND
APPROPRIATE SOFT TISSUE
MANAGEMENT

CLOSED REDUCTION
LONG LEG, STRAIGHT KNEE CAST

Grade I or II
injury

Grade III
injury

(D) Concomitant
injury
(ipsilateral femur
fracture, knee liga-
ment injury, vascular
injury)

Unacceptable
reduction

(A) Acceptable
reduction

(G) EXTERNAL FIXATION
EARLY GRAFTING OF
SEGMENTAL OSSEOUS
DEFECTS

Irreducible
pattern

Major
displacement
or poor bone
apposition

Minor
residual
displacement

REMANIPULATION

WEDGING
OF CAST

(E) Segmental
fracture

Unstable
oblique or
transverse
fracture

(B) Serial check
radiographs

OPEN REDUCTION
INTERNAL FIXATION
WITH PLATE OR
INTRAMEDULLARY ROD

(C) EARLY WEIGHT BEARING
CHANGE TO TOTAL CONTACT
BELOW-KNEE CAST AT
4–8 WEEKS

# COMPARTMENT SYNDROME

## COMMENTS

A. Compartment syndrome is defined as a condition in which increased pressure within a limited space compromises the circulation and function of the tissues within that space.[1] Elevated intracompartmental pressure decreases the local arteriovenous gradient, thereby diminishing blood flow. Prolonged tissue ischemia may result in transient or permanent damage to myoneural elements within the compartment. The only prerequisites for a compartment syndrome are therefore a limiting envelope around neuromuscular tissue and a cause for increased pressure. A variety of clinical entities can initiate a compartment syndrome. The most common traumatic etiologies include (1) bleeding or edema in a compartment following contusion or fracture, (2) thermal and electrical burns, (3) tight casts or dressing, or other exogenous compression, (4) overzealous longitudinal skeletal traction on a traumatized limb, (5) tight surgical closure of facial defects, (6) excessive exercise, and (7) snakebites. The interval between the traumatic event and the development of the syndrome may vary from several hours to a week or more, but usually is around 12 to 48 hours. The most frequent post-traumatic sites for compartment syndromes are the four compartments of the leg, the volar forearm compartments, and the interosseous compartments of the hand.

B. There is significant individual variation in the "critical pressure" necessary to trigger the pathophysiologic cycle leading to a fulminant compartment syndrome. Factors that may lower the tolerance to increased tissue pressure, thus predisposing to the syndrome, are limb elevation, tight circumferential dressings, systemic hypotension, and proximal arterial occlusion.

C. A compartment syndrome is heralded by pain in excess of what is normally expected following the given trauma and local tenderness over the involved compartment. Pain is elicited by passive stretching of the muscles that traverse the compartment. Subsequently, hypesthesia and muscular weakness will be evident. Distal pulses and Doppler signals may be normal. The diagnosis of compartment syndrome is based on these clinical symptoms and signs in the majority of cases. The similar symptoms and signs of peripheral nerve injuries and ischemia from arterial injuries can usually be distinguished from those of compartment syndromes on a clinical basis. Evaluation should be performed quickly and treatment instituted immediately, since irreversible neuromuscular damage can occur within 6 to 8 hours.

D. An ambiguous clinical picture of compartment syndrome occasionally necessitates the direct measurement of intracompartmental pressures. Pressure measurements are also helpful in unconscious patients with limb trauma sufficient to cause a compartment syndrome. The three commonly used methods for measuring tissue pressure are the needle-manometer,[2] the wick catheter,[3] and the continuous infusion techniques.[1] The latter two methods allow for continuous monitoring. Although there is no single absolute critical pressure above which a compartment syndrome is inevitable, there are generally accepted guidelines for proceeding with an immediate fasciotomy. These vary from 30 mg of Hg or more using the wick catheter to 45 mg of Hg using continuous infusion to 50 mg of Hg (or within 20 mg of Hg of the diastolic pressure) using the needle-manometer method.[1,2,3] Accurate calibration and use of any of these systems is imperative, since an erroneous pressure measurement is worse than no measurement at all.

E. Immediate fasciotomy should be performed once the diagnosis of compartment syndrome has been made. Despite the numerous procedures reported for decompression of different compartments, the basic surgical principles are the same.[1,2] The skin and fascia should be opened the entire length of the compartment. All four compartments of the leg routinely should be released. Forearm fasciotomies ought to be extended distally to include a standard carpal tunnel release. Only clearly nonviable muscle is debrided at the time of fasciotomy. The wound is left open and inspected at 5 to 7 days. Closure may be effected by delayed suture or split-thickness skin grafting. Complete fasciotomies may diminish the soft tissue splinting of certain associated fractures, thereby making necessary internal or external frame fixation of the fractures.

## REFERENCES

1. Matsen F. *Compartment Syndromes*. New York: Grune and Stratton, 1980.
2. Whitesides T, Haruda H, Morimoto K. Compartment syndromes and the role of fasciotomy, its parameters and techniques. Instructional Course Lectures, The American Academy of Orthopaedic Surgeons. St. Louis: Mosby. 1977; 26:179.
3. Mubarak S, Owen C, Hargens A, Garetto L, Akeson W. Acute compartment syndromes: diagnosis and treatment with the aid of the Wick catheter. J Bone Joint Surg. 1978; 60A:1091.

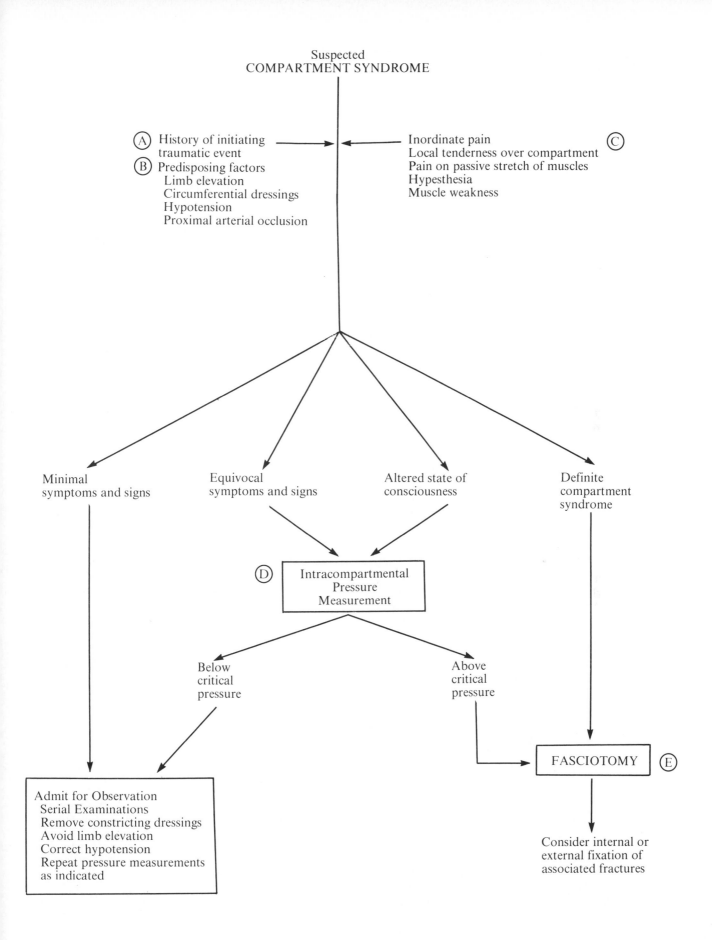

Suspected
COMPARTMENT SYNDROME

Ⓐ History of initiating
traumatic event
Ⓑ Predisposing factors
Limb elevation
Circumferential dressings
Hypotension
Proximal arterial occlusion

Inordinate pain
Local tenderness over compartment
Pain on passive stretch of muscles
Hypesthesia
Muscle weakness
Ⓒ

Minimal
symptoms and signs

Equivocal
symptoms and signs

Altered state of
consciousness

Definite
compartment
syndrome

Ⓓ Intracompartmental
Pressure
Measurement

Below
critical
pressure

Above
critical
pressure

FASCIOTOMY Ⓔ

Admit for Observation
Serial Examinations
Remove constricting dressings
Avoid limb elevation
Correct hypotension
Repeat pressure measurements
as indicated

Consider internal or
external fixation of
associated fractures

# TIBIAL PILON FRACTURE

## COMMENTS

A.  Pilon fractures, distal tibial fractures with extension into the ankle joint, result from severe vertical loads during falls, sporting injuries, and motor vehicle accidents. The position of the foot at the time of impact determines the fracture pattern. Primarily anterior lip fractures of the distal tibia arise when the foot is dorsiflexed, posterior lip fractures when the foot is plantar flexed, and comminuted Y- or T-shaped fractures when the foot is plantigrade. These high-energy injuries may be associated with extensive soft tissue injuries, direct articular cartilage damage, and marked fracture comminution.

B.  Although acute neurovascular injuries are uncommon, delayed neurovascular symptoms and signs may develop with the hemorrhage and edema that invariably accompany these fractures. If surgery is planned but must be postponed, leg elevation and 5 to 15 pounds of longitudinal skeletal traction through a calcaneal pin will minimize soft tissue swelling and fracture shortening.

C.  The rare, minimally displaced fracture with a preserved articular surface may be managed by standard closed techniques. Delayed weight bearing for 6 to 12 weeks will prevent significant displacement of the articular component of the fracture.

D.  The two major questions confronting the orthopaedist in a displaced pilon fracture are whether closed treatment will yield a satisfactory result for the patient's functional needs and if surgical reconstruction with anatomic reduction and rigid internal fixation is possible. The factors that influence the feasibility of surgical fixation include the degree of comminution, the size of the fracture fragments, the status of the soft tissues, the availability of appropriate instrumentation and implants, and the experience of the surgeon. The best results are achieved by operative anatomic restoration of the joint; the worst results follow ill-conceived or inadequate surgery. Limited surgical fixation, such as stabilization of associated fibular fractures only or simple interfragmental fixation of several major articular fragments, offers no predictable benefit over closed treatment.

E.  Technical difficulties in the past have discouraged attempts at surgical repair of these intraarticular fractures. The ASIF group advocates a four-step systematic reconstruction of displaced fractures.[1-3] First, the fibula is anatomically reduced and stabilized, thus restoring normal length to the limb. The fibular escapes fracture in approximately one-fourth of pilon fractures. Second, the disrupted articular surface is reduced and major fragments are temporarily transfixed with multiple Kirschner wires. Third, autologous cancellous bone graft from the iliac crest or greater trochanter of the femur is packed into any metaphyseal defects. Finally, a well-contoured buttress plate is applied medially and/or anteriorly with interfragmental screw fixation of large fragments.

F.  Redisplacement and shortening of a reduced fracture occur after casting alone. Improved alignment is often obtained by os calcis pin traction for 2 to 4 weeks. Early motion of the ankle in traction helps to mold the articular fragments into satisfactory position. Residual fracture displacement of several millimeters may be inconsequential in elderly patients and patients with low functional demands. Irreducible fracture displacement with complete disruption of the articular surfaces is a relative indication for early ankle arthrodesis at 6 to 12 weeks. This technique should be reserved for patients with the most severe fractures judged to be inappropriate for primary open reduction.

G.  Post-traumatic arthritis results from residual joint incongruity, malalignment of the ankle joint with the longitudinal axis of the tibia, cartilage damage at the time of injury, or a combination of these factors. Joint degeneration may therefore be evident even following apparent surgical restoration of the bony anatomy. Ruedi reported 75% good long-term results after open reduction compared with less than 50% following closed treatment.[3] Post-traumatic arthritis usually manifests itself within 2 years of the injury.

## REFERENCES

1.  Ruedi T, Allgower M. Fractures of the lower end of the tibia into the ankle joint. Injury, 1969; 1:92.
2.  Muller M, Allgower M, Schneider R, Willenegger H. (Eds.) *Manual of Internal Fixation.* Berlin: Springer-Verlag, 1979.
3.  Ruedi T, Allgower M. The operative treatment of intra-articular fractures of the lower end of the tibia. Clin Orthop. 1979; 138:105.

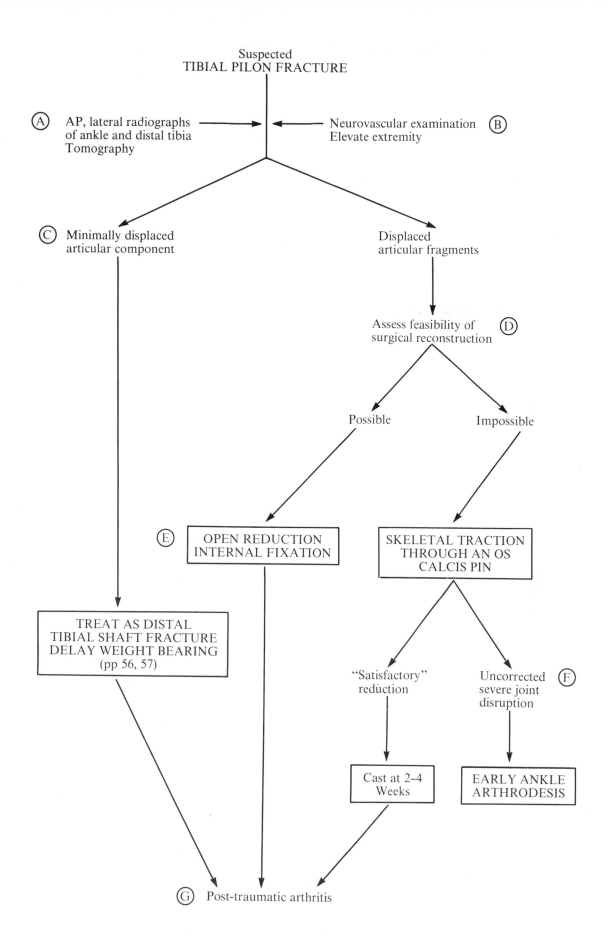

Suspected
**TIBIAL PILON FRACTURE**

Ⓐ AP, lateral radiographs
of ankle and distal tibia
Tomography

Neurovascular examination
Elevate extremity Ⓑ

Ⓒ Minimally displaced
articular component

Displaced
articular fragments

Assess feasibility of
surgical reconstruction Ⓓ

Possible

Impossible

Ⓔ OPEN REDUCTION
INTERNAL FIXATION

SKELETAL TRACTION
THROUGH AN OS
CALCIS PIN

TREAT AS DISTAL
TIBIAL SHAFT FRACTURE
DELAY WEIGHT BEARING
(pp 56, 57)

"Satisfactory"
reduction

Uncorrected
severe joint Ⓕ
disruption

Cast at 2–4
Weeks

EARLY ANKLE
ARTHRODESIS

Ⓖ Post-traumatic arthritis

# EVALUATION OF THE SPRAINED ANKLE

## COMMENTS

A.  A sprain is defined as a partial or complete disruption of the fibers of a ligament. Isolated anterior talofibular ligament ruptures constitute the most common cause of "ankle sprains." More severe adduction injuries may result additionally in calcaneofibular ligament tears. Though swelling may be diffuse over the dorsum of the ankle and foot, point tenderness localizes the injury to the anterior and inferior aspects of the lateral malleolus. Deltoid ligament ruptures usually accompany lateral malleolar fractures and rarely are isolated injuries. The anterior drawer sign is the most sensitive clinical test for major sprains to the lateral ligamentous complex. The heel of the foot is gently pulled forward while the tibia is stabilized by the examiner's opposite hand. Anterior translation of the talar dome on the tibia greater than that in the uninjured contralateral ankle suggests a complete tear of the ante-

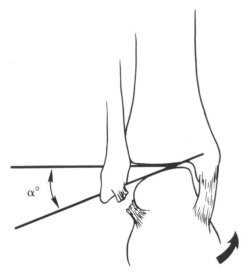

Measurement of Talar Tilt

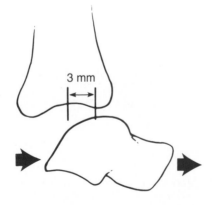

Measurement of Anterior Drawer

rior talofibular ligament. A negative anterior drawer sign implies no significant loss of ankle stability, thus indicating the need for only symptomatic treatment of the sprain with an ankle wrap or short leg cast.

B.  The maximal normal anterior displacement of the talus on the tibia varies from individual to individual. Displacement of greater than 3 mm, however, is abnormal.[1] Stress radiographs are indicated in all patients with positive anterior drawer signs following an acute ankle sprain. Either inversion stress films measuring lateral talar tilt or anterior stress films measuring anterior talar translation can be obtained (see figure). A talar tilt 10° greater than the contralateral ankle or an anterior translation of greater than 3 mm on the lateral radiograph implies major talotibial subluxation.[1] Ankle arthrography may alternatively be used to evaluate the severity of the suspected major sprain. Massive lateral extra-articular extravasation of contrast medium occurs if both the anterior talofibular and calcaneofibular ligaments are completely disrupted.[2]

C.  Satisfactory functional results using careful casting and taping for 6 to 8 weeks can be achieved in patients with documented unstable injuries.[3]

D.  Young active athletes with high functional demands may benefit from surgical reapproximation of the ligaments if complete lateral ligamentous injury is confirmed.[2] Lateral ligamentous ruptures associated with medial or lateral malleolar fractures should be repaired.

E.  Fractures commonly mistaken for ankle sprains include fractures of the fifth metatarsal base, avulsion fractures, and lateral malleolar fractures. Severe ankle sprains may be accompanied by osteochondritis dissecans defects in the talar dome.

F.  Tenderness localized to the posterior aspect of the lateral malleolus should alert the physician to the possibility of peroneal tendon subluxation or Achilles tendon injury.

## REFERENCES

1.  Seligson D, Gassman J, Pope M. Ankle instability: evaluation of the lateral ligaments. Amer J Sports Med. 1980; 8:39–42.
2.  Staples OS. Ruptures of the fibular collateral ligaments of the ankle. J Bone Joint Surg. 1975; 57A:101–107.
3.  Leonard M. Injuries of the lateral ligaments of the ankle—a clinical and experimental study. J Bone Joint Surg. 1949; 31A:373–377.

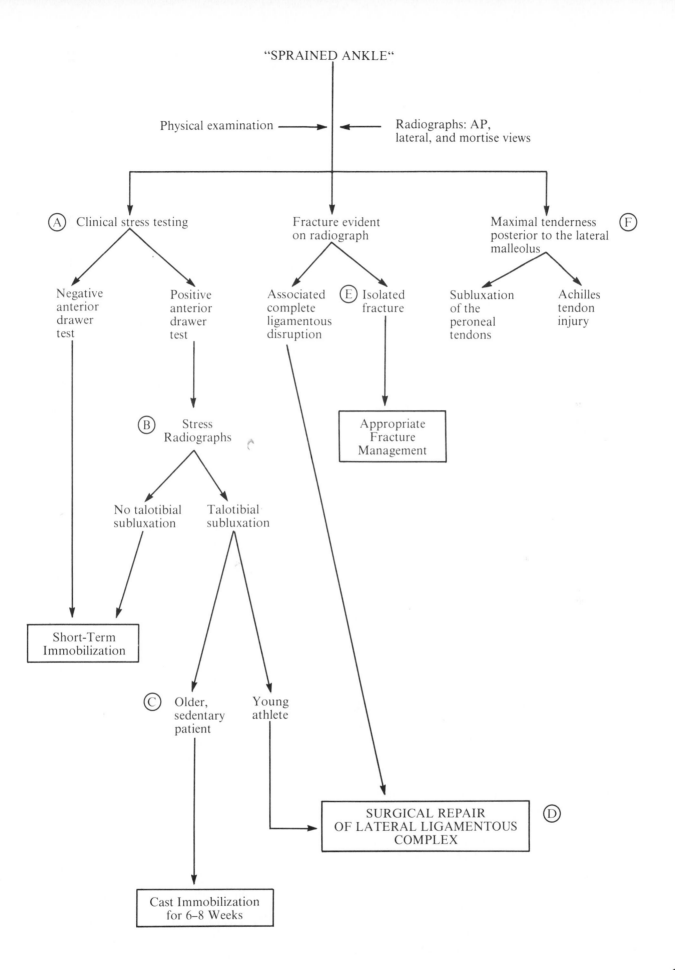

"SPRAINED ANKLE"

Physical examination → ← Radiographs: AP, lateral, and mortise views

Ⓐ Clinical stress testing

Fracture evident on radiograph

Ⓕ Maximal tenderness posterior to the lateral malleolus

Negative anterior drawer test

Positive anterior drawer test

Associated complete ligamentous disruption

Ⓔ Isolated fracture

Subluxation of the peroneal tendons

Achilles tendon injury

Ⓑ Stress Radiographs

Appropriate Fracture Management

No talotibial subluxation

Talotibial subluxation

Short-Term Immobilization

Ⓒ Older, sedentary patient

Young athlete

SURGICAL REPAIR OF LATERAL LIGAMENTOUS COMPLEX Ⓓ

Cast Immobilization for 6–8 Weeks

# ANKLE FRACTURE OR DISLOCATION

**COMMENTS**

A. The stability of the ankle joint depends on the structural integrity of the bones (medial and lateral malleoli, tibial plafond, and talus), the ligaments (lateral collateral, deltoid, and syndesmotic), and, to a lesser degree, the capsular and muscular tissues. A minimum of two breaks, either osseous or ligamentous, in the ankle mortise is necessary for significant talar shift to occur. A weight-bearing line drawn down the center of the tibial shaft should pass through the center of the talus on the AP radiograph.[1] On the lateral radiograph, such a line should intersect the most proximal point of the talar dome. Talar shift of more than 1 or 2 mm in any plane, with or without asymmetry in the articular clear space or evident widening of the distal tibiofibular syndesmosis, is diagnostic of an unstable injury. Stress radiographs and comparable views of the opposite normal ankle may assist in evaluating equivocal fractures.

B. Single breaks in the mortise, commonly isolated fractures of the lateral malleolus, are stable and merely require external immobilization.

C. The goal of surgery is anatomic positioning and stabilization of the talus in the ankle mortise. Radiographs following closed reduction and the use of either the Lauge-Hansen or AO (see figure) classification schemes aid in the preoperative planning for unstable injuries.[2,3] Closed treatment with casting only is unsatisfactory owing to difficulties in achieving acceptable reductions, loss of reductions in plaster necessitating remanipulations, and stiffness and disuse atrophy from prolonged immobilization.

D. Owing to the stout lateral collateral ligament complex and the buttressing role of the lateral malleolus, talar shift correlates directly with the plane and extent of lateral malleolar displacement.[4] Restoration of the length and stability of the lateral malleolus is therefore the first priority of surgery. Anatomic reduction is assured only when intraoperative radiographs show the subchondral bone plate of the distal tibia to be continuous with that of the lateral malleolar articular surface. Interposition of medial malleolar fragments or portions of the deltoid ligament in the joint occasionally blocks the lateral reduction and requires a medial incision for extraction prior to fixation of the lateral malleolus.

E. The joint space must be of equal width throughout the mortise after lateral malleolar stabilization. In the presence of a deltoid ligament rupture, persistent medial widening implies probable infolding of the ligament. Fraying of the ligament makes rigid repair impractical, but reapproximation and apposition of the ligament ends should be achieved.

F. Most posterior malleolar fragments are firmly attached to the lateral malleolus and will reduce with accurate realignment of the lateral malleolar fracture. Potentially unstable fractures involving more than one quarter of the articular surface of the distal tibia warrant interfragmental screw fixation.

G. The syndesmosis consists of the anterior and posterior distal tibiofibular ligaments and the extension of the interosseous membrane. Injury to these ligaments can be deduced from the level of the fibular fracture (see figure). The syndesmosis remains intact with transverse fibular fractures below the joint line. Spiral fibular fractures beginning at the joint line are associated with partial syndesmotic disruption. When the entire fibular fracture is located above the joint, complete rupture can be anticipated. A widened or unstable syndesmosis permits slight lateral displacement of the talus, thereby significantly increasing talotibial joint force and predisposing to degenerative arthritis. Following fixation of all high fractures, the syndesmosis should be evaluated radiographically and manually, using a bone hook to check for excessive laxity. A transfixion or positioning screw is commonly needed to hold the distal tibiofibular joint in a reduced position during the healing of the supporting ligaments. The AO group recommends repair of the syndesmotic ligaments in place of position screws, reserving the latter for the more severe disruptions, e.g., those seen with very proximal (Maisonneuve) fibular fractures.

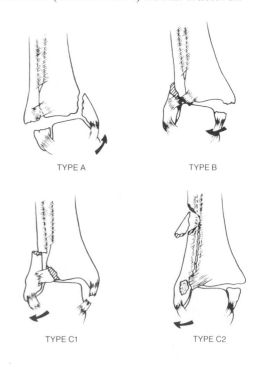

TYPE A          TYPE B

TYPE C1          TYPE C2

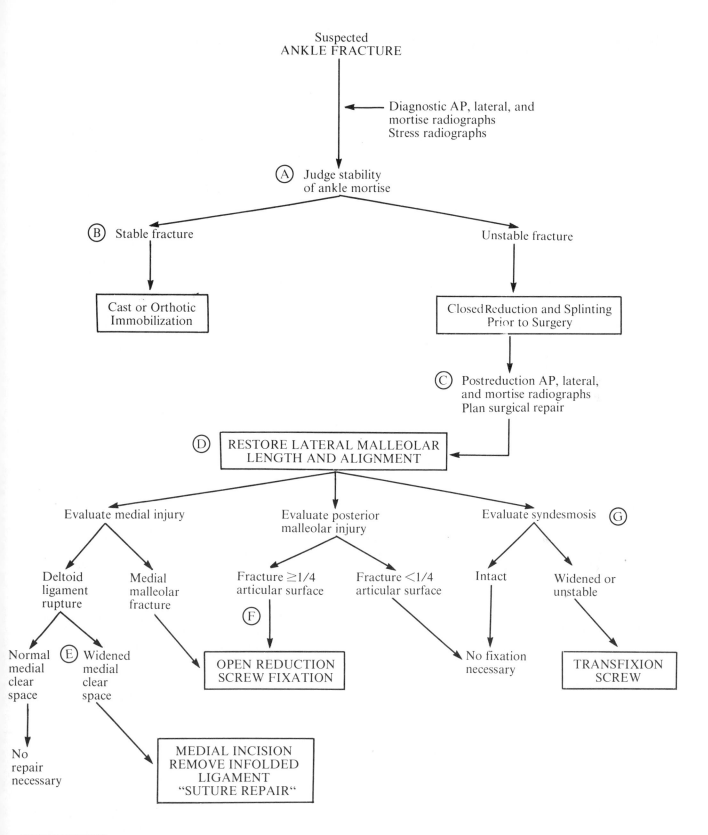

Suspected
ANKLE FRACTURE

Diagnostic AP, lateral, and
mortise radiographs
Stress radiographs

(A) Judge stability
of ankle mortise

(B) Stable fracture

Unstable fracture

Cast or Orthotic
Immobilization

Closed Reduction and Splinting
Prior to Surgery

(C) Postreduction AP, lateral,
and mortise radiographs
Plan surgical repair

(D) RESTORE LATERAL MALLEOLAR
LENGTH AND ALIGNMENT

Evaluate medial injury

Evaluate posterior
malleolar injury

Evaluate syndesmosis (G)

Deltoid
ligament
rupture

Medial
malleolar
fracture

Fracture ≥1/4
articular surface

Fracture <1/4
articular surface

Intact

Widened or
unstable

Normal
medial
clear
space

(E) Widened
medial
clear
space

(F)

OPEN REDUCTION
SCREW FIXATION

No fixation
necessary

TRANSFIXION
SCREW

No
repair
necessary

MEDIAL INCISION
REMOVE INFOLDED
LIGAMENT
"SUTURE REPAIR"

## REFERENCES

1. Joy G, Patzakis M, Harvey J. Precise evaluation of the reduction of severe ankle fractures. J Bone Joint Surg. 1974; 56A:979–993.
2. Lauge-Hansen N. Fractures of the ankle. II. Combined experimental-surgical and experimental-roentgenologic investigations. Arch Surg. 1950; 60:957–985.
3. Muller M, Allgower M, Schneider R, Willenegger H. *Manual of Internal Fixation.* Berlin: Springer-Verlag, 1979; pp. 282–300.
4. Yablon I, Heller F, Shouse L. The key role of the lateral malleolus in displaced fractures of the ankle. J Bone Joint Surg. 1977; 59A:169–173.

# FRACTURE OF THE CALCANEUS

## COMMENTS

A. Accurate delineation of all fracture lines necessitates multiple radiologic views. By demonstrating the extension of fractures into the subtalar joint, the loss of the tuberosity-joint (Bohler's) angle, and the degree of posterior facet depression, the lateral radiograph serves as the basis for most classification schemes.[1,2] The AP radiograph demonstrates the calcaneocuboid joint, while the sustentaculum tali, cortical margins of the tuberosity, and the varus/valgus alignment are seen best on the axial view. Oblique radiographs aid in evaluating the extent of fracture displacement.

B. Since most calcaneal fractures are a result of falls from heights, the 10% incidence of associated compression fractures of the lumbar spine is understandable. A mandatory part of the work-up of all calcaneal fractures is a thorough lumbosacral spine examination, usually including radiographs.

C. Isolated extra-articular chip or avulsion fractures of the tuberosity, sustentaculum tali, or anterior process of the calcaneus and minimally displaced body and tuberosity fractures have an excellent prognosis for full return of function. Treatment is directed at the soft tissues. Following 2 to 3 days of elevation, compressive bulky dressings, and ice, early motion is commenced. Weight bearing is delayed for 6 to 8 weeks on any comminuted fracture with subtalar extension prone to displacement. Cast immobilization leads to muscle atrophy, joint contractures, and slow functional recovery, and therefore should be avoided.

D. Avulsion fractures of the calcaneal tendon insertion comprise less than 5% of all calcaneal fractures. While avulsion fragments displaced less than 5 mm may be treated in plaster casts, those with complete separation from the tuberosity require operative reduction and interfragmental screw fixation.

E. The multitude of recommended approaches in the orthopaedic literature to displaced intra-articular calcaneal fractures attests to the fact that no single treatment regimen is indisputably superior. The loss of Bohler's angle (normally 30 to 40°) implies fracture and impaction of the posterior calcaneal facet. Although specific fracture variants have been classified, it must be recognized that all displaced fractures possess varying degrees of comminution, which makes stabilization of the fracture difficult, if not impossible, in most instances. Since the reported results of all treatment modalities are comparable, it is wise for the minimally experienced surgeon to use the no reduction-early motion treatment recommended for nondisplaced fractures.[3] Weight bearing should not be permitted for 6 to 8 weeks. In most cases the residual distorted morphology, including commonly a broad heel and pronated subtalar joint, is easily compensated. The benefits of this approach include a short hospitalization, full functional weight bearing by 8 to 12 weeks, and early resumption of work.[3] Grossly malaligned fractures with crushing of the subtalar joint are likely to have late complications. Any aggressive surgical approach demands a complete understanding of the pathologic anatomy of a given fracture.[1,4] Using skeletal traction, percutaneous os calcis spikes, and closed manipulations, Essex-Lopresti recommended operative reduction of displaced fractures in patients under 50 years of age.[1] Other authors alternatively have reported improved results by open reduction, fixation and grafting, or primary arthrodesis. The worst long-term results from displaced calcaneal fractures arise from inadequately performed or complicated surgical treatments.

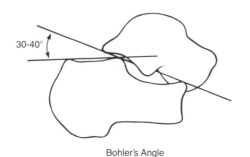

Bohler's Angle

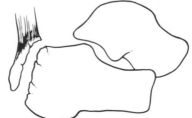

Displaced Avulsion Fracture
of the Calcaneal Tendon Insertion

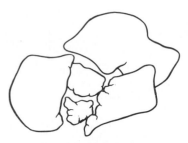

Intra-Articular Fracture with
Loss of Bohler's Angle

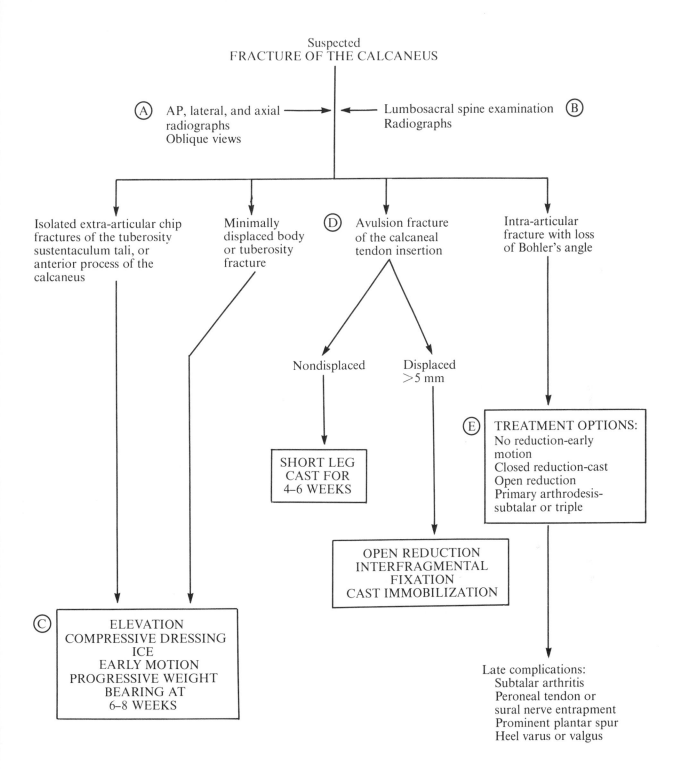

Suspected
FRACTURE OF THE CALCANEUS

(A) AP, lateral, and axial
radiographs
Oblique views

Lumbosacral spine examination
Radiographs (B)

Isolated extra-articular chip
fractures of the tuberosity
sustentaculum tali, or
anterior process of the
calcaneus

Minimally
displaced body
or tuberosity
fracture

(D) Avulsion fracture
of the calcaneal
tendon insertion

Intra-articular
fracture with loss
of Bohler's angle

Nondisplaced

Displaced
>5 mm

(E) TREATMENT OPTIONS:
No reduction-early
motion
Closed reduction-cast
Open reduction
Primary arthrodesis-
subtalar or triple

SHORT LEG
CAST FOR
4–6 WEEKS

OPEN REDUCTION
INTERFRAGMENTAL
FIXATION
CAST IMMOBILIZATION

(C) ELEVATION
COMPRESSIVE DRESSING
ICE
EARLY MOTION
PROGRESSIVE WEIGHT
BEARING AT
6–8 WEEKS

Late complications:
Subtalar arthritis
Peroneal tendon or
sural nerve entrapment
Prominent plantar spur
Heel varus or valgus

**REFERENCES**

1. Essex-Lopresti P. The mechanism, reduction technique, and results in fracture of the os calcis. Br J Surg. 1951; 39:395.
2. Rowe C, Sakellarides H, Freeman P, Sorbie C. Fractures of the os calcis: a long-term follow-up study of 146 patients. JAMA 1963; 184:920.
3. Lance E, Carey E, Wade P. Fractures of the os calcis: treatment by early mobilization. Clin Orthop Rel Res. 1963; 30:76.
4. Warrick C, Bremner A. Fractures of the calcaneum—with an atlas illustrating the various types of fractures. J Bone Joint Surg. 1953; 35B:33.

# FRACTURE OR DISLOCATION OF THE TALUS

## COMMENTS

A. Talar neck fractures are usually secondary to hyperextension forces, whereas body fractures are due to severe axial loads. Nondisplaced neck fractures should be casted with the ankle in neutral or slight equinus.

B. Minimally displaced neck and body fractures occasionally can be manipulated and casted. Maintenance of reductions in casts is difficult, however, and redisplacement frequently occurs. Anatomic reduction and internal fixation yield better functional results in most cases. A medial malleolar osteotomy may assist in exposure of displaced body fractures.

C. A talar neck or body fracture associated with a subtalar or complete dislocation should be treated the same as an isolated neck or body fracture after the dislocation has been reduced.

D. A simple subtalar dislocation commonly can be reduced under general anesthesia by closed manipulation alone. The postreduction radiographs must be inspected carefully to ensure an accurate reduction. The incidence of late subtalar post-traumatic arthritis is low.[1] Associated fractures must be evaluated on the postreduction film and treated appropriately.

E. Closed reduction of complete talar dislocations is usually impossible because of massive soft tissue swelling, triplane displacement and rotation of the talus, and interposed osteochondral fragments.[2] At open reduction, a transcalcaneal pin may be helpful in providing additional distraction of the ankle, thus facilitating talar reduction. If the reduced talus is unstable, a large Steinmann pin through the calcaneus, talus, and distal tibia can supplement the postoperative cast immobilization.

F. In an open complete talar dislocation, the soft tissue should be left open after surgical reduction of the talus. A delayed primary closure or skin grafting can be performed at 5 to 7 days.

G. Transchondral dome fractures are also called flake fractures or osteochondritis dissecans. Lateral dome osteochondral fractures are the most common pattern and can be diagnosed on either the mortise view or tomography of the ankle. Arthroscopy or arthrography occasionally is needed to diagnose pure cartilaginous lesions.

H. Displaced transchondral fractures may mechanically block full joint motion and cause persistent ankle pain. Operative treatment with extraction of all loose fragments, curettage of the defect, and drilling of all exposed subchondral bone has been reported as offering the best long-term results.[3,4] Early postoperative ankle motion stimulates fibrocartilaginous resurfacing of the defect. Lateral dome lesions are usually anterior, but medial lesions are posterior and often necessitate a transmalleolar exposure for adequate debridement.

I. A radiographic zone of bone resorption under the subchondral plate of the dome of the talus at 1 to 2 months postinjury signifies adequate preservation of the vascular supply to the bone (Hawkin's sign). Owing to the tenuous blood supply of the talus,[5] avascular necrosis is a frequent sequela of talar injuries. The incidence of this complication varies from 13% in isolated neck fractures to 50% in subtalar fracture-dislocations to 84% in complete talar fracture-dislocations.[6]

## REFERENCES

1. Monson S, Ryan J. Subtalar dislocation. J Bone Joint Surg. 1981; 63A:1156.
2. Pennal G. Fractures of the talus. Clin Ortho Rel Res. 1963; 30:53.
3. Berndt A, Harty M. Transchondral fractures of the talus. J Bone Joint Surg. 1959; 41A:988.
4. Alexander H, Lichtman D. Surgical treatment of transchondral talar dome fractures (osteochondritis dissecans). J Bone Joint Surg. 1980; 62A:646.
5. Kelly P, Sullivan C. Blood supply of the talus. Clin Ortho Rel Res. 1963; 30:37.
6. Canale T, Kelly F. Fractures of the neck of the talus. J Bone Joint Surg. 1978; 60A:143.

INJURY TO THE TALUS

Assess for vascular
compromise to the foot →

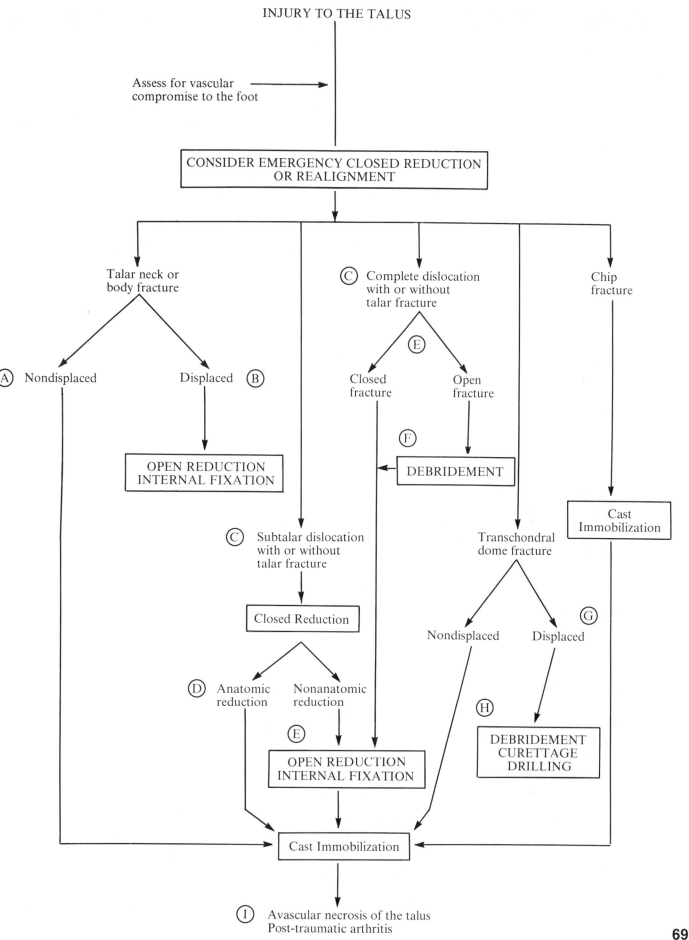

CONSIDER EMERGENCY CLOSED REDUCTION
OR REALIGNMENT

Talar neck or
body fracture

(C) Complete dislocation
with or without
talar fracture

Chip
fracture

(E)

(A) Nondisplaced          Displaced (B)        Closed
fracture

Open
fracture

(F)

OPEN REDUCTION
INTERNAL FIXATION

DEBRIDEMENT

Cast
Immobilization

(C) Subtalar dislocation
with or without
talar fracture

Transchondral
dome fracture

Closed Reduction

Nondisplaced      Displaced (G)

(D) Anatomic      Nonanatomic
reduction      reduction

(H)

(E)

OPEN REDUCTION
INTERNAL FIXATION

DEBRIDEMENT
CURETTAGE
DRILLING

Cast Immobilization

(I) Avascular necrosis of the talus
Post-traumatic arthritis

**69**

# TARSOMETATARSAL FRACTURE-DISLOCATION

## COMMENTS

A. The stability of the tarsometatarsal (Lisfranc) joint is attributable to a thick plantar ligamentous complex and the locking of the second metatarsal base in the cuneiform recess. Disruption of these supporting structures may result from direct or indirect forces applied to the forefoot.[1] Severe abduction or plantar fexion loads are most frequently responsible, but all possible mechanisms have been described. The joint injury may be total, partial, or divergent. The three most common patterns are lateral dislocation of the entire forefoot, lateral dislocation of the second through fifth metatarsals, and medial displacement of the first metatarsal.[2] Divergent injuries with medial dislocation of the first ray and lateral dislocation of the lateral four rays are rare. Radiographic abnormalities may be subtle. A fracture of the base of the second metatarsal or an anterior compression fracture of the cuboid is often the only evidence for significant joint disruption. In such cases, stress radiographs are helpful in detecting spontaneously reduced unstable tarsometatarsal injuries.

B. Complete forefoot dislocations, especially those secondary to direct trauma, can result in injury to the dorsalis pedis artery. Persistent forefoot ischemia after manipulative realignment of the joint is an absolute indication for vessel exploration and internal fixation of the joint.[2]

C. Longitudinal traction through a Chinese finger trap applied to the forefoot aids in obtaining a closed reduction. Closed reduction may fail owing to marked instability of the joint or interposition of soft tissues or osteochondral fragments.

D. Prior to percutaneous Steinmann pin fixation, anatomic reduction in all planes must be confirmed with AP, lateral, and oblique radiographs. Most total fracture-dislocations require two pins, one through the first metatarsal into the medial cuneiform and one through the fifth metatarsal into the cuboid. Modifications in pin placement are individualized for partial and divergent injuries.

E. Residual forefoot displacement or joint widening of greater than one millimeter in active patients and gross instability of a satisfactorily reduced dislocation are indications for open reduction and internal fixation. Two longitudinal skin incisions, one medial and one lateral, usually suffice in exposing the entire disrupted joint. Wide transverse incisions lead to marginal skin necrosis, dorsal sensory loss, and unsightly scarring. Fixation may be secured with multiple Steinmann pins or screws. Late complications, frequently encountered in improperly managed injuries, include joint incongruity with degenerative arthritis, forefoot deformity, and plantar callosities secondary to prominent metatarsal heads. If anatomic reduction is achieved and maintained, excellent functional results can be anticipated.[3]

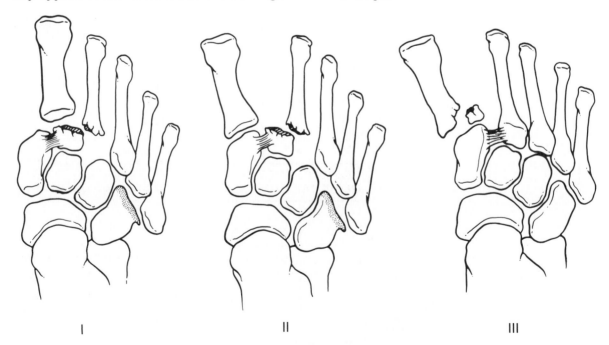

I                    II                    III

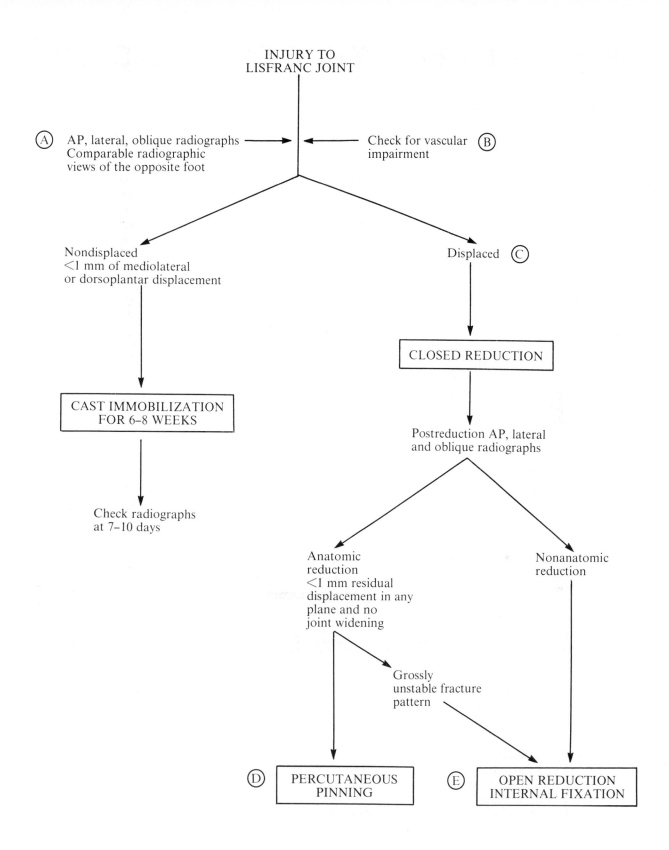

INJURY TO
LISFRANC JOINT

Ⓐ AP, lateral, oblique radiographs → ← Check for vascular Ⓑ
Comparable radiographic impairment
views of the opposite foot

Nondisplaced
<1 mm of mediolateral
or dorsoplantar displacement

Displaced Ⓒ

CLOSED REDUCTION

CAST IMMOBILIZATION
FOR 6–8 WEEKS

Check radiographs
at 7–10 days

Postreduction AP, lateral
and oblique radiographs

Anatomic
reduction
<1 mm residual
displacement in any
plane and no
joint widening

Nonanatomic
reduction

Grossly
unstable fracture
pattern

Ⓓ PERCUTANEOUS
PINNING

Ⓔ OPEN REDUCTION
INTERNAL FIXATION

**REFERENCES**

1. Wiley J. The mechanism of tarsometatarsal joint injuries. J Bone Joint Surg. 1971; 53B:474.
2. Hardcastle P, Reschauer R, Kutacha-Lissberg E, Schoffman W. Injuries to the tarsometatarsal joint— incidence, classification and treatment. J Bone Joint Surg. 1982; 64B:349.
3. Aitken A, Poulson D. Dislocation of the tarsometatarsal joint. J Bone Joint Surg. 1963; 45A:246.

# FOREFOOT FRACTURE OR DISLOCATION

## COMMENTS

A. Direct crush injuries are responsible for most forefoot fractures and dislocations. The evaluation and treatment of the soft tissue injury is therefore of prime importance. An accurate history on the nature of the impact is crucial in anticipating possible neurovascular or skin complications. Control of hemorrhage and edema by immediate splinting, evaluation, and cooling of the foot simplifies subsequent management.

B. A full complement of radiographs is necessary to define the degree of fracture displacement in each plane. Potentially troublesome dorsal or plantar angulation of metatarsal fractures is judged best on true lateral radiographs.

C. Attempts at closed reduction of simple metatarsophalangeal or interphalangeal dislocations may fail owing to tendon or capsule interposition. MTP dislocations of the hallux occasionally are complicated by trapped sesamoid bones. Irreducible dislocations require open reduction.

D. Even when associated with only trivial fractures, major crush injuries to the foot warrant hospitalization. Inpatient management ensures constant elevation of the extremity and prompt recognition of neurovascular and skin complications.

E. Longitudinal traction with Chinese finger traps and careful molding of a short leg cast will achieve a satisfactory reduction of most fractures and a restoration of the arches of the forefoot. Significant translation and angulation of most forefoot fractures are compatible with successful healing and full functional recovery. Metatarsal neck or shaft fractures, which heal with dorsal or plantar angulation of greater than 15 to 20° (or, less commonly, shortening of greater than 5 mm) may lead to uneven pressure distribution under the metatarsal heads, resulting in painful plantar callosities.

F. Open reductions of metatarsal fractures are ideally maintained with intramedullary K–wires or Steinmann pins. Dorsal longitudinal incisions centered between the involved metatarsals will minimize the hazard of skin sloughs in these swollen feet. The pins are easily passed in a retrograde fashion, with care to preserve full length of the bone. Pin removal may be performed at 3 to 6 weeks.

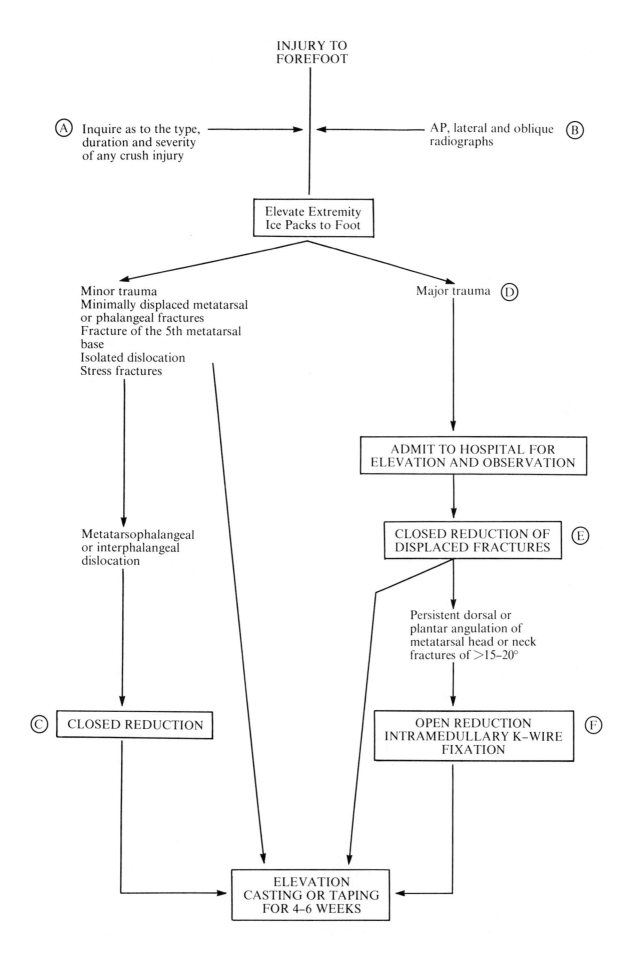

INJURY TO
FOREFOOT

Ⓐ Inquire as to the type,
   duration and severity
   of any crush injury

Ⓑ AP, lateral and oblique
   radiographs

Elevate Extremity
Ice Packs to Foot

Minor trauma
Minimally displaced metatarsal
or phalangeal fractures
Fracture of the 5th metatarsal
base
Isolated dislocation
Stress fractures

Major trauma Ⓓ

ADMIT TO HOSPITAL FOR
ELEVATION AND OBSERVATION

Metatarsophalangeal
or interphalangeal
dislocation

CLOSED REDUCTION OF
DISPLACED FRACTURES Ⓔ

Persistent dorsal or
plantar angulation of
metatarsal head or neck
fractures of >15–20°

Ⓒ CLOSED REDUCTION

OPEN REDUCTION
INTRAMEDULLARY K–WIRE
FIXATION Ⓕ

ELEVATION
CASTING OR TAPING
FOR 4–6 WEEKS

# LONG BONE FRACTURES IN THE CHILD

## COMMENTS

A. The porous nature of pediatric cortical bone accounts for the simple, noncomminuted characteristics of most metaphyseal and diaphyseal fractures in children. Certain fracture patterns unique to children, such as metaphyseal buckle or torus fractures and greenstick fractures, are also attributable to the biomechanical properties of immature bone. Diagnostic radiographs must show the full length of the long bone and its adjacent joints. Frequently missed associated joint injuries include radial head subluxations or dislocations with apparent isolated ulnar shaft fractures (Monteggia lesion) and hip fractures or epiphyseal separations with femoral shaft fractures. The degree of angulation from seemingly trivial greenstick fractures of the proximal tibia may be underestimated unless a full length anteroposterior radiograph is obtained.

B. The potential for growth remodeling should not be used as an excuse for a cavalier attitude toward pediatric fractures. All angulation and displacement of long bone fractures ideally should be corrected by that means with the least risk and discomfort to the patient. The listed criteria for unacceptable rotation, varus/valgus, and anterior/posterior angulation necessitating a formal closed reduction are not absolute. While rotatory malalignment will not correct in any age group, greater degrees of varus/valgus and anterior/posterior angulation are allowable in metaphyseal fractures near a growth plate, fractures displaced in the same plane as the movement of the adjacent joint, and all long bone fractures in infants and younger children. The need for precise reduction increases with the age of the child. Older children demonstrate little more than rounding off of the apex of a malunited diaphyseal fracture. All pediatric fractures, especially those in a juxtaphyseal location, induce longitudinal growth. Although this anticipated overgrowth of an injured bone can compensate for fracture shortening, the limits of growth stimulation are unpredictable. Other than certain femur fractures mentioned below, all long bone fractures in children should be held out to length during the healing process.

C. Nearly all humeral, forearm, and tibial fractures are readily managed by cast immobilization. Rotational alignment can be evaluated by comparison of the casted limb with the contralateral extremity and careful scrutiny of the postreduction radiographs. Greenstick fractures of the proximal tibial metaphysis tend to progressively angulate during healing in children from 3 to 10 years of age. Unless complete correction of all tibial angulation is achieved, open reduction with extraction of any interposed soft tissue in the fracture is recommended by some authors.[1]

D. Femoral shaft fractures traditionally are treated by skin or skeletal traction for approximately 3 weeks or until there is early callus consolidation, followed by hip spica casting. Various modifications of Thomas splint suspension are used for midshaft and distal fractures, whereas 90–90 skeletal traction is preferred for proximal fractures. The acceptable limits of angulation vary with the patient's age. Overriding of 1 cm is desirable in patients under 10 years of age, though end-to-end apposition of the fracture fragments causes only a minimal, unnoticeable overgrowth. The recently popularized immediate spica treatment shortens the period of hospitalization, but requires close radiographic follow-up.[2]

E. Most residual angulation after a closed reduction is correctable by repeat manipulation or wedging of the cast. Irreducible long bone fractures are rarely encountered. Both bone forearm fractures in adolescents (girls over 10 years and boys over 12 years of age) should be treated as adult injuries with open reduction and internal fixation unless an anatomic closed reduction is achieved and maintained. The AO group recommends serious consideration of surgical stabilization of femur fractures in cases with major soft tissue injuries, ipsilateral hip fractures, or bilateral fractures in the adolescent.[1]

F. Femur fractures in children with severe spasticity from a closed head injury are often impossible to keep aligned, even with the use of 90–90 skeletal traction. Internal fixation with a compression plate or intramedullary nail may be indicated.

G. Kirschner wires, Steinmann pins, and lag screws usually suffice in the fixation of metaphyseal fractures. Bulkier fixation devices are not warranted. Compression plates, or intramedullary nails in cases where the proximal and distal physes are surgically avoidable, are preferred for diaphyseal fractures.

H. The rapid healing of fractures of long bones in children demands radiographic confirmation of the retention of reduction at 5 to 10 days after injury and at frequent subsequent intervals. Closed reduction of a reangulated fracture is not feasible after 2 to 3 weeks.

## REFERENCES

1. Weber B, Brunner B, Freuler F (Eds.). *Treatment of Fractures in Children and Adolescents.* Berlin: Springer-Verlag, 1980.
2. Irani R, Nicholson J, Chung S. Long-term results in the treatment of femoral-shaft fractures in young children by immediate spica immobilization. J Bone Joing Surg. 1976; 58A:945.
3. Rang M. *Children's Fractures.* Philadelphia: JB Lippincott, 1974.

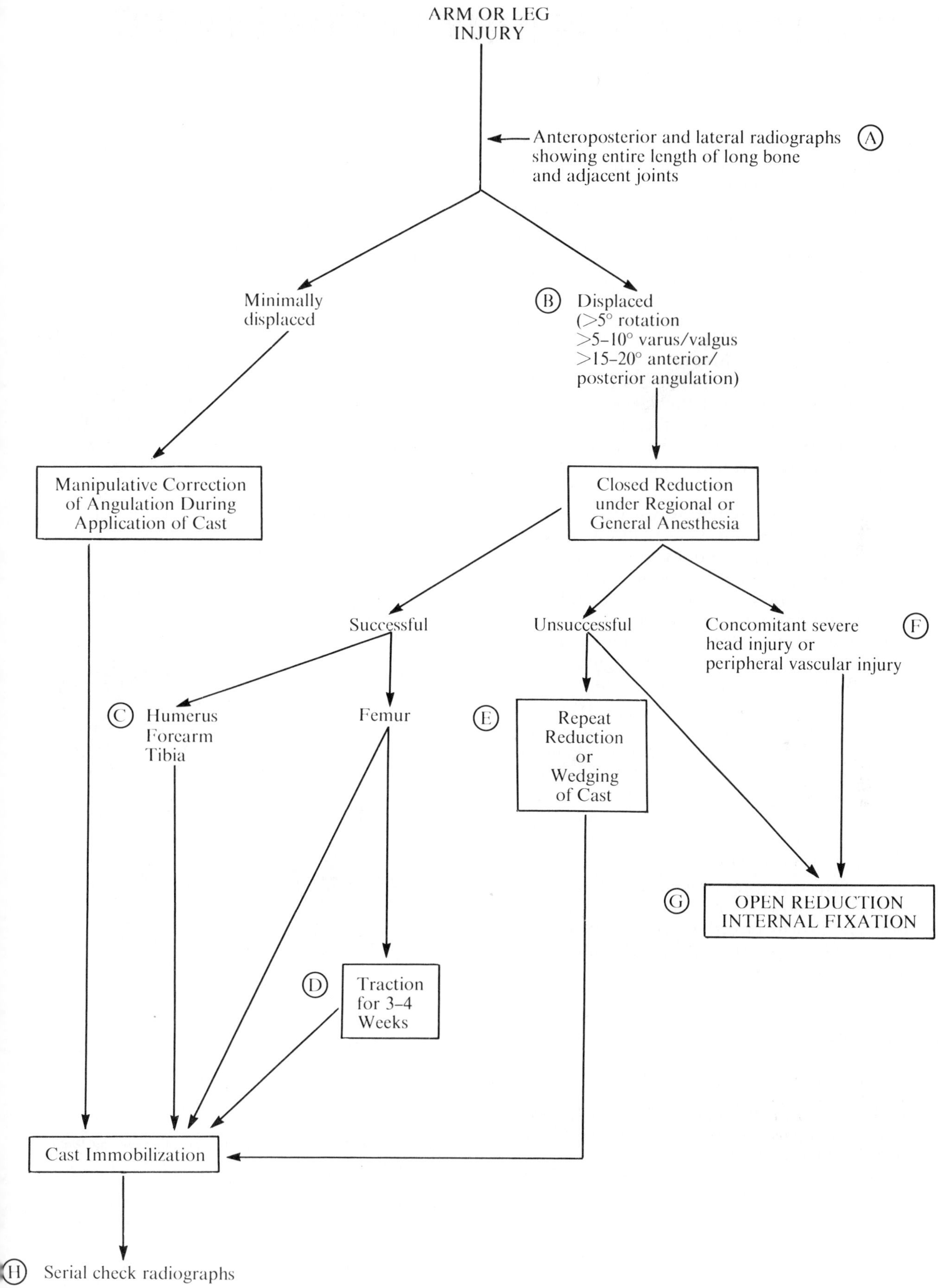
ARM OR LEG INJURY
Anteroposterior and lateral radiographs showing entire length of long bone and adjacent joints
A
Minimally displaced
B
Displaced (>5° rotation >5–10° varus/valgus >15–20° anterior/ posterior angulation)
Manipulative Correction of Angulation During Application of Cast
Closed Reduction under Regional or General Anesthesia
Successful
Unsuccessful
Concomitant severe head injury or peripheral vascular injury
F
C
Humerus Forearm Tibia
Femur
E
Repeat Reduction or Wedging of Cast
G
OPEN REDUCTION INTERNAL FIXATION
D
Traction for 3–4 Weeks
Cast Immobilization
H
Serial check radiographs

# GROWTH PLATE INJURY IN THE CHILD

**COMMENTS**

A. Gentle stress radiographs assist in detecting occult physeal injuries in "sprained" joints with normal plain radiographs.

B. The prognosis for Salter-Harris[1] type I and II injuries (see figure) is good except in cases with concomitant interruption of epiphyseal vessels (e.g.,the proximal femur). The guarded prognosis of type III and IV injuries arises from the potential for joint incongruity, and occasional nonunions (e.g., type IV lateral condyle fractures of the humerus). Crushing injury of the rare type V fracture often goes unrecognized until the inevitable partial or total physeal closure results in clinical deformity. Other factors influencing the long-term outcome include the age of the patient and the growth contribution of the injured physis.

C. The criteria for acceptable displacement, with or without reduction, are more rigid for fractures about the knee, ankle, and elbow joints than they are around a multiplanar joint, such as the shoulder. Except for nondisplaced fractures, all injuries should be gently reduced before or during cast application. Anteroposterior angulation of less than 30° and varus/valgus angulation less than 10° may be accepted in most cases.

D. Anatomic reduction of displaced type III and IV fractures usually require an operative procedure. Threaded pins, screws, and plates should not be inserted across the growth plate. Nondisplaced fractures managed with cast immobilization must be followed closely with serial radiographs. Early fracture displacement in a cast may necessitate surgical correction.

E. Specific fracture patterns have higher incidences of varied complications.[2] Parent education of possible growth disturbances is crucial in the long-term follow up that all growth plate injuries warrant.

**REFERENCES**

1. Salter K, Harris W. Injuries involving the epiphyseal plate. J Bone Joint Surg. 1963; 45A:587–621.
2. Ogden JA. Injury to the immature skeleton. In *Pediatric Trauma*. Edited by RJ Touloukian. New York: John Wiley and Sons, 1978; pp. 473–547.

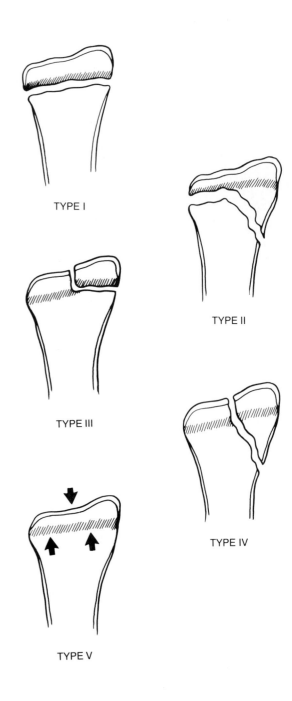

TYPE I

TYPE II

TYPE III

TYPE IV

TYPE V

Salter-Harris Classification of Injuries to the Epiphyseal Plate

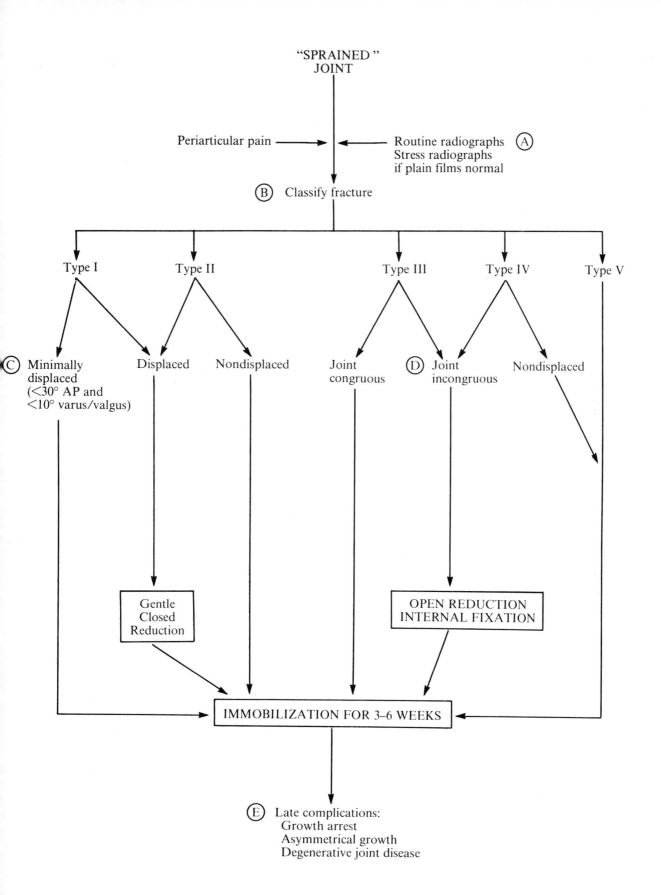

# DISTAL HUMERAL FRACTURES IN CHILDREN

### COMMENTS

A. The secondary ossification centers of the elbow appear in a predictable sequence—capitellum, radial head, internal or medial epicondyle, trochlea, olecranon, external or lateral epicondyle (mnemonic CRITOE)—at approximate 2–year intervals beginning with the capitellum at 6 to 12 months of age. Familiarity with these ossification centers and routine requisition of comparable radiographic views of the contralateral normal elbow will minimize both over- and underdiagnosis of injuries. Oblique radiographs are required in suspicious cases such as those with a "fat pad" sign on the lateral radiograph.

B. Ten percent of all displaced supracondylar fractures present with neurologic signs, usually involving the median or radial nerve. Vascular compromise occurs most frequently with severely displaced supracondylar fractures, especially when the elbow is splinted in flexion.

C. These three fracture patterns constitute 99% of all distal humeral fractures in children. Rarer fractures, such as Salter-Harris type I and II epiphyseal separations, occasionally are sustained in infants and young children.

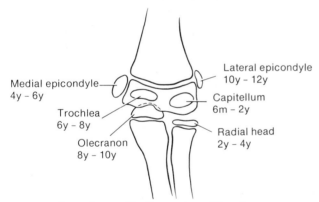

Medial epicondyle 4y – 6y
Trochlea 6y – 8y
Olecranon 8y – 10y
Lateral epicondyle 10y – 12y
Capitellum 6m – 2y
Radial head 2y – 4y

Secondary ossification centers of the elbow

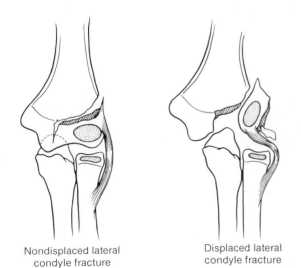

Nondisplaced lateral condyle fracture

Displaced lateral condyle fracture

D. Emergency closed reduction under anesthesia should be performed to relieve any neurovascular compression by fracture fragments. Most hyperextension injuries (90% of all supracondylar fractures) have an intact posterior periosteal hinge, which aids in achieving a satisfactory manipulative reduction. Elbow flexion beyond 90° is imperative to hold the reduction. Although perfect anatomic reduction is not necessary in the AP plane, complete correction of varus/valgus and rotatory displacement is mandatory.[1] The stability of the reduction can be tested by stressing the reduced fracture under fluoroscopic control in both medial-lateral and AP planes. All children with displaced fractures should be admitted to the hospital for observation.

E. Never immobilize the elbow in maximal flexion for more than 2 to 3 weeks. Serial check radiographs are important to detect, as early as possible, any varus or internal rotational malalignment, which may result in a permanent cubitus varus (gunstock) deformity.

F. Medial epicondyle fractures, often associated with elbow dislocations, may be unstable by virtue of complete loss of all soft tissue attachments to the distal humerus. Such displaced fractures often fail to unite and result in loss of elbow extension and potential late elbow instability. Open reduction and internal fixation with smooth K-wires is therefore the preferred treatment for all displaced fragments.[2]

G. This Salter-Harris type IV fracture extends from the lateral distal humeral metaphysis down across the physis, exiting in the lateral aspect of the trochlea. Multiple oblique radiographic views are often needed to distinguish displaced from nondisplaced fractures. True nondisplaced fractures with an intact articular cartilaginous hinge may be treated with a long arm cast for 4 weeks.[3] Displaced fractures have a propensity for nonunion and resultant cubitus valgus with tardy ulnar nerve palsy. Open reduction and internal fixation with several smooth K-wires is thus the conservative treatment for all displaced lateral condyles. The K-wires should routinely be removed at 3 to 5 weeks.

### REFERENCES

1. Ogden J. Injury to the immature skeleton. In *Pediatric Trauma*. Edited by R. Touloukian. New York: Wiley & Sons, 1978; pp. 473–547.
2. Rang M. Children's Fractures. Philadelphia: JB Lippincott. 1974; pp. 93–123.
3. Jakob R, Fowles J, Rang M, Kassab M. Observations concerning fractures of the lateral humeral condyle in children. J Bone Joint Surg. 1975; 57B:430–436.

DISTAL HUMERUS FRACTURE

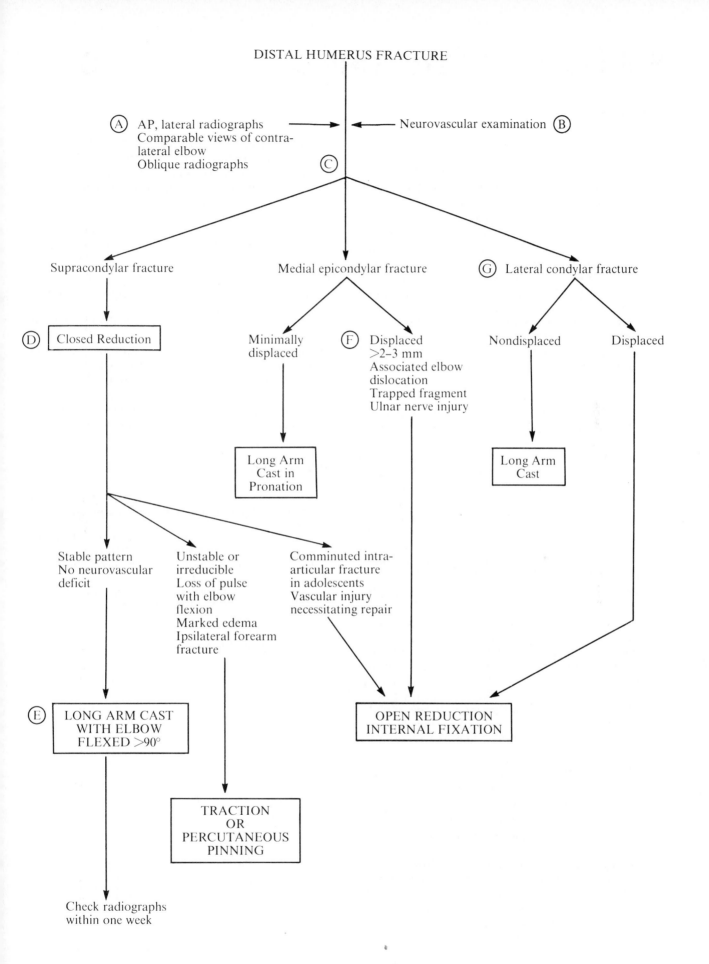

Ⓐ AP, lateral radiographs
Comparable views of contra-
lateral elbow
Oblique radiographs

Neurovascular examination Ⓑ

Ⓒ

Supracondylar fracture

Medial epicondylar fracture

Ⓖ Lateral condylar fracture

Ⓓ Closed Reduction

Minimally
displaced

Ⓕ Displaced
>2–3 mm
Associated elbow
dislocation
Trapped fragment
Ulnar nerve injury

Nondisplaced

Displaced

Long Arm
Cast in
Pronation

Long Arm
Cast

Stable pattern
No neurovascular
deficit

Unstable or
irreducible
Loss of pulse
with elbow
flexion
Marked edema
Ipsilateral forearm
fracture

Comminuted intra-
articular fracture
in adolescents
Vascular injury
necessitating repair

Ⓔ LONG ARM CAST
WITH ELBOW
FLEXED >90°

OPEN REDUCTION
INTERNAL FIXATION

TRACTION
OR
PERCUTANEOUS
PINNING

Check radiographs
within one week

# HIP INJURY IN THE CHILD

## COMMENTS

A. Hip fractures and dislocations in children are sustained from high-energy impacts. Associated pelvic (hemipelvis or triradiate cartilage) and visceral trauma is commonly encountered with these relatively rare bone and joint injuries.

B. The diagnosis of a Salter-Harris type I or II traumatic separation of the proximal femoral epiphysis often can be made with certainty only in the young child. Its distinction from an idiopathic or pathologic slipped capital femoral epiphysis depends upon a clear history of immediate hip pain after major trauma to a young child without pre-existing endocrine abnormalities (pp 194, 195). Most separations can be reduced easily and held in a spica cast. Concomitant dislocation of the femoral head or loss of reduction in plaster is an indication for operative intervention. Varus displacement must be avoided. Despite satisfactory treatment, permanent residual deformity from avascular necrosis or premature growth plate closure results in over half of these hips.[1]

C. Transcervical and base of femoral neck fractures are frequently nondisplaced, with the thick soft tissue sleeve of the neck maintaining an anatomic position. Spica immobilization in internal rotation and abduction should be checked with serial radiographs. Any loss of fracture alignment in plaster within the first 3 weeks of injury should be reduced and internally fixed.

D. Deforming muscle forces invariably cause displaced neck fractures to settle into a varus malalignment. Internal fixation yields improved results. Once an anatomic reduction is accomplished by gentle manipulation on a fracture table or under direct visualization through a capsulotomy, multiple threaded pins are used to hold the corrected position. When technically possible, multiple lag screw fixation with the threads of the screw purchased in the cancellous bone of the metaphysis is preferred to pins crossing the growth plate.[2]

E. Management of the rare intertrochanteric fracture in the child is similar to that for a femoral shaft fracture, with 2 to 3 weeks of skeletal traction followed by a hip spica cast.

F. Traumatic hip dislocations usually are easily distinguishable from longstanding congenital or paralytic dislocations. Immediate closed reduction under a general anesthesia should be performed. Hip spica immobilization for 4 to 6 weeks or early motion at 2 to 3 weeks are both reasonable treatment alternatives.

G. In Pearson's series of 24 hip dislocations, only two necessitated open reduction, one for a failed manipulative reduction and one for a large fracture fragment.[3] Associated femoral neck fracture or separation of the proximal femoral epiphysis should also be treated operatively. Avascular necrosis occurs in less than 10 percent of all promptly treated traumatic dislocations in children.

H. Nearly three-fourths of all displaced proximal femoral fractures in children develop complications.[4] Avascular necrosis of all or a portion of the femoral head and neck is evident in 45% of cases. Premature physeal closure is usually a sequel of avascular necrosis. Failure to stabilize internally a displaced femoral neck fracture may lead to delayed union or nonunion. The late surgical reconstruction of these complicated hips is based in the same principles as those used in common pediatric hip disorders (pp 186–195).

## REFERENCES

1. Ratliff A. Traumatic separation of the upper femoral epiphysis in young children. J Bone Joint Surg. 1968; 50B:757.
2. Boitzy A. Fractures of the proximal femur. In *Treatment of Fractures in Children and Adolescents*. Edited by B Weber, C Brinner, F Freuler. Berlin: Springer-Verlag, 1980.
3. Pearson D, Mann R. Traumatic hip dislocation in children. Clin Orthop Rel Res. 1973; 92:189.
4. Ratliff A. Complications after fractures of the femoral neck in children and their treatment. J Bone Joint Surg. 1970; 52B:175.

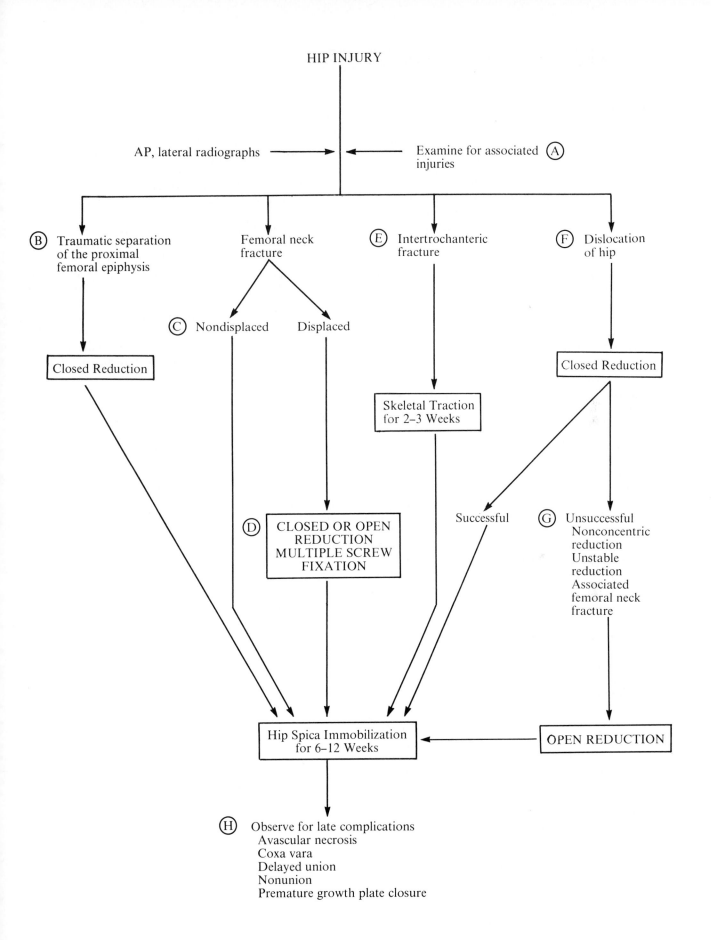

HIP INJURY

AP, lateral radiographs → ← Examine for associated (A) injuries

(B) Traumatic separation of the proximal femoral epiphysis

Femoral neck fracture

(E) Intertrochanteric fracture

(F) Dislocation of hip

(C) Nondisplaced     Displaced

Closed Reduction

Closed Reduction

Skeletal Traction for 2–3 Weeks

(D) CLOSED OR OPEN REDUCTION MULTIPLE SCREW FIXATION

Successful

(G) Unsuccessful
Nonconcentric reduction
Unstable reduction
Associated femoral neck fracture

Hip Spica Immobilization for 6–12 Weeks ← OPEN REDUCTION

(H) Observe for late complications
Avascular necrosis
Coxa vara
Delayed union
Nonunion
Premature growth plate closure

# PATHOLOGIC FRACTURE

## COMMENTS

A. Pathologic fractures occur in areas of structural weakness of bones with pre-existing disease. Patients often relate a history of only trivial trauma. Plain radiographs demonstrate isolated or generalized areas of abnormal bone density or distorted bone architecture. Bone scans are more sensitive than radiographic skeletal surveys in identifying additional osseous lesions.

B. The diagnosis of the pre-existing disease must be established. In addition to biopsy, bacteriologic culture of lesional tissue should be obtained in cases of suspected osteomyelitis (pp 166, 167). Certain benign bone tumors with pathognomonic radiographic changes (e.g., unicameral bone cyst, enchondroma of the hand, nonossifying fibroma) do not require biopsy.

C. Pathologic fractures through benign osseous lesions occur mainly in children. Treatment is simplified by allowing the fracture to heal prior to definitive management of the bone tumor. Most isolated lesions in adults must be assumed malignant until proved otherwise.

D. Biopsy of pathologic fractures secondary to possible primary malignant tumors of bone must be done carefully. The callus of a healing fracture may be mistaken histologically for primary osteosarcoma. The biopsy surgical wound may also interfere with future radical excision of a histologically proved malignant lesion. It is therefore preferable to refer patients with presumptive primary malignant bone tumors to centers specializing in the multidisciplinary diagnosis and treatment of these problems.

E. Biopsy is seldom necessary in systemic or metabolic bone disease when the laboratory and radiographic changes are diagnostic. In patients with multiple discrete osseous lesions without an evident primary tumor, biopsy of the most accessible lesion is warranted.

F. Patients with advanced osteoporosis present with vertebral compression fractures, hip fractures, and metaphyseal fractures of long bones. Specific fracture patterns are also commonly seen with other systemic diseases, such as osteogenesis imperfecta, osteomalacia, and Paget's disease.

G. Pathologic fractures of long bones other than the femur, tibia, and humerus are rare and usually manageable with casting or splinting. Vertebral body lesions may result in spinal cord compromise, necessitating surgical decompression. Pathologic fracture through the acetabulum presents an especially difficult reconstructive problem.[1]

H. Approximately half of all pathologic fractures requiring orthopedic care arise from metastatic breast carcinoma. The advantages of surgical stabilization of long bone pathologic fractures include relief of pain, the procurement of biopsy tissue in cases without a definitive preoperative diagnosis, and improved function of the extremity. Periarticular fractures often require prosthetic replacement of the involved portion of bone, whereas diaphyseal lesions are stabilized ideally with intramedullary devices and adjunctive methylmethacrylate.[2,3] The prerequisites for surgical intervention are a projected life expectancy of the patient sufficiently long to warrant a major operation, a stable general medical condition of the patient, and a high probability of achieving a rigid surgical construct.

## REFERENCES

1. Harrington K. The management of acetabular insufficiency secondary to metastatic malignant disease. J Bone Joint Surg. 1981; 63A:653
2. Parrish R, Murray J. Surgical treatment for secondary neoplastic fractures. J Bone Joint Surg. 1970; 52A:664.
3. Harrington K, Johnston J, Turner R, Green D. The use of methylmethacrylate as an adjunct in the internal fixation of malignant neoplastic fractures. J Bone Joint Surg. 1972; 54A:1665.

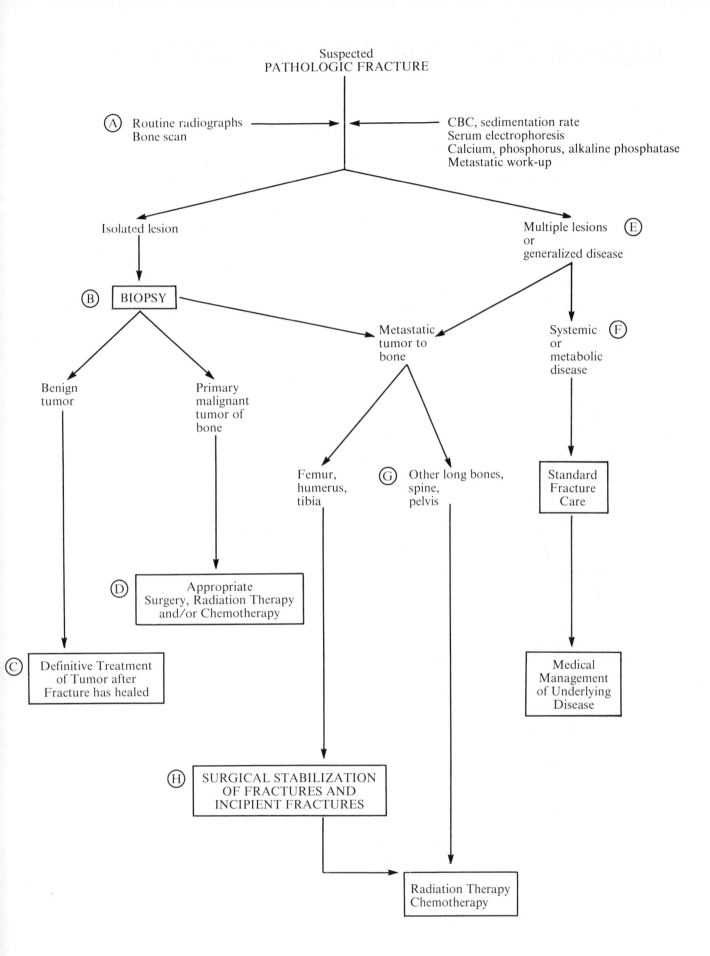

Suspected
PATHOLOGIC FRACTURE

(A) Routine radiographs
Bone scan

CBC, sedimentation rate
Serum electrophoresis
Calcium, phosphorus, alkaline phosphatase
Metastatic work-up

Isolated lesion

Multiple lesions (E)
or
generalized disease

(B) BIOPSY

Metastatic
tumor to
bone

Systemic (F)
or
metabolic
disease

Benign
tumor

Primary
malignant
tumor of
bone

Femur,
humerus,
tibia

(G) Other long bones,
spine,
pelvis

Standard
Fracture
Care

(D) Appropriate
Surgery, Radiation Therapy
and/or Chemotherapy

Medical
Management
of Underlying
Disease

(C) Definitive Treatment
of Tumor after
Fracture has healed

(H) SURGICAL STABILIZATION
OF FRACTURES AND
INCIPIENT FRACTURES

Radiation Therapy
Chemotherapy

# GUNSHOT WOUND TO THE EXTREMITY

## COMMENTS

A. The kinetic energy and thus wounding potential of a missile vary with the square of its velocity. Low-velocity gunshots are defined as having a muzzle velocity of less than 600–700 m/sec. Most civilian handguns and rifles, including .22, .38, .32, .25, and .45 caliber weapons, inflict low-velocity injuries. Only certain hunting and military rifles have muzzle velocities over 700 m/sec and are classified as high-velocity weapons. In addition to the missile tract damage of a low-velocity bullet, a high-velocity bullet causes extensive wound cavitation and distant tissue necrosis. Fracture fragments may act as significant secondary missiles.

B. Because soft tissue damage of most handgun injuries is minimal in civilian practice, local wound care with skin cleansing and ellipsing of the skin edges is sufficient. Few cases of deep wound infection have been reported.[1] Definitive fracture treatment may proceed regardless of the retained missile fragments and the bullet tract.

C. Joints traversed by missile fragments should be surgically debrided. The risk of infection in the potential intra-articular dead space is high unless arthrotomy and thorough irrigation and drainage are performed. Retained lead bullets bathed in synovial fluid may also result in lead intoxication[2] or chronic synovitis.

D. Although shotgun pellets are technically low-velocity projectiles, close range shotgun blasts produce wounds similar to those produced by high-velocity bullets. Shot wadding consisting of animal hair, jute, cardboard, plastic, or a variety of other materials may be found in wounds sustained at ranges up to 30 feet.[3] Similarly, clothing and other substances may be embedded in the wound.

E. Radical debridement of all devitalized bone and soft tissues minimizes the opportunity for infection.[4,5] Occasionally, counterincisions are necessary for thorough debridement of all foreign bodies, especially shotgun wadding. Nerve and tendon repairs must wait until soft tissue healing is completed.

F. Fractures from high-velocity bullets or close-range shotgun blasts must be meticulously debrided with excision of all free osseous fragments. Traction, casts, or external fixation devices temporarily stabilize the fracture during the management of the soft tissue wound. Definitive fracture management, with bone grafting of segmental defects, may proceed subsequent to successful wound healing.

## REFERENCES

1. Howland W, Ritchey S. Gunshot fractures in civilian practice. J Bone Joint Surg. 1971; 53A:47–55.
2. Dillman R, Brumb C, Lidsky M. Lead poisoning from a gunshot wound. Am J Med. 1979; 66:509–514.
3. Paradies L, Gregory C. The early treatment of close-range shotgun wounds to the extremities. J Bone Joint Surg. 1966; 48A:425–435.
4. DeMuth W, Smith J. High velocity bullet wounds of muscle and bone: the basis of rational early treatment. J Trauma. 1966; 744–755.
5. Carr C, Stevenson C. The treatment of missile wounds of the extremities. Instructional Course Lectures of the American Academy of Orthopaedic Surgeons. 1954; 11:189–210.

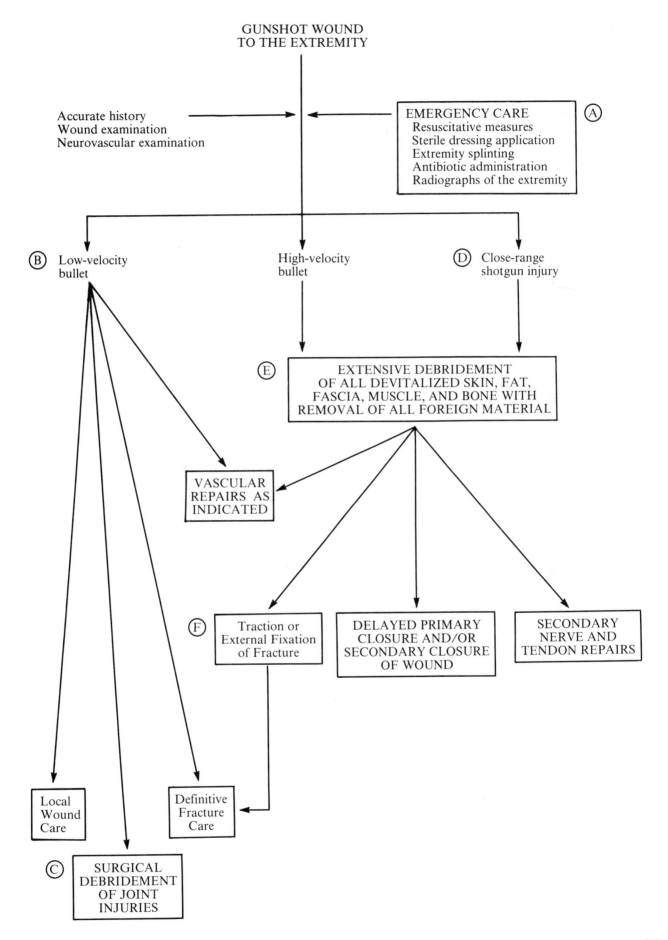

GUNSHOT WOUND
TO THE EXTREMITY

Accurate history
Wound examination
Neurovascular examination

EMERGENCY CARE    Ⓐ
Resuscitative measures
Sterile dressing application
Extremity splinting
Antibiotic administration
Radiographs of the extremity

Ⓑ Low-velocity
bullet

High-velocity
bullet

Ⓓ Close-range
shotgun injury

Ⓔ EXTENSIVE DEBRIDEMENT
OF ALL DEVITALIZED SKIN, FAT,
FASCIA, MUSCLE, AND BONE WITH
REMOVAL OF ALL FOREIGN MATERIAL

VASCULAR
REPAIRS AS
INDICATED

Ⓕ Traction or
External Fixation
of Fracture

DELAYED PRIMARY
CLOSURE AND/OR
SECONDARY CLOSURE
OF WOUND

SECONDARY
NERVE AND
TENDON REPAIRS

Local
Wound
Care

Definitive
Fracture
Care

Ⓒ SURGICAL
DEBRIDEMENT
OF JOINT
INJURIES

85

# EVALUATION OF BACK PAIN

## INTRODUCTION

Back pain, in most cases, is in the region of the lumbar spine. Almost everyone at some time experiences low back pain, and in 85% of cases, recovery occurs within 3 months. The source of the back pain is frequently difficult to identify because of such contributing factors as emotional overlay and secondary gain. Not to be overlooked, however, is the pathology that needs immediate treatment, such as cauda equina syndrome, infection, or neoplasm. Initially, most mechanical and disc-related low back pain requires conservative treatment, including weight reduction, postural improvement, reduction of lumbar lordosis, pelvic tilting exercises, and activity and life-style changes. Nonsteroidal anti-inflammatory drugs, analgesics, muscle relaxants, and lumbosacral corsets are also important.

## COMMENTS

A.  First, establish whether the problem is acute (3 to 6 months) or chronic (longer than 6 months) and whether there is neurologic involvement, as indicated by such symptoms as muscular weakness or bladder dysfunction. Note the relationship of the pain to ambulatory activity, posture, recumbency, and Valsalva and sciatic tension-producing maneuvers. Pain that is constant at night suggests a tumor.[1] In chronic cases, a long period of unemployment suggests secondary gain factors. Multiple joint involvement, particularly in the hips and knees, may signify spondyloarthropathy. A pain drawing by the patient, depicting the location and type of discomfort, will readily distinguish anatomic from hysterical patterns. Relate complaints to observations by watching the patient walk, undress, and move. Distract the patient during the examination to sort out pain behavior from real pathology. Objective physical findings include dysrhythmic motion, list, muscle spasm, contralateral positive straight leg raising, and muscle atrophy. Also, check for other joint involvement and decreased chest expansion.

B.  AP, lateral, and oblique radiographic views of the spine are studied for alignment and structural changes. Traction spurs and disc space narrowing point toward degenerative disc disease. A CT scan and myelogram done together are valuable when spinal stenosis is suspected. Sedimentation rate, alkaline phosphatase, calcium, phosphorus, uric acid, Bence-Jones proteins, protein electrophoresis, and HLA-B-27 determinations help to identify multiple myeloma, the spondyloarthropathies, or metabolic bone disease. An MMPI and psychologic evaluation are always important in interpreting low back pain.

Patients with a conversion V fare poorly after surgery even with prolapsed discs.[10] An EMG helps to localize the involved root level. Urologic evaluation of bladder dysfunction is important when a cauda equina syndrome is suspected. A differential spinal is valuable in cases of intractable pain when the source of pain is obscure.[3] If pain is still felt by the patient after complete muscle paralysis of the involved area, a central pain problem is present.

C.  Acute low back pain may either be event-related or occur with gradual but recent onset. Rule out cauda equina syndrome, tumor, and infection.

D.  Osteoporosis and compression fractures may be the only indication of primary or metastatic disease of the spine.

E.  Tension signs are objective findings of nerve root irritation, usually caused by a herniated nucleus pulposus.

F.  A new job or sport, soft mattress, or recent lifting activity may cause lumbar strain with minimal findings.

G.  A long history of low back pain should be assessed carefully for objective findings and secondary gain factors.

H.  Pain behavior out of proportion to the findings suggests a secondary gain component. An MMPI and psychologic evaluation are indicated to identify personality patterns that predispose to pain behavior.[12]

I.  Large joint involvement associated with intestinal symptoms is suggestive of spondyloarthropathy, which is often associated with a positive HLA-B-27 and elevated sedimentation rate.

J.  There may be no objective physical findings,[5] but a history of walking or even standing claudication, relieved by squatting or lying down, is usually diagnostic. Vascular claudication is different in that stopping without squatting or lying down relieves the symptoms. A CT scan and myelogram can show the area of stenosis.

K.  Osteoporosis and anterior wedging of the vertebral bodies out of proportion to age, together with abnormalities of calcium metabolism, suggest metabolic bone disease.

L.  Osteoarthritis of the spine is typically associated with restricted range of motion and symptoms that improve with rest, but increase with activity. X-ray findings show osteophytes, loss of facet joint spaces, and even spondylolisthesis.

M.  Intermittent low back pain, with or without tension signs, together with anterior vertebral body traction spurs and disc space narrowing suggests degenerative disc disease as a contributing factor.[8,13] Osteoarthritis usually coexists.

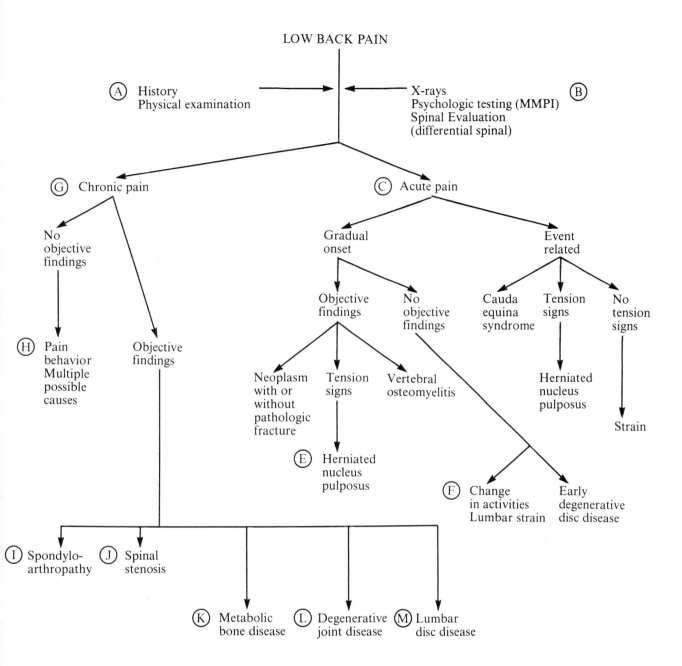

LOW BACK PAIN

(A) History
Physical examination

(B) X-rays
Psychologic testing (MMPI)
Spinal Evaluation
(differential spinal)

(G) Chronic pain

(C) Acute pain

No objective findings

Gradual onset

Event related

(H) Pain behavior
Multiple possible causes

Objective findings

Objective findings

No objective findings

Cauda equina syndrome

Tension signs

No tension signs

Neoplasm with or without pathologic fracture

Tension signs

Vertebral osteomyelitis

Herniated nucleus pulposus

Strain

(E) Herniated nucleus pulposus

(F) Change in activities
Lumbar strain

Early degenerative disc disease

(I) Spondylo-arthropathy

(J) Spinal stenosis

(K) Metabolic bone disease

(L) Degenerative joint disease

(M) Lumbar disc disease

## REFERENCES

1. Boland PJ, Lane JM, Sundaresan N. Metastatic disease of the spine. Clin Ortho Rel Res. 1982; 169:95–102.
2. Ling CM. Pyogenic osteomyelitis of the spine. Orthop Rev. 1975; 4:23.
3. McCollum DE, Stephen CR. The use of graduated spinal anesthesia in the differential diagnosis of pain in the back and lower extremities. S Med J. 1964; 57:410.
4. Newman PH. Surgical treatment for spondylolisthesis in the adult. Clin Orthop Rel Res. 1976; 117:107.
5. Paine KWE. Clinical features of lumbar spinal stenosis. Clin Orthop Rel Res. 1976; 115:77.
6. Parfitt AM, Duncan H. Metabolic bone disease affecting the spine. In *Acute Low Back Pain*. Philadelphia: WB Saunders, 1975.
7. Ross PM, Flemming JL. Vertebral body osteomyelitis spectrum and natural history. A retrospective analysis of thirty-seven cases. Clin Orthop Rel Res. 1976; 118:190.
8. Rothman RH, Simeone FA. Lumbar disc disease. In *The Spine*. Edited by RH Rothman and FA Simeone. Philadelphia: WB Saunders, 1975.
9. Rothman RH, Simeone FA. Cauda equina syndrome. In *The Spine*. Edited by RH Rothman and FA Simeone. Philadelphia: WB Saunders, 1975.
10. Spengler DM, Freeman CW. Patient selection for lumbar discectomy. Spine. 1979; 2:192.
11. Stauffer RN. Pyogenic vertebral osteomyelitis. Orthop Clin N Amer. 1975; 6:4.
12. Sternbach RA, Wolf SR, Murphy RW, Akeson WH. Traits of pain patients: the low back loser. Psychosomatics 1973; 14:226–229.
13. Verbiest H. Radicular syndrome from developmental narrowing of the lumbar vertebral canal. J Bone Joint Surg. 1954; 230–237.

# MANAGEMENT OF ACUTE LOW BACK PAIN

## INTRODUCTION

The treatment of back pain must begin with a specific diagnosis (pp. 86, 87). For nonprogressive conditions, much can be done in the initial period with bed rest, anti-inflammatory medication, analgesics, and local measures such as hot moist heat. As symptoms improve, gradual mobilization is begun. At that time, a long-term back maintenance program should be initiated under supervision. This program includes: (1) postural training, (2) lifting biomechanics, (3) alignment and conditioning exercises, and (4) activity precautions.

## COMMENTS

A. In the absence of a progressive neurologic deficit and bladder dysfunction, the initial treatment of a herniated nucleus pulposus is conservative;[8] and 85% will recover without surgery. Disc excision is indicated in psychiatrically stable individuals who have objective evidence of a prolapsed disc with neuropathy.[10] The role of chymopapain has been the subject of much controversy, and its use has recently been approved by the FDA. Carefully controlled studies are under way to document both its safety and efficacy.

B. The treatment of vertebral osteomyelitis is rest, appropriate antibiotics, and a spinal jacket. Drainage is not necessary unless an abscess forms and causes systemic or spinal cord symptoms.[2,7,11]

C. The treatment of pathologic fractures of the spine is directed at preventing spinal cord compression. Treatment consists of disease-specific measures including chemotherapy in the case of tumor and local measures such as radiation, acrylic replacement of eroded vertebrae, and internal reinforcement with hardware and bone graft.[1] A spinal orthotic or cast may provide temporary protection and pain relief. Stabilization should take place before cord symptoms develop.

D. Acute back strains require the same conservative measures outlined above for herniated nucleus pulposus. A common pitfall is to return to previous activity levels too soon, aggravating symptoms and prolonging recovery.

E. Short-term treatment of an arthritic flare consists of anti-inflammatory medication and rest. The long-term problem of progressive deformity and contractures can be reduced by a life-long program of postural training and stretching exercises.

## REFERENCES

1. Boland PJ, Lane JM. Sundaresan N. Metastatic disease of the spine. Clin Orthop Rel Res. 1982; 169:95–102.
2. Ling CM. Pyogenic osteomyelitis of the spine. Orthop Rev. 1975; 4:23.
3. McCollum DE, Stephen CR. The use of graduated spinal anesthesia in the differential diagnosis of pain in the back and lower extremities. S Med J. 1964; 57:410.
4. Newman PH. Surgical treatment for spondylolisthesis in the adult. Clin Orthop Rel Res. 1976; 117:107.
5. Paine KWE. Clinical features of lumbar spinal stenosis. Clin Orthop Rel Res. 1976; 115:77.
6. Parfitt AM, Duncan H. Metabolic bone disease affecting the spine. In *Acute Low Back Pain*. Philadelphia: WB Saunders, 1975.
7. Flemming JL. Vertebral body osteomyelitis spectrum and natural history. A retrospective analysis of thirty-seven cases. Clin Orthop Rel Res. 1976; 118:190.
8. Rothman RH, Simeone FA. Lumbar disc disease. In *The Spine*. Edited by RH Rothman and FA Simeone. Philadelphia: WB Saunders, 1975.
9. Rothman RH, Simeone FA. Cauda equina syndrome. In *The Spine*. Edited by RH Rothman and FA Simeone. Philadelphia: WB Saunders, 1975.
10. Spengler DM, Freeman CW. Patient selection for lumbar discectomy. Spine. 1979; 2:192.
11. Stauffer RN. Pyogenic vertebral osteomyelitis. Orthop Clin N Amer. 1975; 6:4.
12. Sternbach RA, Wolf SR, Murphy RW, Akeson WH. Traits of pain patients: the low back loser. Psychosomatics. 1973; 14:226–229.
13. Verbiest H. Radicular syndrome from developmental narrowing of the lumbar vertebral canal. J Bone Joint Surg. 1954; 230–237.

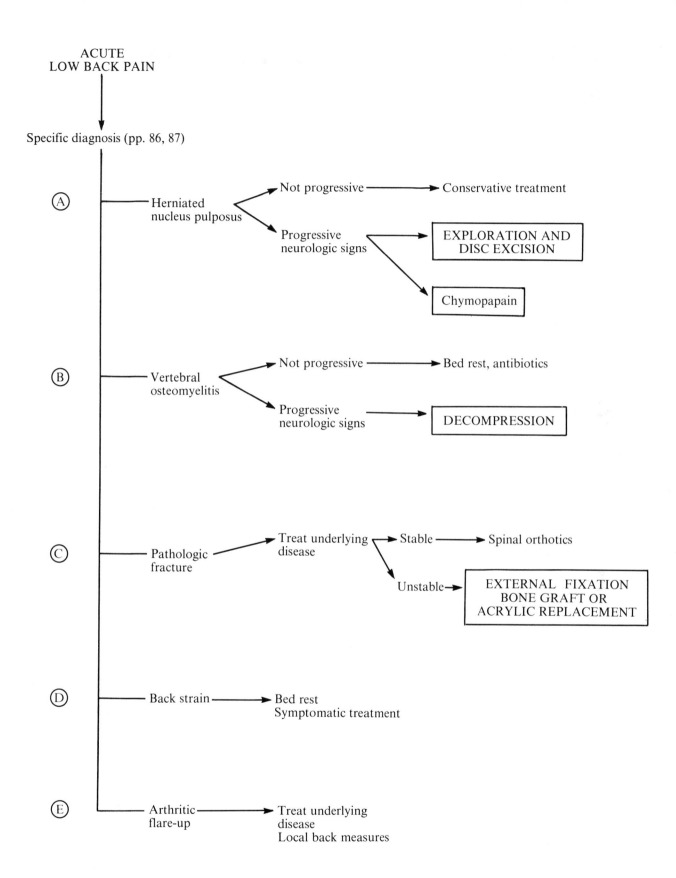

ACUTE
LOW BACK PAIN

Specific diagnosis (pp. 86, 87)

Ⓐ — Herniated nucleus pulposus
- Not progressive ——→ Conservative treatment
- Progressive neurologic signs
  - → EXPLORATION AND DISC EXCISION
  - → Chymopapain

Ⓑ — Vertebral osteomyelitis
- Not progressive ——→ Bed rest, antibiotics
- Progressive neurologic signs ——→ DECOMPRESSION

Ⓒ — Pathologic fracture
- Treat underlying disease
  - Stable ——→ Spinal orthotics
  - Unstable ——→ EXTERNAL FIXATION BONE GRAFT OR ACRYLIC REPLACEMENT

Ⓓ — Back strain ——→ Bed rest / Symptomatic treatment

Ⓔ — Arthritic flare-up ——→ Treat underlying disease / Local back measures

# MANAGEMENT OF CHRONIC LOW BACK PAIN

## INTRODUCTION

Chronic low back pain is pain that has been present for 6 months or longer and usually causes changes in the patient's life style and behavior. Unfortunately, our society rewards patients with chronic pain problems and low work incentive by disability payments. Recovery is more difficult the longer the pain has been present. A careful assessment of these patients and their functioning environment is needed. The multidisciplinary approach is a helpful way to share responsibility, validate the patient's findings, and develop an individually tailored rehabilitation program.[8,10,12]

## COMMENTS

A. Many questions remain unanswered regarding the etiology of spinal stenosis and the long-term residua when the condition is untreated. A CT scan done after a myelogram helps to correlate anatomic pathology with the clinical picture. Decompression in patients who are severely limited affords relief and return of function. The extent of the decompression required is dependent on the operative findings.[4,5]

B. Osteoarthritis of the facet joints causes pain and decreased range of motion. Activity tends to aggravate the symptoms, whereas rest relieves them. Surgery is rarely required. Most patients achieve a tolerable life style by a carefully adjusted program of weight control, rest, analgesics, and anti-inflammatory medications.

C. Osteoporosis with varying degrees of vertebral body collapse is a sequel of metabolic bone disease. Treatment is directed at correcting the underlying metabolic abnormality and reducing activities and postures that produce deforming stresses on the anterior spine. Spinal orthotics, avoidance of lifting, and the use of a firm back support when recumbent or sitting are essential measures.[6]

D. Spondylolisthesis, or forward displacement of one vertebra on the other, is due to a pars interarticularis defect. It is usually treated conservatively in adults. In some cases, the fibrocartilaginous mass at the pars interarticularis defect together with forward displacement of the vertebrae cause nerve root compression and/or traction resulting in sciatica. Spinal stenosis may occur later. When it is confirmed by a CT scan and myelogram, decompression of stenotic areas in symptomatic patients is warranted. Older patients tolerate this type of decompressive surgery well, and so it should not be withheld because of age alone.[4]

## REFERENCES

1. Boland PJ, Lane JM, Sundaresan N. Metastatic disease of the spine. Clin Orthop Rel Res. 1982; 169:95–102.
2. Ling CM. Pyogenic osteomyelitis of the spine. Orthop Rev. 1975; 4:23.
3. McCollum DE, Stephen CR. The use of graduated spinal anesthesia in the differential diagnosis of pain in the back and lower extremities. S Med J. 1964; 57:410.
4. Newman PH. Surgical treatment for spondylolisthesis in the adult. Clin Orthop Rel Res. 1976; 117;107.
5. Paine KWE. Clinical features of lumbar spinal stenosis. Clin Orthop Rel Res. 1976; 115:77.
6. Parfitt AM, Duncan H. Metabolic bone disease affecting the spine. In *Acute Low Back Pain*. Philadelphia: WB Saunders, 1975.
7. Ross RM, Flemming JL. Vertebral body osteomyelitis spectrum and natural history. A retrospective analysis of thirty-seven cases. Clin Orthop Rel Res. 1976; 118:190.
8. Rothman RH, Simeone FA. Lumbar disc disease. In *The Spine*. Edited by RH Rothman and FA Simeone. Philadelphia: WB Saunders, 1975.
9. Rothman RH, Simeone FA. Cauda equina syndrome. In *The Spine*. Edited by RH Rothman and FA Simeone. Philadelphia: WB Saunders, 1975.
10. Spengler DM, Freeman CW. Patient selection for lumbar discectomy. Spine. 1979; 2:192.
11. Stauffer RN. Pyogenic vertebral osteomyelitis. Orthop Clin N Amer. 1975; 6:4.
12. Sternbach RA, Wolf SR, Murphy RW, Akeson WH. Traits of pain patients: the low back loser. Psychosomatics. 1973; 14:226–229.
13. Verbiest H. Radicular syndrome from developmental narrowong of the lumbar vertebral canal. J Bone Joint Surg. 1954; 230–237.

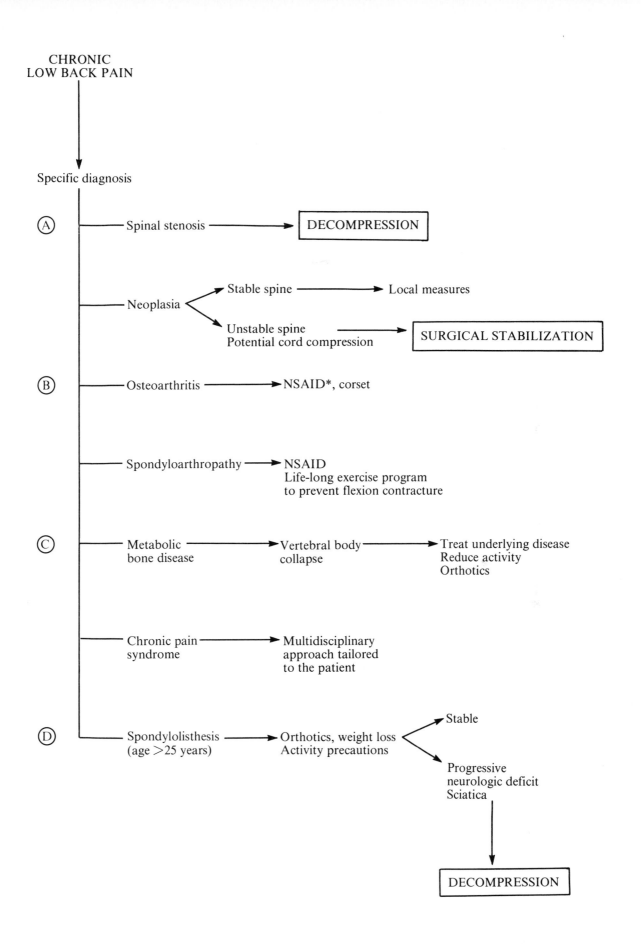

CHRONIC
LOW BACK PAIN

Specific diagnosis

(A) —— Spinal stenosis ——————→ [ DECOMPRESSION ]

—— Neoplasia

Stable spine ——————→ Local measures

Unstable spine ————→ [ SURGICAL STABILIZATION ]
Potential cord compression

(B) —— Osteoarthritis ——————→ NSAID*, corset

—— Spondyloarthropathy ——→ NSAID
Life-long exercise program
to prevent flexion contracture

(C) —— Metabolic ————→ Vertebral body ————→ Treat underlying disease
bone disease        collapse                Reduce activity
Orthotics

—— Chronic pain ————→ Multidisciplinary
syndrome              approach tailored
to the patient

(D) —— Spondylolisthesis ————→ Orthotics, weight loss
(age >25 years)            Activity precautions

Stable

Progressive
neurologic deficit
Sciatica

[ DECOMPRESSION ]

*Nonsteroidal anti-inflammatory drug

# NONTRAUMATIC DISORDERS OF THE CERVICAL SPINE

## INTRODUCTION

Cervical spine problems may be clouded by a functional overlay. Recovery from sprains and cervical disc problems may take many months and tax the patience of the physician as well as the patient. Most cervical spine problems of a nontraumatic nature can be treated nonoperatively. Treatment consists of a variable period of immobilization in a cervical collar, attention to neck posture, and night-time support on a cervical pillow. Anti-inflammatory drugs, analgesics, and muscle relaxants are also helpful.

## COMMENTS

A. Ask about previous trauma or activities requiring extreme neck postures. With radiating pain into the extremities, look for radiculopathy. If the picture is one of neurologic progression, surgical decompression and/or stabilization may be necessary. Nontraumatic cervical spine problems present in five typical patterns:[3] (1) as the residua from a recent neck sprain; (2) as a crick in the neck which occurred on awakening in the morning; (3) as a recurrence of symptoms in a patient with a previous neck injury; (4) as one of many flare-ups related to a long-standing problem such as rheumatoid arthritis; and (5) as an acute exacerbation of chronic neck pain. Inspect the general posture of the patient and the way in which the head is held. With straightening of the normal cervical lordosis, a forward neck posture is often adopted. Palpation of the back of the neck frequently reveals tight paraspinal muscles or areas of pain in the paraspinal region. The patient should be asked to move his own head to the limits of comfortable motion. Apply compression and traction on the head while it is tilted in different planes to elicit radicular symptoms. A thorough neurologic examination should be performed. The sensory examination should be recorded graphically.

B. AP, odontoid, oblique, and flexion and extension films are taken to show the presence of any segmental instability, skeletal lesions, foraminal encroachment, degenerative changes, and residua from previous trauma. Cineradiography can show whether neck motion is symmetrical and at what level dysrhythmia occurs. There is frequently a poor correlation between symptoms and the pathology seen on the x-ray film. Myelography helps to localize a protruded cervical disc. The EMG will indicate which roots are involved and should be correlated with the clinical and x-ray examinations.

C. Some patients continue to have neck pain months after a sprain injury. There may be radiating pain with no neurologic pattern. Symptoms usually respond to heat, analgesics, trigger point injection, and home traction. A soft collar is also helpful. A poor prognosis has been associated with the following factors:[2] arm pain, sharp reversal of the cervical curve, decreased motion at one cervical level, the need to wear a collar longer than 12 weeks, the need for home traction, and the necessity of repeating a course of physical therapy.

D. A patient may present with excruciating pain localized to one side of the neck. The head is typically tilted away from the painful side with the chin rotated toward the involved side. The cause of this problem is probably a unilateral facet subluxation or synovial impingement. The mechanism is unclear, but the crick may occur during the night as the patient turns his head. Treatment consists of soft collar immobilization and motorized traction if a subluxation is suspected. A traction program may be necessary until symptoms subside.[3]

E. The inflammatory process of the rheumatoid arthritis involves the apophyseal joints, which become eroded and irregular. The cervical joint spaces thin out, making the cervical spine subject to subluxation. Approximately 25% go on to develop atlantoaxial subluxation. This is seen on a lateral x-ray film as a separation of 3 mm or more between the anterior margin of the odontoid and the posterior margin of the atlas. When long track signs such as hyperreflexia and clonus develop, atlantoaxial or occipitocervical fusion is indicated. Patients with any atlantoaxial subluxation need cervical collar protection and avoidance of axial loading conditions, such as riding in cars on bumpy roads.[1] Cervical spondylosis occurs because of disc degeneration and the formation of osteophytic protrusions which may encroach upon the nerve root foramen.[4] The midcervical region is the most common site. Treatment consists of immobilization in a soft collar holding the neck in slight flexion. Sometimes a period of traction in bed is required to control symptoms. Anti-inflammatory medication, analgesics, and muscle relaxants provide symptomatic relief. Activity modification should be part of the rehabilitation program. Indications for anterior disc excision and interbody fusion include a neurologic deficit that is progressing, progressive long track signs, vertebral artery compression, and intractable pain. The

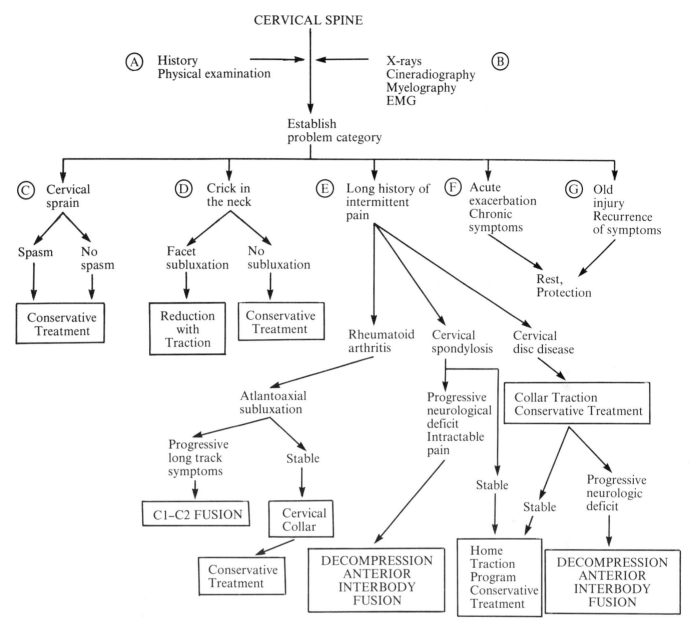

CERVICAL SPINE

Ⓐ History
Physical examination → ← X-rays
Cineradiography
Myelography
EMG Ⓑ

Establish problem category

Ⓒ Cervical sprain

Ⓓ Crick in the neck

Ⓔ Long history of intermittent pain

Ⓕ Acute exacerbation Chronic symptoms

Ⓖ Old injury Recurrence of symptoms

Spasm   No spasm

Facet subluxation   No subluxation

Rest, Protection

Conservative Treatment

Reduction with Traction   Conservative Treatment

Rheumatoid arthritis   Cervical spondylosis   Cervical disc disease

Atlantoaxial subluxation

Progressive neurological deficit Intractable pain

Collar Traction Conservative Treatment

Progressive long track symptoms   Stable

Stable

Stable   Progressive neurologic deficit

C1–C2 FUSION   Cervical Collar

Conservative Treatment

DECOMPRESSION ANTERIOR INTERBODY FUSION

Home Traction Program Conservative Treatment

DECOMPRESSION ANTERIOR INTERBODY FUSION

rationale of the interbody fusion of unstable segments is that the osteophytes about the neuro-central joints gradually resorb relieving compression. Cervical disc degeneration may lead to herniation and pressure upon the cervical cord as well as foraminal compression of emerging nerve roots. The majority of patients respond to conservative therapy, which consists of rest and immobilization using a soft cervical collar. As long as 6 weeks may be necessary to recuperate from the initial episode of pain, with final recovery taking as long as 4 to 6 months. Symptomatic measures include the use of anti-inflammatory medication, analgesics, and muscle relaxants as well as local hot moist heat. As the pain subsides, a program of cervical isometric exercises helps the patient to wean away from the collar. Surgery is indicated when there are progressive neurologic signs secondary to root or cord compression as well as intractable pain in an otherwise emotionally stable patient.

F. Acute exacerbations of old problems usually
G. respond to a period of soft collar immobilization and symptomatic measures. A careful history often reveals that the patient was involved in some unusual activity or minor injury.

**REFERENCES**

1. Bateman JE. Arthritis and Related Diseases, The Shoulder and Neck. Philadelphia: WB Saunders, 1972, p. 526.
2. Hohl M. Soft tissue injuries of the neck. Clin Orthop. 1975; 109:42.
3. Jackson R. The Cervical Syndrome. Springfield, Il: Charles C Thomas, 1978.
4. McNab I. Cervical spondylosis. Clin Orthop Rel Res. 1975; 109:69.
5. Rothman RH, Marvel JP. The acute cervical disc. Clin Orthop Rel Res. 1975; 109:59.

# SHOULDER PAIN

## INTRODUCTION

Problems affecting the shoulder can be broadly classified as intrinsic or extrinsic.[1,4] Localized pain and radiation patterns are not always typical. A carpal tunnel syndrome, for instance, may radiate as high as the shoulder. Usually, a careful history and physical examination with appropriate x-ray studies can make this initial distinction. Treatment depends on a careful analysis of the patient's needs, his ability to cooperate with a rehabilitation program, and the surgeon's experience.

## COMMENTS

A. A history of trauma or overuse should point toward rotator cuff, A/C joint or glenohumeral subluxation problems. Activities with overhead positioning, such as painting, cleaning, and wiring, frequently cause impingement.[3] Pain that is not related to shoulder movement is probably extrinsic. Radiation patterns are helpful. The pain of rotator cuff lesions usually radiates downward into the upper arm, whereas the pain of cervical spine disease radiates from the neck into the upper extremity and often into the hand. Important objective findings of intrinsic disease include atrophy of the spinati and deltoid, shrugging on active abduction, and restricted passive motion. A clunking or crepitus during passive range of motion points to glenohumeral diseases. The test for weakness may be falsely positive owing to pain inhibition and should be correlated with atrophy and EMG changes. Site of local pressure tenderness is helpful in distinguishing acromioclavicular joint pain from glenohumeral pain.

B. AP, lateral, and axillary views show the condition and position of the joint surfaces. Stress views, with weights and during forced abduction and external rotation, demonstrate abnormal positions of the joint expected with A/C separations and glenohumeral subluxation. Arthrograms of the shoulder illustrate dye extravasation into the subacromial bursa with rotator cuff tears and decreased capsular space in frozen shoulders.[2,3] Tomograms are useful to define glenohumeral changes such as avascular necrosis or loose bodies.

C. Intrinsic lesions hurt with active or passive range of motion and involve the A/C joint, rotator cuff, and glenohumeral articulation.

D. Full passive motion with motor weakness suggests a massive rotator cuff tear or neuropathy, i.e., brachial neuritis. An EMG will help to make the distinction.[4]

E. Restricted passive motion is caused by mechanical problems. A frozen shoulder is restricted in all ranges of motion, whereas impingement syndromes tend to cause maximal restriction in forward flexion. Intra-articular loose bodies cause shifting obstructions to motion, which may be elicited by circumduction motion or stress testing in external rotation in abduction.

F. Extrinsic shoulder lesions are suspected when there is no restriction of motion or local tenderness. Cervical spine pain referred to the shoulder region is most common. Degenerative changes in the cervical spine, positive EMG findings, and restricted cervical motion are typical.

G. The real trap is a sulcus tumor irritating the brachial plexus.[1] Sometimes there is fullness in the supraclavicular region. A history of smoking and multiple peripheral nerve involvement should make the examiner suspicious. Apical lordotic x-rays and diffuse EMG changes are diagnostic.

H. Brachial neuritis appears insidiously and is associated not only with pain and weakness, but also with sensory loss and reflex changes.[4]

I. When no pathologic conditions can be found and pain persists, one should look to visceral causes.

## REFERENCES

1. Brown C. Referred pain to the shoulder. Clin Orthop Rel Res. 1983; 173:55.
2. Golman AB, Ghelman B. The double-contrast shoulder arthrogram. Radiology. 1978; 127:655.
3. Neer CS, II. Impingement lesions. Clin Orthop Rel Res. 1983; 173:70.
4. Neviaser RJ. Painful conditions affecting the shoulder. Clin Orthop Rel Res. 1983; 173:63.

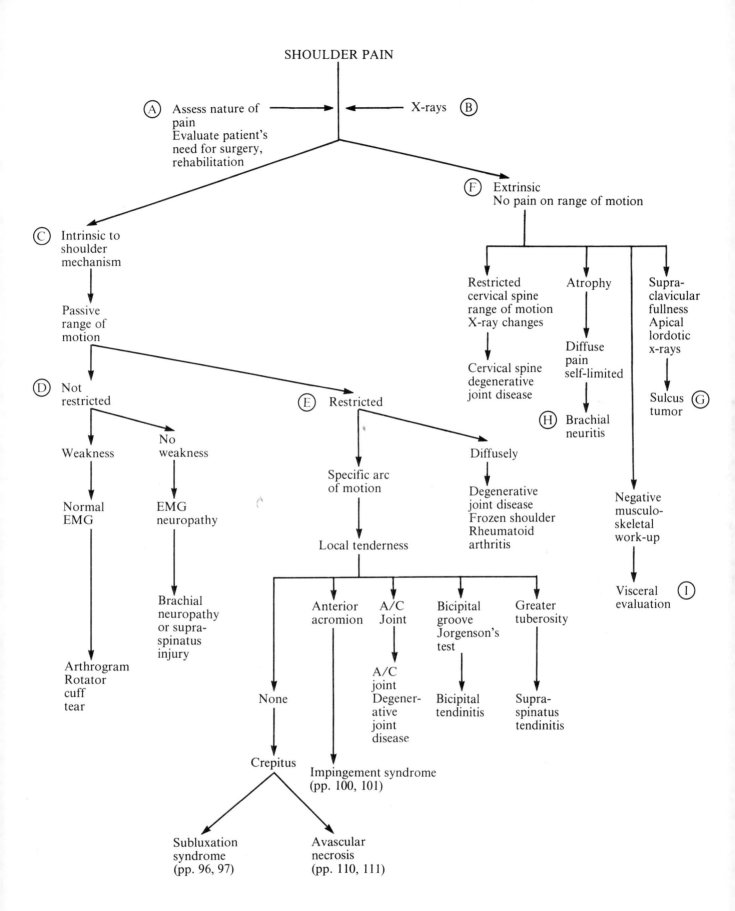

SHOULDER PAIN

Ⓐ Assess nature of pain
Evaluate patient's need for surgery, rehabilitation

X-rays Ⓑ

Ⓒ Intrinsic to shoulder mechanism

Passive range of motion

Ⓓ Not restricted

Weakness

No weakness

Normal EMG

EMG neuropathy

Arthrogram Rotator cuff tear

Brachial neuropathy or supra-spinatus injury

Ⓔ Restricted

Specific arc of motion

Local tenderness

Anterior acromion

A/C Joint

Bicipital groove Jorgenson's test

Greater tuberosity

A/C joint Degener-ative joint disease

Bicipital tendinitis

Supra-spinatus tendinitis

None

Crepitus

Impingement syndrome (pp. 100, 101)

Subluxation syndrome (pp. 96, 97)

Avascular necrosis (pp. 110, 111)

Diffusely

Degenerative joint disease
Frozen shoulder
Rheumatoid arthritis

Ⓕ Extrinsic
No pain on range of motion

Restricted cervical spine range of motion X-ray changes

Atrophy

Supra-clavicular fullness
Apical lordotic x-rays

Cervical spine degenerative joint disease

Diffuse pain self-limited

Sulcus tumor Ⓖ

Ⓗ Brachial neuritis

Negative musculo-skeletal work-up

Visceral evaluation Ⓘ

# SHOULDER INSTABILITY

## INTRODUCTION

Shoulder instability may be uni- or multidirectional.[2] The instability may be manifested by subluxation or dislocation.[3] Generalized ligamentous laxity may be a predisposing factor in an active individual or in one who develops a habit of voluntary shoulder subluxation. Trauma is the most common cause. When the humeral head has been pushed anteriorly out of the glenoid cavity, the following lesions may result: (1) a tear of the fibrocartilaginous labrum; (2) a defect in the posterolateral aspect of the humeral head; (3) erosion of the anterior glenoid; (4) capsular stretching, and, (5) intra-articular loose bodies.

Conservative treatment consists of strengthening the subscapularis and modifying activities to avoid excessive external rotation activities. Operative treatment is lesion-specific. The surgeon makes the final decision at surgery when the full extent of the pathology has been identified. Posterior dislocations are less common and not uncommonly missed. The treatment principles are the same.[1,2]

## COMMENTS

A.  The direction of instability is not always obvious. A description of the initial injury mechanism and subsequent maneuvers causing dislocation will help to establish the direction of instability. Apprehension with maneuvers requiring external rotation and abduction typically reflect anterior instability. The motor and sensory branches of the axillary nerve may be injured during the initial dislocation. Check for deltoid atrophy and sensory changes. Check for generalized ligamentous laxity. The ability to voluntarily sublux the shoulder often accompanied by grotesque maneuvers indicates that an underlying personality disorder may be present. Excessive ligamentous laxity or a poorly controlled seizure disorder predisposes to a poor surgical result. Palpating the involved shoulder during active circumduction movements will frequently reveal crepitus. With the patient supine, the examiner can frequently detect the presence of instability by inducing anterior posterior translatory movements of the humeral head. An examination under anesthesia comparing shoulders together with x-ray studies is helpful for establishing the presence of subluxation.

B.  Both AP and axillary views should be obtained. A 70° internal rotation view shows posterolateral defects in the humeral head.[3] The axillary view show glenoid erosion and humeral head subluxation during stress testing. An arthrogram will help to detect the presence of a rotator cuff tear and reveal any capsular stretching.

C.  In acute dislocations, the first dislocation should be treated by 3 weeks of immobilization in internal rotation followed by internal rotator exercises. One or two additional dislocations are still compatible with successful conservative treatment, depending on the reasons for the dislocation. With an established pattern of dislocations some form of repair is necessary, not only for the comfort and function, but also for the safety of the patient. The surgical reconstruction should be lesion-specific. Posterior dislocations are usually managed by glenoid osteotomy and capsular reinforcement, whereas anterior dislocations involve reconstituting the glenoid cavity by labral repairs, capsular tightening, and bone graft if necessary. With large posterolateral humeral defects, limiting external rotation may also be necessary. The extent of the reconstructive surgery for instability depends on the functional requirements and age of the patient.

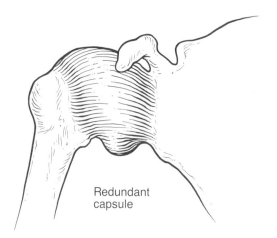

Redundant capsule

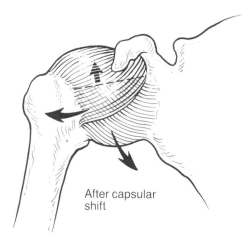

After capsular shift

Elimination of capsular laxity by pullup, overlap and reinforcement. (After Neer)

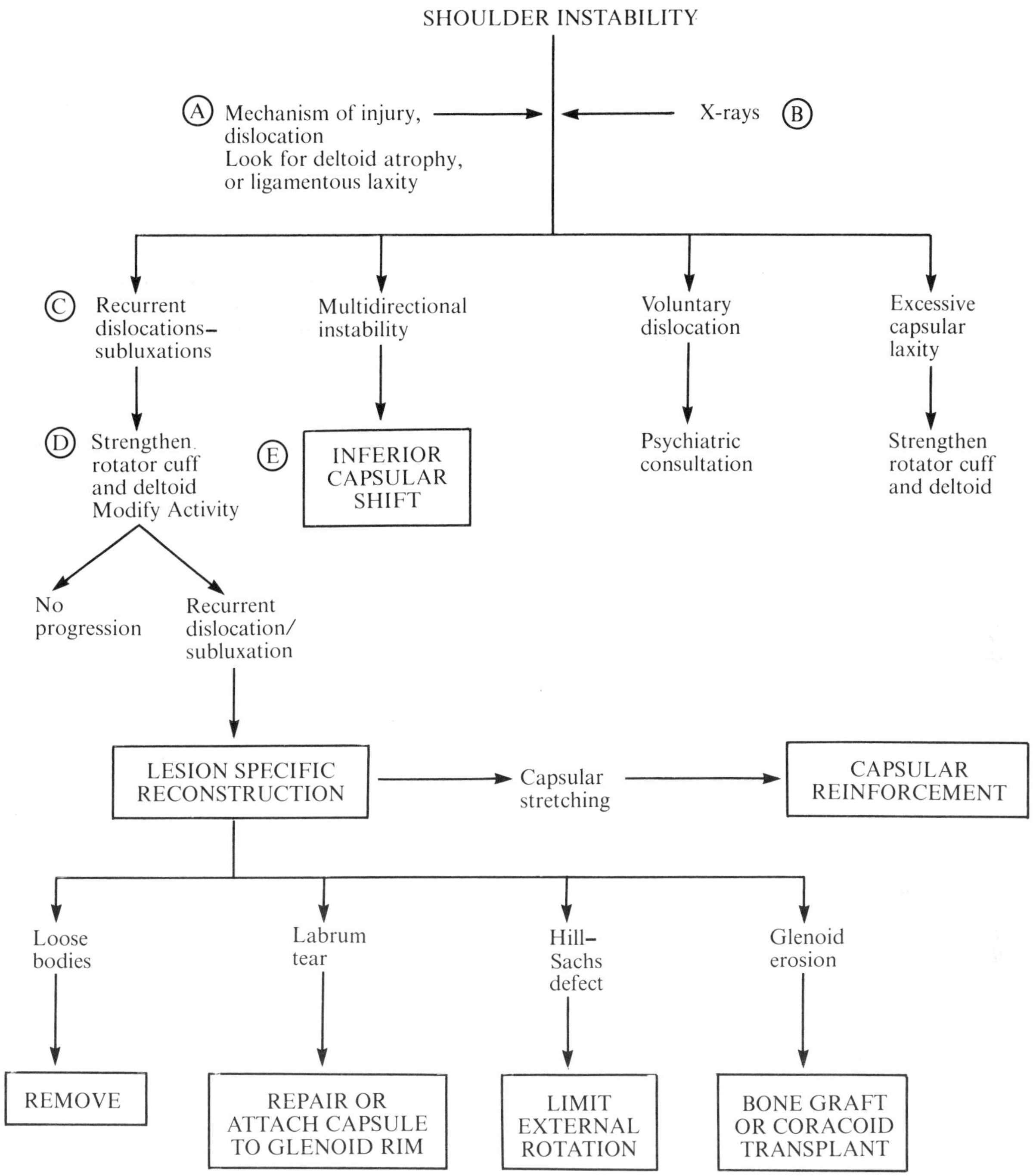

## SHOULDER INSTABILITY

(A) Mechanism of injury, dislocation
Look for deltoid atrophy, or ligamentous laxity

(B) X-rays

(C) Recurrent dislocations–subluxations

Multidirectional instability

Voluntary dislocation

Excessive capsular laxity

(D) Strengthen rotator cuff and deltoid
Modify Activity

(E) INFERIOR CAPSULAR SHIFT

Psychiatric consultation

Strengthen rotator cuff and deltoid

No progression

Recurrent dislocation/subluxation

LESION SPECIFIC RECONSTRUCTION → Capsular stretching → CAPSULAR REINFORCEMENT

Loose bodies

Labrum tear

Hill–Sachs defect

Glenoid erosion

REMOVE

REPAIR OR ATTACH CAPSULE TO GLENOID RIM

LIMIT EXTERNAL ROTATION

BONE GRAFT OR CORACOID TRANSPLANT

---

D. Rotator cuff strengthening exercises, particularly those involved in internal rotation, are often successful. With continued pain and subluxation on external rotation maneuvers, surgical reconstruction is indicated. The treatment should be lesion-specific, but often requires only limitation of external rotation.[3]

E. For multidirectional instability[2] the inferior capsular shift is designed to eliminate capsular incompetencies.

## REFERENCES

1. Boyd HB, Sisk TD. Recurrent posterior dislocation of the shoulder. J Bone Joint Surg. 1972;54-A:779.
2. Neer CS, Foster CR. Inferior capsular shift for involuntary inferior and multidirectional instability of the shoulder. J Bone Joint Surg. 1980;62-A:897-908.
3. Protzman RR. Anterior instability of the shoulder. J Bone Joint Surg. 1980;62-A:909-918.
4. Rowe R. Prognosis in dislocations of the shoulder. J Bone Joint Surg. 1956;38-A:957-977.

# ARTHRITIS OF THE SHOULDER

## INTRODUCTION

The shoulder joint is rarely involved in systemic disease. In rheumatoid arthritis, the shoulder will eventually be involved.[1] Degenerative joint disease is relatively rare and usually secondary to trauma. The wide range of mobility predisposes the shoulder to minor injury, which over time leads to degenerative joint disease. Heavy construction workers and athletes are unusually susceptible. Treatment is directed at relieving the pain and maintaining motion so that the hand can reach the face, hair, buttocks, and feet. Conservative treatment is always tried first. For severe disease and persistent symptoms, a total shoulder replacement can be done if the rotator cuff is reparable. Septic joints require arthrodesis.

## COMMENTS

A. Osteoarthritic pain is especially annoying at night, whereas rheumatoid disease is associated with morning stiffness. Since treatment is largely directed at relief of pain and maintaining function, a careful description of the pain and its response to various treatments should be elicited. Range of motion of the shoulder—particularly as it permits the hand to reach face, hair, buttocks, and feet—should be assessed. Note any crepitus and loss of strength. Rotator cuff function is an important prerequisite to total joint arthroplasty. Joint effusion present in inflammatory disease usually points anteriorly and can be easily aspirated.

B. A shoulder effusion can be easily aspirated anteriorly. This allows division into four major categories, noninflammatory, inflammatory, septic, and traumatic. Sedimentation rate, uric acid, rheumatoid factor, and antinuclear antibody studies are helpful in assessing the presence and activity of inflammatory disease. X-ray studies of the shoulder include AP of the shoulder in internal and external rotation as well as 40° posterior oblique to show the glenohumeral joint space and joint surfaces. With avascular necrosis, a humeral head crescent sign or segmental collapse is noted. A cold technetium pyrophosphate scan of the humeral head indicates avascular necrosis.

C. Osteoarthritis, both primary and secondary, of the shoulder should be treated initially with nonsteroidal, anti-inflammatory agents, rest, and activity modification. Occasionally a direct steroid injection will bring relief for several months. Most patients respond to conservative treatment. When symptoms are progressive and result in continuous night and rest pain, total shoulder arthroplasty is recommended. The unconstrained total shoulder replacement is the procedure of choice, but needs a functioning rotator cuff. Cuff repair can be done at the time of surgery. The role of constrained total shoulder replacement in patients with nonreparable rotator cuff is still controversial.

D. Symptoms and functional disability frequently do not parallel the radiographic changes. Symptoms are dependent on the general status of the disease and fluctuate widely. Nonsteroidal anti-inflammatory agents and intra-articular steroid injections may suffice for long periods of time despite severe radiographic changes. One should follow the patient and the course of the disease before deciding whether a total shoulder replacement is appropriate.

E. Septic joints occur in patients with a decreased immunocompetency and with a history of injections in and around the shoulder, particularly by members of the drug subculture who do not take sterile precautions. The result is a painful and incomplete fibrous ankylosis. Arthrodesis with compression screw fixation is usually attainable and offers relief of pain. The position of arthrodesis should be 20 to 25° of abduction, 30° of flexion, and 45° of internal rotation.[3]

F. The most common condition causing Charcot joint arthropathy in the shoulder is cervical syringomyelia. Conservative treatment described under degenerative joint disease is appropriate.[2]

G. Avascular necrosis is half as common in the shoulder as in the hip and is caused by similar factors. Steroids and trauma probably account for the greatest incidence. When involvement is minimal, conservative treatment with activity modification suffices. However, as disease progresses with collapse of part of the humeral head, symptoms are more intense. Arthrotomograms and arthroscopy help to evaluate the extent of the lesion. With minimal involvement, excision of the involved articular surface and drilling subchondral bone may be all that is required. However, with more extensive involvement and mechanical impingement, a hemiarthroplasty is usually necessary. Total shoulder replacement is reserved for advanced cases of glenohumeral arthritis.[2]

## REFERENCES

1. Curran JF, Ellman MH, Brown NL. Rheumatologic aspects of painful conditions about the shoulder. Clin Orthop Rel Res. 1983; 173:27.
2. Neer CS II. Replacement arthroplasty for glenohumeral arthritis. J Bone J Surg. 1974; 56-A:1.
3. Rowe CR. Arthrodesis of the shoulder used in treating painful conditions. Clin Orthop Rel Res. 1983; 173:92.

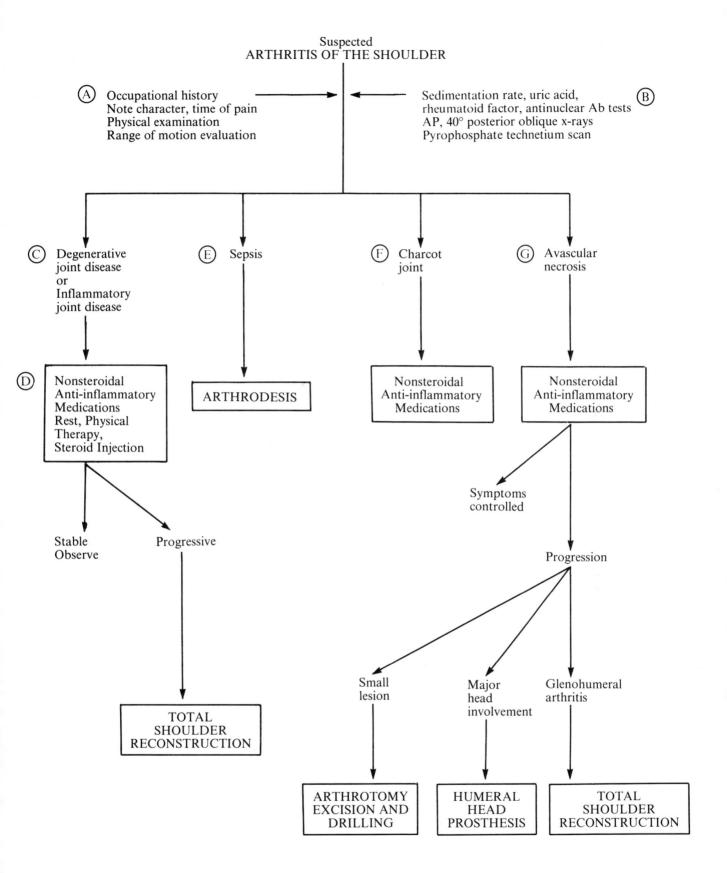

Suspected
**ARTHRITIS OF THE SHOULDER**

Ⓐ Occupational history
Note character, time of pain
Physical examination
Range of motion evaluation

Ⓑ Sedimentation rate, uric acid,
rheumatoid factor, antinuclear Ab tests
AP, 40° posterior oblique x-rays
Pyrophosphate technetium scan

Ⓒ Degenerative
joint disease
or
Inflammatory
joint disease

Ⓔ Sepsis

Ⓕ Charcot
joint

Ⓖ Avascular
necrosis

Ⓓ Nonsteroidal
Anti-inflammatory
Medications
Rest, Physical
Therapy,
Steroid Injection

ARTHRODESIS

Nonsteroidal
Anti-inflammatory
Medications

Nonsteroidal
Anti-inflammatory
Medications

Stable
Observe

Progressive

Symptoms
controlled

Progression

TOTAL
SHOULDER
RECONSTRUCTION

Small
lesion

Major
head
involvement

Glenohumeral
arthritis

ARTHROTOMY
EXCISION AND
DRILLING

HUMERAL
HEAD
PROSTHESIS

TOTAL
SHOULDER
RECONSTRUCTION

# IMPINGEMENT SYNDROME AND ROTATOR CUFF TEARS

## INTRODUCTION

Neer has made a major contribution to the understanding of shoulder pathology with his concepts of rotator cuff impingement.[1,2] The functional arc of movement of the humerus is forward, not lateral. The supraspinatus is impinged against the outer lateral aspect of the acromion with forward elevation. This area of the rotator cuff has a poor blood supply and when injured heals slowly. Occupational and recreational activities involving overhead movement predispose to impingement injury. Once formed, the injury lesions persist and may extend with subsequent activity or trauma. Treatment consists of reducing inflammation, eliminating impingement-producing activities and anatomy, and repairing cuff tears in suitable patients.

## COMMENTS

A.  A history of overhead activities and trauma should be sought. With careful questioning, a history of an episodic pattern of shoulder pain can be elicited. Complaints of weakness should always make one suspect a cuff tear. Local tenderness at the anterior lateral edge of the acromion is a common sign. Forward flexion of the shoulder will accentuate this pain. Injection of 10 ml 1% xylocaine under the acromion eliminates the impingement sign. Carefully observe for supraspinatus and deltoid atrophy along with rotator cuff weakness. Test both biceps and supraspinatus tendon for inflammation by the impingement test, plus abduction, flexion, supination against resistance. Forearm flexion and supination against resistance will cause pain in the bicipital groove with bicipital irritation.

B.  AP x-rays of the shoulder in internal and external rotation will show the bicipital groove region as well as the greater tuberosity. Changes associated with the impingement syndrome include A/C joint spurs, enlargement and sclerosis of the greater tuberosity, acromial erosion, and a high-riding humeral head.[1] The arthrogram is an important adjunct to x-ray studies in that it will show the presence of, and to some extent the degree of, cuff tear. Dye extravasation into the subacromial bursa is pathognomonic of a cuff tear, while the thickness of the supraspinatus tendon is a measure of the amount of intact cuff.

C.  Stage I impingement consists of edema and hemorrhage of the rotator cuff occurring mainly in young athletes.[1] Response to rest, anti-inflammatory agents, and careful range of motion is usually good. The condition may be recurrent, with continued impingement-related activity. The use of steroids under the acromion is controversial and certainly should not be used more than once or twice.

D.  Stage II impingement is characterized by a thickening of the bursa, which causes more impingement and leads to chronicity of symptoms.[1,2] Typically, symptoms decrease with inactivity, but return with overhead sports and tasks. This tends to occur in the middle-aged individual. Sectioning of the coracoacromial ligament and resection of the thickened bursa may be all that is necessary. At the time of surgery, acromioplasty can be performed if the aforementioned mechanical lesions are demonstrated radiographically.

E.  Stage III impingement[2] lesions frequently include complete tears of the rotator cuff along with spur formation, which adds to mechanical impingement. When conservative treatment fails and more function is required by the patient, anterior acromioplasty and A/C joint resection eliminate the mechanical impingement. When feasible, a rotator cuff repair will reduce the high-riding humeral head and further eliminate impingement. One must carefully balance the condition and needs of a given patient with the effects of the extensive surgery and length of recovery period in repair of massive cuff tears.

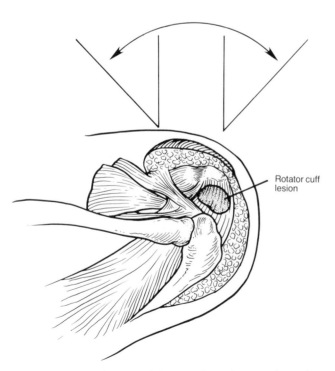

Rotator cuff lesion

The site of impingement is just anterior to the acromion and occurs with forward flexion.

100

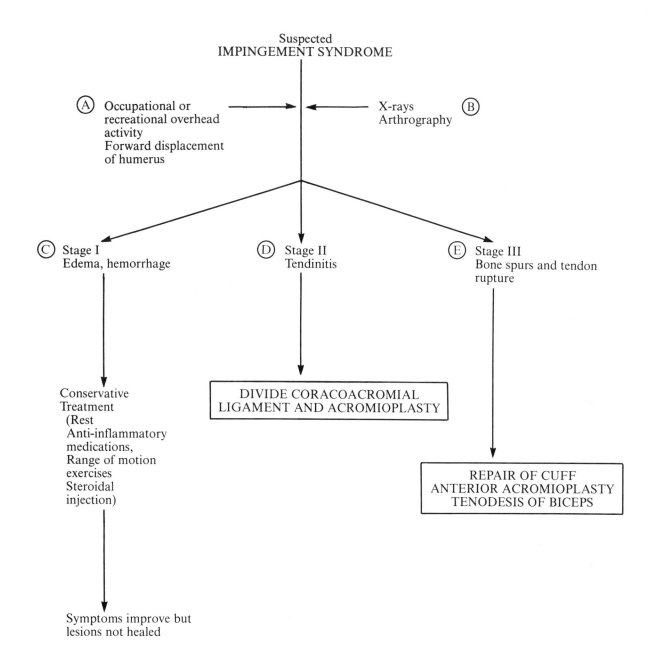

Suspected
IMPINGEMENT SYNDROME

(A) Occupational or
recreational overhead
activity
Forward displacement
of humerus

X-rays
Arthrography (B)

(C) Stage I
Edema, hemorrhage

(D) Stage II
Tendinitis

(E) Stage III
Bone spurs and tendon
rupture

Conservative
Treatment
(Rest
Anti-inflammatory
medications,
Range of motion
exercises
Steroidal
injection)

DIVIDE CORACOACROMIAL
LIGAMENT AND ACROMIOPLASTY

REPAIR OF CUFF
ANTERIOR ACROMIOPLASTY
TENODESIS OF BICEPS

Symptoms improve but
lesions not healed

**REFERENCES**

1. Neer CS II. Impingement lesions. Clin Orthop.
   1983:173:70.

2. Neer CS II: Anterior acromioplasty for the chronic
   impingement syndrome in the shoulder. A preliminary
   report. J Bone Joint Surg. 1972; 54-A:41.

# ELBOW PAIN

## INTRODUCTION

The most common complaints about the elbow are related to the musculotendinous structures—origins and insertions. Like the shoulder, the elbow is rarely involved with primary inflammatory arthritic affections. It is frequently involved with osteoarthritis following sports trauma, heavy labor, and unusual activities. Preservation of good function is still consistent with the loss of full flexion and extension. Treatment is usually conservative. The main problems requiring surgery are *catching* due to loose bodies and instability secondary to rheumatoid arthritis. The clinical picture does not always correlate with the x-ray findings.

## COMMENTS

A. Elbow problems are intrinsic or extrinsic to the joint. Extrinsic problems are caused by activities such as tennis or carrying heavy briefcases and suitcases, which cause traction on the epicondylar muscle origins. Intrinsic problems are related more to long-term occupation or previous trauma, and involve the elbow joint itself. Check range of motion for loss of full flexion and extension. Palpate the radial head and both epicondyles, which are tender in tennis or pitcher's elbow. Dorsiflexing and supinating the wrist against resistance will usually aggravate the pain. An elbow effusion is best noted, with the elbow flexed, by inspecting and palpating just beneath the lateral epicondyle.

B. AP and lateral radiographic views will demonstrate degenerative changes, loose bodies, and osteophytic impingement. An arthrotomogram will show loose bodies and osteochondritis dissecans of the capitellum.[1] Arthroscopy through the lateral portal allows inspection of the radiocapitellar joint, but in my experience it is of limited value.

C. Intrinsic elbow pain refers to pain within the elbow joint itself.

D. Osteophytic impingement, loss of joint surface, and loose bodies are the hallmark of degenerative joint disease. The exact etiology of a severely affected elbow may not be clear. A careful history may point to an occupational or recreational cause. Limitation of full flexion and extension is still compatible with good function.

E. Involvement of the elbow joint by inflammatory joint diseases such as rheumatoid arthritis causes flexion contractures, destruction of joint surfaces, ligamentous laxity, and sometimes considerable instability. Crepitation at the radiocapitellar joint and diffuse synovial thickening are common findings. An elbow joint effusion can be seen and palpated beneath the lateral epicondyle of the flexed elbow.

F. The most common cause of upper extremity neuropathic joints is cervical syringomyelia.[2] A neuropathic joint is crepitant, warm, and swollen. Considerable destruction may be seen on x-ray examination despite the minimal or absent pain.

G. Extrinsic problems arise from the musculotendinous structures about the elbow and from pain that is referred from the shoulder and cervical spine.

H. Musculotendinous pain at the flexor and extensor origins about the elbow are common to many occupational and sporting activities. Palpation of the radial head and epicondylar areas causes pain, which is also aggravated by dorsiflexion and supination/pronation against resistance.

I. Pain may be referred distally to the elbow from shoulder impingement syndromes and cervical spine radiculopathy.[3] A superior sulcus or Pancoast tumor also causes diffuse ill-defined pain, sometimes felt as aching in and around the elbow.

J. When the ulnar nerve at the level of the cubital tunnel becomes irritated, it produces local discomfort as well as distal paresthesias. The nerve may be swollen, tender, and easily displaced from its cubital tunnel.

## REFERENCES

1. Woodward AH, Bianco AJ. Osteochondritis dissecans of the elbow. Clin Orthop Rel Res. 1975;110:35.
2. Kornberg M. Neuropathic arthropathy. Orthop Rev. 1983;12:45.
3. Spengler DM, Kirsh MW, Kaufer H. Orthopaedic aspects and early diagnosis of superior sulcus tumor of lung (Pancoast). J Bone Joint Surg. 1973;55-A:1645.

ELBOW PAIN

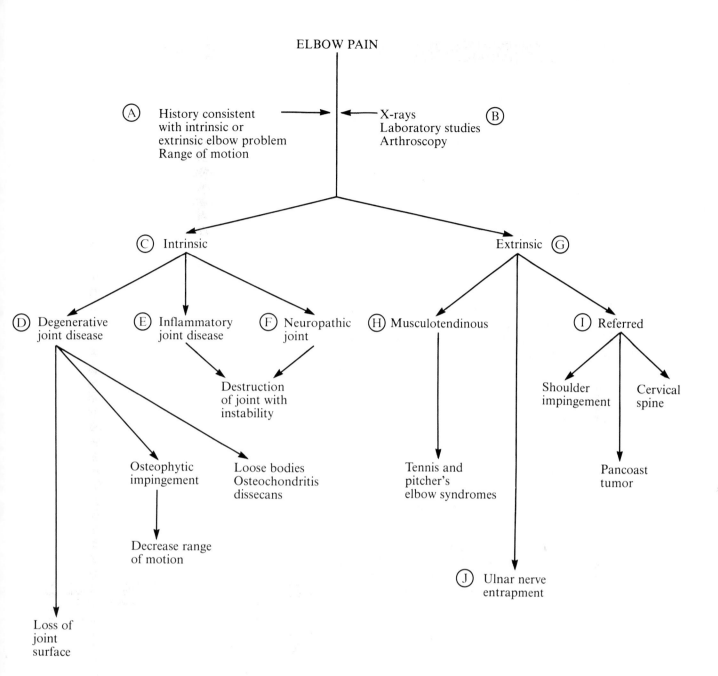

Ⓐ History consistent with intrinsic or extrinsic elbow problem Range of motion

Ⓑ X-rays Laboratory studies Arthroscopy

Ⓒ Intrinsic

Ⓖ Extrinsic

Ⓓ Degenerative joint disease

Ⓔ Inflammatory joint disease

Ⓕ Neuropathic joint

Ⓗ Musculotendinous

Ⓘ Referred

Destruction of joint with instability

Osteophytic impingement

Loose bodies Osteochondritis dissecans

Shoulder impingement

Cervical spine

Tennis and pitcher's elbow syndromes

Pancoast tumor

Decrease range of motion

Ⓙ Ulnar nerve entrapment

Loss of joint surface

# ARTHRITIS OF THE ELBOW

## COMMENTS

A. Degenerative joint disease typically results from occupational or recreational stresses over a long period of time. The treatment is symptomatic with anti-inflammatory and analgesic medications. If loose bodies produce locking symptoms, they should be excised. Occasionally, severe intractable pain follows degenerative joint disease. A fusion of the elbow at 90° provides relief and reasonable function.

B. A proliferative synovitis causes pain and gradually destroys the joint. The ulnar nerve may become involved in this process, causing peripheral symptoms. Synovectomy is a pain-relieving measure as well as one that may retard destruction of the joint. Usually, both synovectomy and radial head excision are done,[3] through a medial and lateral incision. With progressive joint destruction and instability, total elbow replacement is possible, although still experimental.[2,3] Arthrodesis is probably better suited to the osteoarthritic elbow.

C. Osteochondritis dissecans[4] is relatively uncommon, but it is important because it may present as locking due to loose bodies. The disease usually affects the capitellum, causing pain and loss of elbow motion. Once the osteochondral fragment has been shed, loose bodies will be seen on x-ray examination and cause locking of the elbow clinically. From published studies, excision of the loose bodies alone is probably sufficient.

## REFERENCES

1. Ewald FC, Scheinberg RD, Porth R, Thomas WH, Scott RD, Sledge CB. Capitellocondylar total elbow arthroplasty: two to five-year follow up in rheumatoid arthritis. J Bone Joint Surg. 1980; 62-A:1259.
2. Inglis AE, Pellici PM. Total elbow replacemnt, J Bone Joint Surg. 1980; 62A:1253.
3. Petty W. Synovectomy in rheumatoid arthritis. Orthop Surg, a Weekly Update. 1979;1:1.
4. Woodward, AH, Bianco AJ. Osteochondritis dissecans of the elbow. Clin Orthop Rel Res. 1975; 110:35.

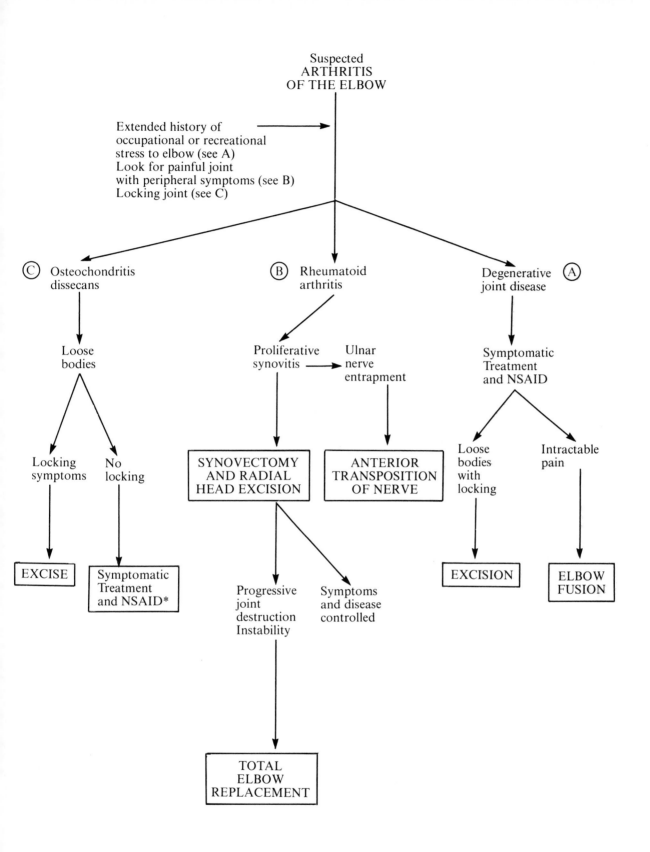

Suspected
ARTHRITIS
OF THE ELBOW

Extended history of
occupational or recreational
stress to elbow (see A)
Look for painful joint
with peripheral symptoms (see B)
Locking joint (see C)

Ⓒ Osteochondritis
dissecans

Ⓑ Rheumatoid
arthritis

Degenerative Ⓐ
joint disease

Loose
bodies

Proliferative
synovitis → Ulnar
nerve
entrapment

Symptomatic
Treatment
and NSAID

Locking
symptoms

No
locking

SYNOVECTOMY
AND RADIAL
HEAD EXCISION

ANTERIOR
TRANSPOSITION
OF NERVE

Loose
bodies
with
locking

Intractable
pain

EXCISE

Symptomatic
Treatment
and NSAID*

Progressive
joint
destruction
Instability

Symptoms
and disease
controlled

EXCISION

ELBOW
FUSION

TOTAL
ELBOW
REPLACEMENT

*Nonsteroidal Anti-Inflammatory Medications

# ULNAR NERVE ENTRAPMENT

## INTRODUCTION

Compression of the ulnar nerve within the cubital tunnel occurs secondary to a variety of causes.[3] Contusion may result from a direct blow. Hospital patients in the supine position and resting the elbows on the bed, particularly after anesthesia, may develop cubital tunnel compression symptoms. With the elbow flexed, the ulnar nerve is stretched tightly within the tunnel and causes similar symptoms. The nature of the pathologic changes within the affected nerve segment is not completely clear, but beyond a certain point, full recovery is not possible. The exact turning point is not readily detectable. Therefore, treatment should be aggressive, with surgical release and transposition being done early enough to allow maximal recovery.[2,4] Whether or not to do a neurolysis and the choice of method to secure the nerve in its new position are subjects of continuing controversy. In my opinion, neurolysis should be withheld for extremely scarred nerves and the anterior transposition should be held in place by a fascial dermal sling.

## COMMENTS

A. Typical complaints include paresthesias in the ring and little finger, weakness, and clumsiness in performing tasks requiring manual dexterity, such as buttoning a shirt, and picking up small objects. The onset of symptoms may be insidious, in which case patients delay seeking help for as long as 6 months to a year. The carrying angle of the elbow involved should be compared to the opposite side. Increased cubitus valgus following previous injury may be causing a traction effect on the nerve. Palpate the nerve in the cubital tunnel for irritability, excessive mobility, and coverage by the tunnel. Advanced involvement causes interosseous wasting, weakness, clawing, and sensory loss. Tinel's sign is positive early on. Two-point discrimination is greater than 2 mm.

B. Examine the AP and lateral radiographic views for supracondylar spurs and degenerative changes, which may be directly affecting the nerve. Nerve conduction velocity is slowed across the elbow, compared to the opposite side. Denervation changes of ulnar nerve innervated muscles appear over time on EMG studies.

C. In the presence of positive electrical studies, such as nerve conduction slowing across the elbow, release and anterior transposition of the nerve are indicated to avoid permanent damage. With minimal changes, the inciting cause should be determined and eliminated. A sheepskin elbow pad and attention to the position of the elbow in the case of desk workers may eliminate the cubital tunnel compression early enough to avoid surgery.

D. The ulnar nerve should be released from its exit point at the medial intermuscular septum down to the site of penetration into the flexor carpi ulnaris. Several articular branches may need to be sacrificed in order to gain adequate mobility for the anterior transposition. Once the nerve is released, a fascial flap, based either distally or at the medial epicondyle, is fashioned to provide a sling to prevent the nerve from returning to its former position.[1] The approach has the advantage of minimal scarring about the nerve, such as might be incurred when burying it in a muscle tunnel.

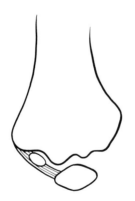

Perineural fibrosis

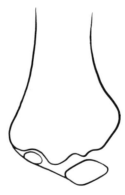

Lateral shift of ulna

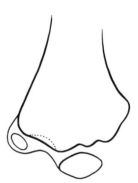

Shallow groove
Excessive mobility of ulnar nerve

Cubital Tunnel Compression Syndrome

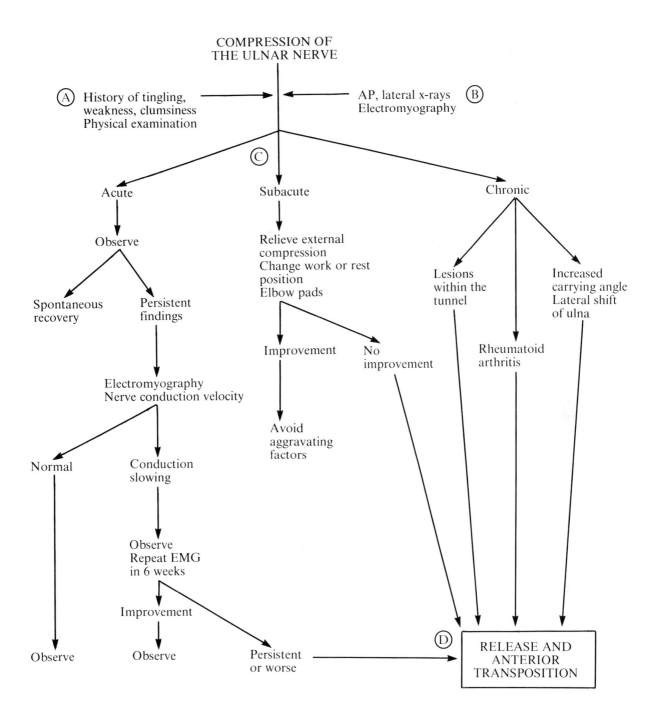

COMPRESSION OF
THE ULNAR NERVE

(A) History of tingling, weakness, clumsiness Physical examination

(B) AP, lateral x-rays Electromyography

(C)

Acute

Subacute

Chronic

Observe

Relieve external compression
Change work or rest position
Elbow pads

Lesions within the tunnel

Increased carrying angle
Lateral shift of ulna

Spontaneous recovery

Persistent findings

Improvement

No improvement

Rheumatoid arthritis

Electromyography
Nerve conduction velocity

Avoid aggravating factors

Normal

Conduction slowing

Observe

Observe
Repeat EMG in 6 weeks

Improvement

Observe

Observe

Persistent or worse

(D) RELEASE AND ANTERIOR TRANSPOSITION

## REFERENCES

1. Eaton RG, Crowe JF, Parkes JC, III. Anterior transposition of the ulnar nerve using a non-compressing fasciodermal sling. 1980; 62–A:820.
2. Harrison MJG, Nurick S. Results of anterior transposition of the ulnar nerve for ulnar neuritis. Br Med J. 1970; 1:27.
3. Wadsworth TG, Williams JR. Cubital tunnel external compression syndrome. Br Med J. 1973; 1:662–666.
4. Tayin J. Anterior transposition of the ulnar nerve: An electrophysiological study. J Neurol Neurosurg Psychiat. 1970; 33:157–165.

# HIP PAIN

## INTRODUCTION

The term "hip pain" is interpreted differently by the clinician and patient. The patient should be asked to point to the location of the pain. The pain of true hip disease usually presents in the groin, although it may radiate laterally and sometimes posteriorly. Back-related disorders refer pain to the buttock and down the back of the leg, but occasionally this pain may be felt in the groin. A symptomatic trochanteric bursa presents as lateral buttock pain. Hardware from previous hip surgery may cause trochanteric pain when lateral migration has occurred, but this pain may also herald a nonunion, which will declare itself once the hardware is removed. In summary, when presented with a chief complaint of hip pain, determine the site specifically.

## COMMENTS

A.  Establish the relationship of the pain to ambulation, rest, sleep, and any therapeutic measures such as anti-inflammatory medication. Establish whether there has been any recent activity change or traumatic episode in the past. Gradual device migration after previous hip surgery could cause hip pain. Increased or unusual activity may cause a stress fracture of the femoral neck. An old dislocation may have caused avascular necrosis. The presence of any factors contributing to avascular necrosis, such as alcohol abuse, use of steroids, inflammatory joint disease, any of the reticuloendothelioses, or unusual occupations, should be sought. Cancer of the prostate, multiple myeloma, and other metastases can produce persistent pain, even at night while the patient is recumbent.

B.  Watch the patient undress and walk in the corridor at normal ambulatory speed. An abductor lurch, positive Trendelenberg test and antalgic gait indicate a hip problem. Restricted lumbar spine motion distinguishes hip from low back disease. With the patient sitting, test range of motion of the hips for guarding. With the patient in the supine position, positive straight leg raising indicates sciatic nerve tension. Stress the sacroiliac (SI)joints with Patrick's test. Percussion on the heel or over the trochanter will induce groin discomfort if there is hip disease. Palpate the sciatic notch, trochanteric bursa, and deeply in the groin in search of extracapsular disease such as femoral aneurysm, inguinal adenopathy, or inflamed trochanteric bursa. Pulled muscles and iliopsoas bursitis can cause groin pain. The pain is increased when the patient resists or initiates motion against resistance. A rectal examination helps to identify prostate cancer, which can cause hip pain from pelvic metastases. Decreased chest expansion suggests a spondyloarthropathy. Obtain specific tests such as ESR and HLA B-27.

C.  X-ray views include AP and lateral of both hips for comparison and AP and lateral of lumbar spine.

D.  Routine laboratory tests include determination of sedimentation rate, alkaline phosphatase, urinalysis, calcium, phosphorus, protein electrophoresis, and uric acid.

E.  Even after a thorough work-up, the source of hip pain may be obscure. Instill 2 cc of 1% xylocaine into the hip joint under image intensifier control, using Renografin as a dye marker to ensure intra-articular injection. This will temporarily relieve most hip joint-related pain. I use this technique frequently and find it to be a great help in distinguishing between the hip, back, and knee as the primary referral source for the pain.

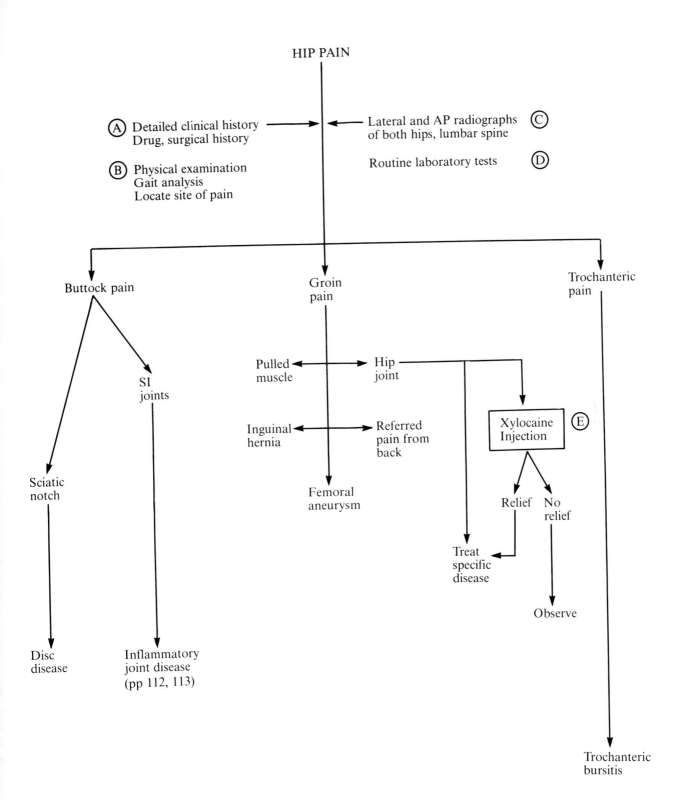

HIP PAIN

Ⓐ Detailed clinical history
Drug, surgical history

Lateral and AP radiographs
of both hips, lumbar spine  Ⓒ

Routine laboratory tests  Ⓓ

Ⓑ Physical examination
Gait analysis
Locate site of pain

Buttock pain

Groin
pain

Trochanteric
pain

SI
joints

Pulled
muscle

Hip
joint

Xylocaine
Injection  Ⓔ

Inguinal
hernia

Referred
pain from
back

Sciatic
notch

Femoral
aneurysm

Relief    No
relief

Treat
specific
disease

Observe

Disc
disease

Inflammatory
joint disease
(pp 112, 113)

Trochanteric
bursitis

# AVASCULAR NECROSIS

## INTRODUCTION

Degenerative joint disease, inflammatory joint disease, and trauma account for most hip pain. Avascular necrosis ranks fourth as a cause of hip pain. The exact cause of this condition is not known. It is related to fractures, dislocations, alcohol abuse, steroids, gout, decompression sickness, systemic lupus erythematosis, leukemia, reticuloendothelioses, sickle cell anemia, and other conditions.[4-6] In general, the condition can be classified as secondary to macrovascular abnormality, such as that resulting from trauma, or secondary to microvascular abnormality caused by emboli. The result is either a local or a diffuse necrosis of subchondral bone. Treatment is directed at relief of pain, and preservation of a normal articular surface as long as possible. With eventual progression, total hip replacement must be considered.

## COMMENTS

A. Symptoms of avascular necrosis may not occur for as long as six months to several years following a traumatic event such as dislocation. Early symptoms include groin pain with activity, for which there appears to be no explainable reason. Sometimes the onset of pain is sudden, corresponding to collapse of cartilage and subchondral bone over the involved area. The patient demonstrates an antalgic gait, positive Trendelenberg, and some guarding on rotation, but otherwise a remarkably preserved range of motion.

B. Radiographs initially may show radiolucency, followed by coalescence of these lucencies and a crescent sign as the subchondral bone separates through the necrotic area. This can be made more prominent by traction on the affected leg during the study. Involved areas are radiodense, and with time and collapse a step deformity and flattening appears. Eventually, the head becomes more and more deformed, with secondary changes occurring in the acetabulum. End-stage avascular necrosis is the typical picture of severe degenerative joint disease. Scintigraphy performed early, using radioactive technetium diphosphonate, reveals a cold scintiscan.[2] With time and revascularization, this can again become hot.

C. Avascular necrosis can be classified into six stages:[4] Stage I—subtle mottled densities throughout the femoral head. Stage 2—well-demarcated infarct. Stage 3—subtle flattening of

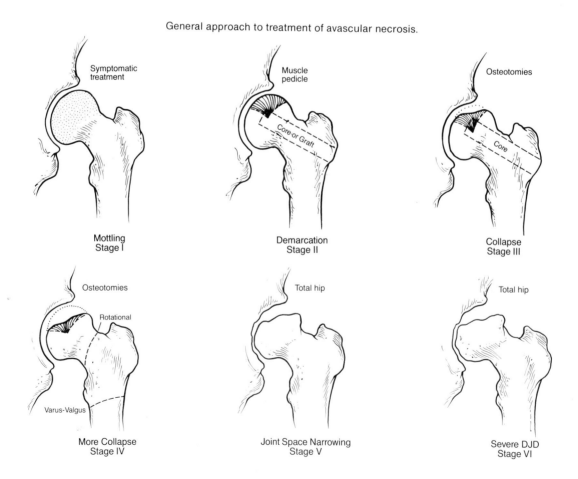

General approach to treatment of avascular necrosis.

Symptomatic treatment

Mottling
Stage I

Muscle pedicle

Core or Graft

Demarcation
Stage II

Osteotomies

Core

Collapse
Stage III

Osteotomies

Rotational

Varus-Valgus

More Collapse
Stage IV

Total hip

Joint Space Narrowing
Stage V

Total hip

Severe DJD
Stage VI

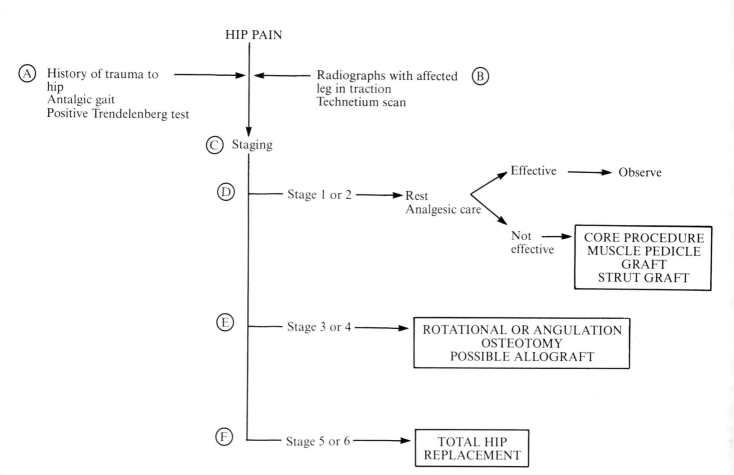

HIP PAIN

(A) History of trauma to hip
Antalgic gait
Positive Trendelenberg test

(B) Radiographs with affected leg in traction
Technetium scan

(C) Staging

(D) Stage 1 or 2 → Rest Analgesic care
- Effective → Observe
- Not effective →

CORE PROCEDURE
MUSCLE PEDICLE GRAFT
STRUT GRAFT

(E) Stage 3 or 4 →

ROTATIONAL OR ANGULATION OSTEOTOMY
POSSIBLE ALLOGRAFT

(F) Stage 5 or 6 →

TOTAL HIP REPLACEMENT

the overlying area, crescent sign. Stage 4—femoral head flattening with increased asymmetry and flattened area. Stage 5—narrowing of the joint space. Stage 6—more marked degenerative changes. Treatment is directed at relief of pain and preservation of a normal articular surface as long as possible. With eventual progression, total hip replacement must be considered but young patients are not good candidates for total hip surgery.

D. Analgesics, activity modification, and crutches are the mainstay of initial treatment for stage 1 or 2 disease. When the pain progresses and becomes unbearable, coring of the femoral neck and head up to subchondral bone is frequently a good pain-relieving measure.[4] Even when some flattening has occurred, substantial relief is possible. The duration of results, however, is unpredictable. A muscle pedicle graft has also been advocated as a method to restore blood supply to the femoral head.[5] The use of strut grafts to prevent eventual collapse has been extensively described, but results are unpredictable.[1,6]

E. When the disease has progressed to stages 3 and 4, flattening and collapse have occurred. If sufficient articular surface remains, an osteotomy such as described by Sugioka places a better joint surface under the weight-bearing dome.[7] Such operations are technically difficult and long term results are controversial. The allograft replacement of the diseased portion of the femoral head has been described, but substantial experience with this technique has not been reported.[5]

F. When the disease has progressed to stages 5 and 6, considerable degenerative joint disease has occurred. At this point, total hip replacement is the treatment of choice.[3]

**REFERENCES**

1. Boettcher WG, Bonfiglio M, Smith K. Non-traumatic necrosis of the femoral head. Part II Experiences and treatment. J Bone Joint Surg. 1970; 52-A:322–329.
2. D'Ambrosia R, Shoji H, Riggins RS, Stadalnik RC, DeNardo GL. Scintigraphy in the diagnosis of osteonecrosis. Clin Orthop Rel Res. 1978; 131:139–143.
3. Dutton RO, Amstutz HC, Thomas BJ, Higley AK. Theories of surface replacement for osteonecrosis of the femoral head. J Bone Joint Surg. 1982; 64-A:1225–1237.
4. Hungerford WG, Bonfiglio M, Smith K. Non-traumatic necrosis of the femoral head. Early diagnosis and treatment. Clin Orthop Rel Res. 1978; 131:144–153.
5. Meyers, M. The treatment of osteonecrosis of the hip with fresh osteo-allografts and with muscle pedicle graft technique. Clin Orthop 1978; 130:202–209.
6. Springfield DS, Enneking WJ. Surgery for aseptic necrosis of the femoral head. Clin Orth Rel Res. 1978; 130:175–185.

# ARTHRITIS OF THE HIP

## INTRODUCTION

Arthritis produces pain, restricted motion, and gradual destruction of the hip joint. The main causes of arthritis of the hip are trauma, degenerative joint disease, inflammatory joint disease, avascular necrosis, and infection. Untreated, the natural history of the disease is one of gradual progression and disability. Treatment is directed at diminishing the inflammatory response to arthritis while maintaining motion and weight-bearing function.

## COMMENTS

A.  Since there is a wide spectrum of pain and disability for various stages of the disease, a careful history is important. Patients with severe changes on radiographs may have very little pain and vice versa. Determine the extent of the pain, at night and at rest as well as the limitations it imposes on activities of daily living. Ask about the effects of previous medication. Anti-inflammatory medication sometimes brings about miraculous relief for 6 months to a year. Because treatment is dependent on the impact of the disease on the patient's life, observing the patient as he walks, sits, and undresses is an important part of the examination. The presence of an abductor lurch and a positive Trendelenberg are objective findings of hip disease. A hip flexion and adduction contracture limit range of motion and are important to correct at the time of total hip replacement.

B.  Since the treatment of inflammatory arthritis of the hip joint is the treatment of the underlying disease process, a specific diagnosis is important. Such screening studies as sedimentation rate, WBC, protein electrophoresis, uric acid, HLA-B27, rheumatoid factor are helpful, depending on the presenting picture.[1] With previous sepsis, a joint aspiration for identification of causative organisms should be attempted. An AP view of the pelvis and a lateral view of each hip should be obtained in order to compare the affected to the normal side. One should assess the extent of involvement to determine whether an osteotomy is appropriate. Look for irregularities in anatomy, which are potential technical problems for total hip replacement. Acetabular protrusion is a typical problem requiring careful preoperative planning.

C.  Conservative treatment of degenerative joint disease of the hip includes loss of weight, use of a cane, anti-inflammatories, and activity modification.[1] When these measures are no longer effective, surgery is indicated. If any femoral head cartilage is still present, a rotational or angulatory osteotomy can theoretically put this cartilage under the weight-bearing dome of the acetabulum.[2,3] When the arthritis has advanced to the point of intractable pain and disability, total hip replacement is the procedure of choice.

D.  Previous infection may obliterate the joint with resulting ankylosis. The presence of previous infections strongly contraindicates a total joint replacement unless the organism is *Staphylococcus epidermidis*. In the latter case, a total hip replacement may be attempted after debridement and under prolonged antibiotic protection. The alternatives to total hip replacement in the septic joint are resection arthroplasty and hip fusion. A hip fusion provides a stable pain-free limb for the younger patient who must work, but may result in lumbar spine discomfort later.[5] A resection arthroplasty is a good alternative for the sedentary patient.[4] The result is some motion with reasonable pain relief. Ambulatory aids are usually necessary.

E.  The treatment of inflammatory hip disease is the treatment of the underlying disease plus the conservative measures just described. When conservative measures no longer work, a total hip replacement is the procedure of choice.[4]

## REFERENCES

1.  Guidelines for Rheumatic Disease Management. Bull Rheum Dis Arthritis Foundation. 1981; 31:11–14.
2.  McMurray TP. Osteoarthritis of the hip joint. Br J Bone Joint Surg. 1935; 22:716.
3.  Muller MD. Intertrochanteric osteotomy in the treatment of arthritic hip pain. In Tronzo RG (Ed) *Surgery of the Hip Joint*. Philadelphia: Lea & Febiger, 1973.
4.  Parr PL, Croft C, Enneking WF. Resection of the head and neck of the femur with and without ambulation osteotomy. J Bone Joint Surg. 1971; 53A:935–;944.
5.  Stinchfield FE, Cavallaro WA. Arthrodesis of the hip joint: a follow-up study. J Bone Joint Surg. 1950; 32-A:48.

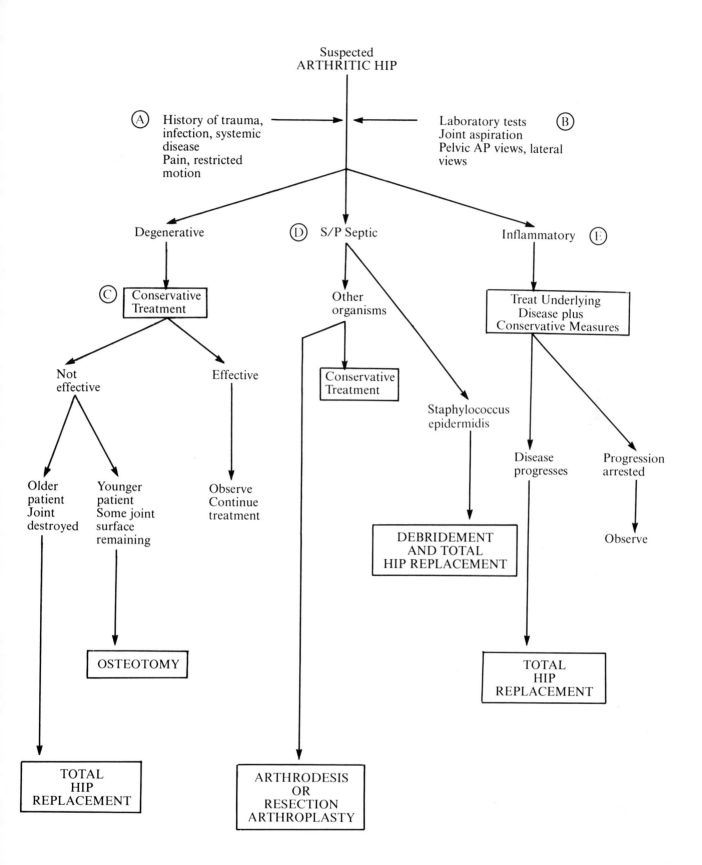

Suspected
ARTHRITIC HIP

(A) History of trauma,
infection, systemic
disease
Pain, restricted
motion

(B) Laboratory tests
Joint aspiration
Pelvic AP views, lateral
views

Degenerative

(D) S/P Septic

Inflammatory (E)

(C) Conservative
Treatment

Other
organisms

Treat Underlying
Disease plus
Conservative Measures

Not
effective

Effective

Conservative
Treatment

Staphylococcus
epidermidis

Disease
progresses

Progression
arrested

Older
patient
Joint
destroyed

Younger
patient
Some joint
surface
remaining

Observe
Continue
treatment

Observe

OSTEOTOMY

DEBRIDEMENT
AND TOTAL
HIP REPLACEMENT

TOTAL
HIP
REPLACEMENT

TOTAL
HIP
REPLACEMENT

ARTHRODESIS
OR
RESECTION
ARTHROPLASTY

# HIP PAIN FOLLOWING TOTAL HIP RECONSTRUCTION

## INTRODUCTION

Total hip replacement has been a major breakthrough for patients with arthritic affections of the hip joint. Although early follow-up results suggested an extremely optimistic prognosis, long-term studies show a progressive increase in the loosening rate, particularly after 15 years.[1] Complications include infection, loosening, chronic pain of undetermined etiology, non-union of the trochanter, recurrent subluxation or dislocation, leg-length discrepancy, stress fracture, component failure, and others. The patient with complications usually presents with pain, drainage from around the hip, or recurrent subluxation and dislocation.

## COMMENTS

A. The location of the pain is informative. Acetabular problems present with groin pain, whereas femoral component problems present with thigh pain. A specific traumatic incident may have caused cement failure. The heavy individual who has not complied with activity precautions is a prime candidate for early loosening. Trochanter removal and reattachment is associated with 20% non-union. Inspect the operative site for local tenderness, induration, and warmth suggestive of an inflammatory or infectious process. Keep in mind that deep sepsis may exist in the absence of abnormal superficial findings.

B. Aspirate the hip for culture and sensitivity studies when sepsis is suspected. The sedimentation rate is a useful indicator of septic activity. Weight-bearing and non-weight-bearing x-ray studies are done to elicit motion and the presence of loosening. A radiolucent line at the bone cement interface, which shows progressive widening over time, is strongly suggestive of loosening.

C. Two key questions arise when loosening has been diagnosed. First, is the condition progressive with loss of bone stock? Second, is sepsis present? Ongoing subsidence or migration with dissolution of bone stock must be dealt with even if no sepsis is present. An early revision is indicated to avoid component or cortical failure. When sepsis is present, if the organism is treatable, a two-stage revision may be considered (debridement and closure followed 6 weeks later by revision).[3] Otherwise, a resection arthroplasty with complete removal of components and cement is preferable. When loosening is not progressive and the pain is tolerable, conserva-

tive treatment may suffice. Long-term antibiotic therapy is an alternative to revision in low-grade nonprogressive sepsis.[2,3]

D. The incidence of trochanteric non-unions after reattachment is approximately 20%. Besides the presence of pain, the main issue is whether or not the trochanter functions competently as part of the abductor mechanism. Proximal migration compromises this function, permitting subluxation or dislocation. Painful non-unions can be bone grafted. Non-unions with proximal migration should be mobilized, brought down, and reattached with bone grafting.

## REFERENCES

1. Harris WH. Revision surgery for failed, non-septic total hip arthroplasty. Clin Orthop Rel Res. 1982; 170:8–20.
2. Hunter G, Dandy D. The natural history of the patient with an infected total hip replacement. J Bone Joint Surg. 1977; 59-B:293.
3. Salvati EA, Chefkofslay KW, Brause BD, Wilson PD. Reimplantation in infection—12 year experience. Clin Orthop Rel Res. 1982; 170:62–75.
4. Woo RY, Money BF. Dislocation after total hip arthroplasty. J Bone Joint Surg. 1982; 64-A:1295–1306.

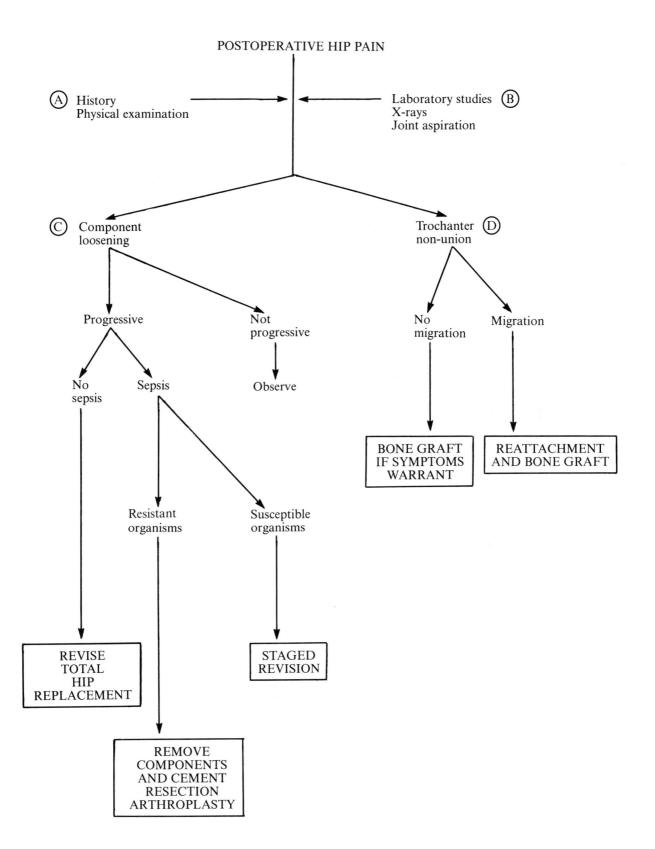

POSTOPERATIVE HIP PAIN

A History
Physical examination

B Laboratory studies
X-rays
Joint aspiration

C Component loosening

D Trochanter non-union

Progressive

Not progressive

No sepsis

Sepsis

Observe

No migration

Migration

Resistant organisms

Susceptible organisms

BONE GRAFT
IF SYMPTOMS
WARRANT

REATTACHMENT
AND BONE GRAFT

REVISE
TOTAL
HIP
REPLACEMENT

STAGED
REVISION

REMOVE
COMPONENTS
AND CEMENT
RESECTION
ARTHROPLASTY

# DISLOCATION FOLLOWING TOTAL HIP RECONSTRUCTION

## COMMENTS

A. Establish the circumstances surrounding the first dislocation. It is important to know whether the patient is compliant and follows instructions or whether dislocation occurs because of excessive flexion and internal rotation of the hip. Examine the operative note for comments regarding observed stability and range of motion at surgery. In chronic dislocations, determine the activities that predispose to dislocation. Careful range of motion of the hip will usually allow the examiner to feel the point at which impingement and subluxation begins.

B. X-ray studies will show the component geometry. Dynamic stability can be further assessed by ranging the hip under an image intensifier and noting the position at which subluxation begins.

C. Acute dislocations occur in the immediate postoperative period during patient transfers or unsupervised physical therapy. The first assessment should be whether the component geom-

etry is stable. With stable geometry, the patient can be treated in a spica for 6 weeks. Then start careful motion allowing the capsule to heal. Unstable components usually require revision. A trial spica immobilization for 6 weeks is warranted when the degree of instability is not great.

## REFERENCES

1. Harris WH. Revision surgery for failed, non-septic total hip arthroplasty. Clin Orthop Rel Res. 1982; 170:8–20.
2. Hunter G, Dandy D. The natural history of the patient with an infected total hip replacement. J Bone Joint Surg. 1977; 59-B:293.
3. Salvati EA, Chefkofslay KW, Brause BD, Wilson PD. Reimplantation in infection—12-year experience. Clin Orthop Rel Res. 1982; 170:62–75.
4. Woo RY, Money BF. Dislocation after total hip arthroplasty. J Bone Joint Surg. 1982; 64-A:1295–1306.

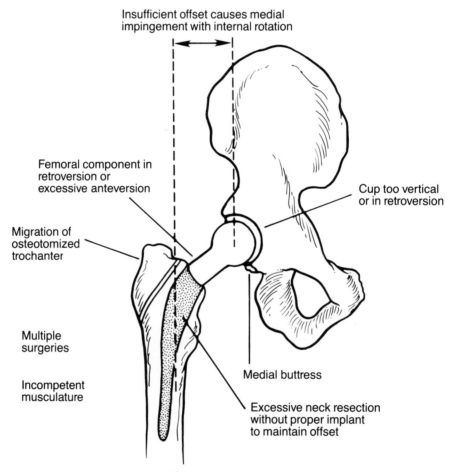

Insufficient offset causes medial impingement with internal rotation

Femoral component in retroversion or excessive anteversion

Migration of osteotomized trochanter

Multiple surgeries

Incompetent musculature

Cup too vertical or in retroversion

Medial buttress

Excessive neck resection without proper implant to maintain offset

Mechanical factors contributing to total hip dislocation.

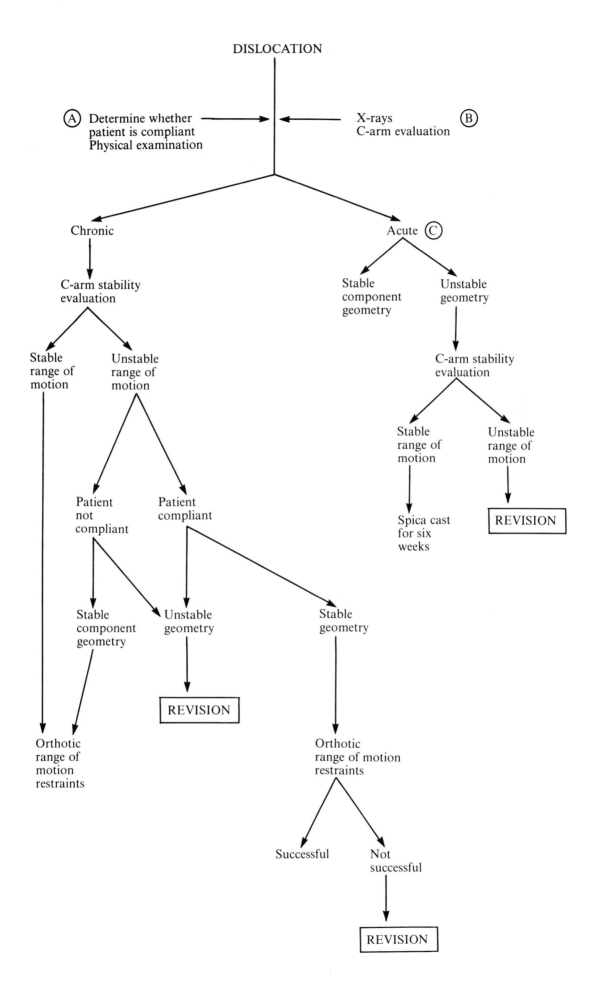

DISLOCATION

Ⓐ Determine whether
patient is compliant
Physical examination

X-rays
C-arm evaluation Ⓑ

Chronic

Acute Ⓒ

C-arm stability
evaluation

Stable
component
geometry

Unstable
geometry

Stable
range of
motion

Unstable
range of
motion

C-arm stability
evaluation

Patient
not
compliant

Patient
compliant

Stable
range of
motion

Unstable
range of
motion

Stable
component
geometry

Unstable
geometry

Stable
geometry

Spica cast
for six
weeks

REVISION

REVISION

Orthotic
range of
motion
restraints

Orthotic
range of motion
restraints

Successful

Not
successful

REVISION

**117**

# SEPTIC TOTAL HIP REPLACEMENT

## COMMENTS

A. When sepsis has been established, the pattern of drainage and febrile episodes must be determined. A knowledge of response to previous treatment and the identification of responsible organisms are helpful before secondary infection obscures the primary organism. The presence of erythema, induration, or sinus tracts should be noted. They are indicators of the extent of the infection and thus determine the management plan.

B. Cultures taken from sinus tract drainage, as well as hip joint aspirations, establish the causative organisms. X-ray studies include AP and lateral of the hip to detect endosteal resorption, arthrograms to assess interface separation, and sinograms to identify sinus tracts.

C. Acute sepsis typically occurs within the first 2 to 3 weeks after hip replacement. Deep infections are insidious and may not be accompanied by surface signs. Sinus tracts through the skin should be assumed to communicate deeply unless otherwise proven. Aggressive antibiotics may slow the infection process, but do not eradicate the infection. Early debridement is mandatory. If components are not loose, a trial of antibiotics and spica immobilization is reasonable. It is my practice to give IV antibiotics for 2 weeks, and then oral antibiotics for 6 weeks. The patient is immobilized in a spica cast for 6 weeks to allow the scar tissue to heal without shear forces and under the protection of bactericidal antibiotic levels. After removal of the spica, if wound healing has occurred and no drainage is present, gradual mobilization is started. The sedimentation rate is a guide to the degree of septic activity. With recurrence of inflammation and drainage, components and cement should be removed. If the organism is susceptible to antibiotics, a staged revision may be successful. For most organisms other than Staphylococcus, removal of components and cement followed by a resection arthroplasty is the safest course. The use of antibiotic cement in staged revisions has been advocated, but routine use, in my opinion, is controversial.[3]

D. If chronic sepsis is present, but not progressive, and there are no febrile episodes, drainage, or bone dissolution, treatment with long-term antibiotics alone is an acceptable alternative.[3] On the other hand, with progressive bone destruction, components and cement should be completely removed. A resection arthroplasty or a staged revision can be done, depending upon the nature of the organism and the amount of bone stock remaining.

## REFERENCES

1. Harris WH. Revision surgery for failed, non-septic total hip arthroplasty. Clin Orthop Rel Res. 1982; 170:8–20.
2. Hunter G, Dandy D. The natural history of the patient with an infected total hip replacement. J Bone Joint Surg. 1977; 59–B:293.
3. Salvati EA, Chefkofslav KW, Brause BD, Wilson PD. Reimplantation in infection—12-year experience. Clin Orthop Rel Res. 1982; 170:62–75.
4. Woo RY, Money BF. Dislocation after total hip arthroplasty. J Bone Joint Surg. 1982; 64–A:1295–1306.

POSTOPERATIVE
SEPSIS

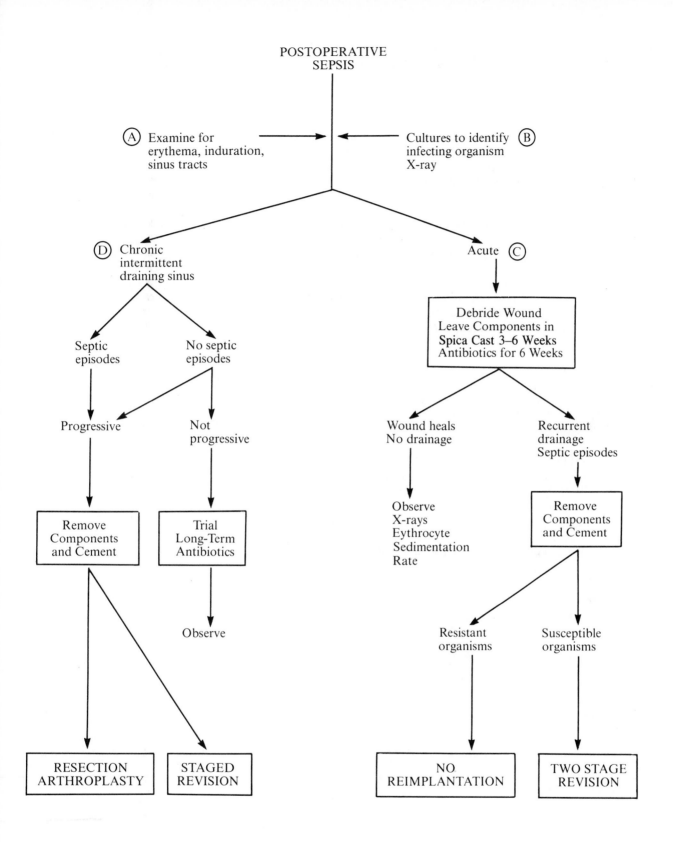

Ⓐ Examine for
erythema, induration,
sinus tracts

Ⓑ Cultures to identify
infecting organism
X-ray

Ⓓ Chronic
intermittent
draining sinus

Acute Ⓒ

Septic
episodes

No septic
episodes

Debride Wound
Leave Components in
**Spica Cast 3–6 Weeks**
Antibiotics for 6 Weeks

Progressive

Not
progressive

Wound heals
No drainage

Recurrent
drainage
Septic episodes

Remove
Components
and Cement

Trial
Long-Term
Antibiotics

Observe
X-rays
Eythrocyte
Sedimentation
Rate

Remove
Components
and Cement

Observe

Resistant
organisms

Susceptible
organisms

RESECTION
ARTHROPLASTY

STAGED
REVISION

NO
REIMPLANTATION

TWO STAGE
REVISION

# THE CATCHING KNEE

## INTRODUCTION

The term "catch" refers to the sensation interpreted by patients to mean everything from a mometary "click" to mechanical locking of the knee. The angle of knee flexion at which the catch occurs is diagnostic. Meniscus pathology affects extension during the mid-range and prevents terminal extension. Patellar subluxation occurs during the last 30° of extension without true locking. A loose body moves about the joint and may cause impingement in different locations. The physical examination confirms the presence of terminal extension loss, patellar alignment, tracking abnormalities, audible and palpable clicks, the presence of meniscal entrapment to specific maneuvers, effusion, shifting, or subluxation of the knee during stress testing.

## COMMENTS

A.  Little may be found on physical examination despite a convincing history. In the absence of objective findings, a course of quadriceps exercises and periodic observation is recommended. If objective findings appear, a more aggressive work-up is warranted.

B.  "Snapping tendons" may be caused by the iliotibial band or medial hamstrings snapping across a bony spur. The presenting complaint may be more one of concern rather than actual disability. Many snapping sensations and sounds are asymptomatic. In the absence of objective findings, aggressive work-up probably is not indicated.

C.  Patellofemoral subluxation during the last 30° of knee extension produces a catching sensation. The alignment of the patellofemoral mechanism and a lateral tracking pattern will suggest a subluxing tendency. A course of conservative treatment, including quadriceps rehabilitation, is always indicated before proceeding with an operative approach.

D.  The features of giving way, locking, and the objective findings described above are consistent with abnormal mechanical function. These features point to an internal derangement. Since an internal derangement is potentially dangerous to the structural integrity of the joint, prompt work-up should be completed. Arthrography, arthrotomography, and arthroscopy may be required to fully define the problem before definitive treatment can be initiated.

## REFERENCE

Smillie IS. *Injuries of the Knee Joint*. 4th ed; Edinburgh: Churchill-Livingston, 1970.

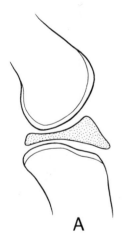 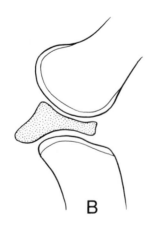 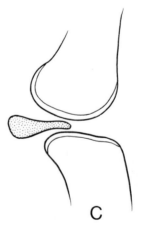 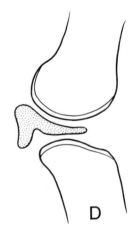

Discoid lateral meniscus, "snapping knee".
A and B. Relation of femoral condyle to meniscal ridge.
C and D. Displacement of meniscus by condyle against meniscal ridge. (After Smilie)

CLICKING OR
LOCKING KNEE

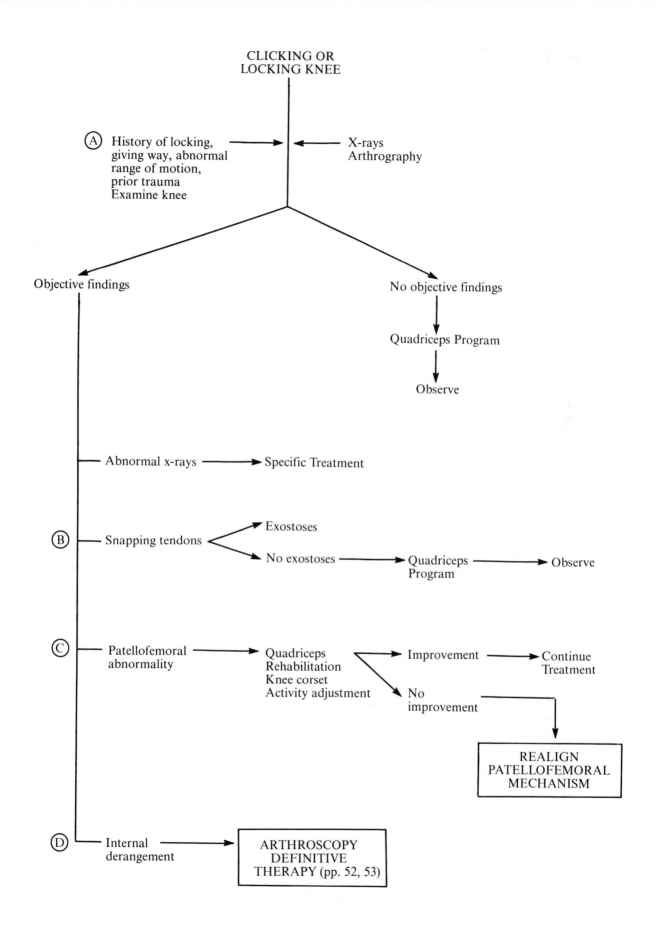

Ⓐ History of locking,
giving way, abnormal
range of motion,
prior trauma
Examine knee

X-rays
Arthrography

Objective findings

No objective findings

Quadriceps Program

Observe

Abnormal x-rays ⟶ Specific Treatment

Ⓑ Snapping tendons

Exostoses

No exostoses ⟶ Quadriceps
Program ⟶ Observe

Ⓒ Patellofemoral
abnormality ⟶ Quadriceps
Rehabilitation
Knee corset
Activity adjustment

Improvement ⟶ Continue
Treatment

No
improvement

REALIGN
PATELLOFEMORAL
MECHANISM

Ⓓ Internal
derangement ⟶ ARTHROSCOPY
DEFINITIVE
THERAPY (pp. 52, 53)

# CHRONIC KNEE EFFUSION

## INTRODUCTION

Chronic knee effusion is a manifestation of many pathologic conditions affecting the knee joint. The emphasis should be on diagnosing the cause for the knee effusion rather than on treating the effusion itself. The presence of an effusion signifies synovial irritation. Fluid in the knee joint causes quadriceps inhibition and reduces the ability of the quadriceps mechanism to adequately protect the knee. The patient with a knee effusion should not walk unprotected. During the work-up period, the knee should be immobilized in a splint. Crutches should be used for any prolonged walking in order to protect both knees.

## COMMENTS

A. A careful history will often reveal the precipitating event, such as a twisting episode, locking, giving way, or instability. Details of previous surgery should be sought for a full understanding of the nature of the internal derangement and the rehabilitation accomplished by the patient. An insufficiently rehabilitated knee will develop a chronic effusion, even though the underlying pathology has been corrected. One should also assess the life style and activity profiles of the patient because the asymptomatic, normally functioning knee is dependent on a balance between the activity demands and the mechanical integrity of the knee. When the balance is upset, an effusion develops. In evaluating the swollen knee, first confirm that the effusion is in the knee and not in the prepatellar bursa. Next, establish whether the effusion is primarily fluid or a combination of proliferative synovitis and synovial effusion. The inflamed knee is warm in contrast to the temperature of the knee with a mechanical derangement. Palpate quadriceps tone and measure the thighs for atrophy; the quadriceps deficient knee will develop a chronic effusion. Carefully assess the patellar mechanism for tracking abnormalities; which will be accentuated by quadriceps atrophy. Ligamentous instability causes knee irritation, which produces an effusion. Since a chronic knee effusion may represent an internal derangement, careful examination for meniscal injuries is important.

B. An AP, lateral, and sunrise view will allow inspection of all three compartments of the knee. Degenerative arthritis, loose bodies, malalignment and osteochondritis dissecans are causes easily identifiable radiographically. An arthrogram will identify the extent of any synovial cysts and the integrity of the menisci. A chronic effusion for which there is no obvious explanation should be aspirated and the aspirate sent for culture, sensitivity, cell count, and crystal examination. A sedimentation rate and disease-specific tests for inflammatory conditions are ordered, depending on the indications. A synovial biopsy should be performed for inflammatory conditions when the diagnosis is in doubt and particularly when the fluid is serosanguinous.

C. A cool, chronic knee effusion usually represents a mechanical derangement. Treat the underlying abnormality first and then have the patient begin supervised quadriceps rehabilitation. A common pitfall is to inadequately rehabilitate the knee after correcting the internal derangement.

D. A warm effusion signifies an inflammatory synovitis. Exquisite pain on range of motion suggests a septic joint. Other inflammatory conditions are less painful than a septic joint, but more painful then an internal derangement. Lesions of the distal femur, such as osteomyelitis, often cause a sympathetic effusion.

## REFERENCE

1. Exam of Joint Fluid, Primer on Rheumatic Diseases: p. 140 7th Edition, 1973.

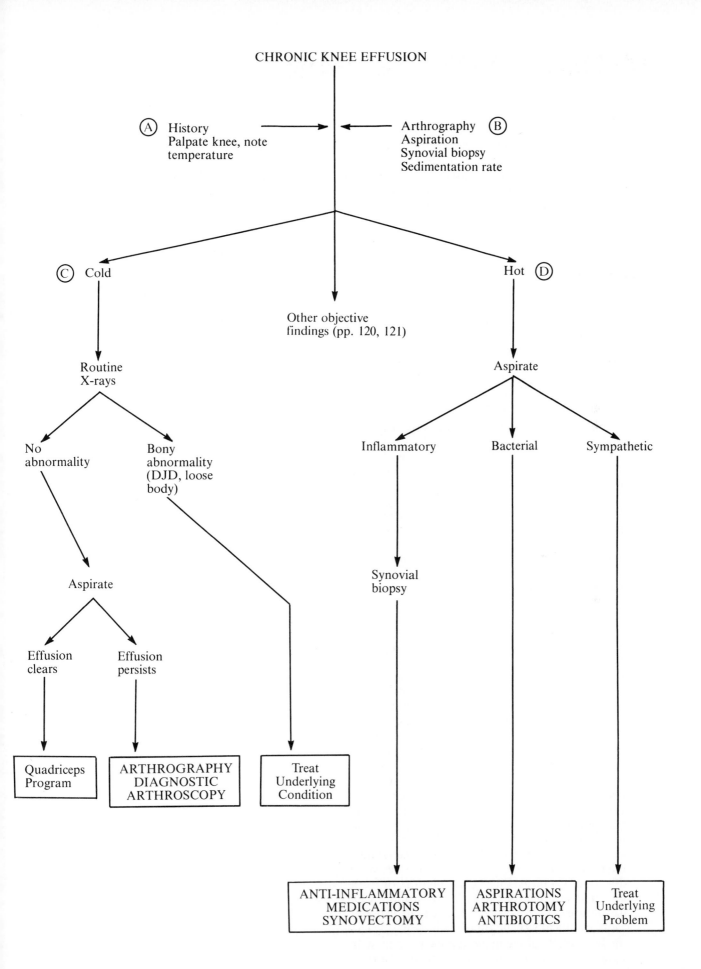

CHRONIC KNEE EFFUSION

(A) History
Palpate knee, note temperature

(B) Arthrography
Aspiration
Synovial biopsy
Sedimentation rate

(C) Cold

Other objective findings (pp. 120, 121)

Hot (D)

Routine X-rays

Aspirate

No abnormality

Bony abnormality (DJD, loose body)

Inflammatory

Bacterial

Sympathetic

Aspirate

Synovial biopsy

Effusion clears

Effusion persists

Quadriceps Program

ARTHROGRAPHY DIAGNOSTIC ARTHROSCOPY

Treat Underlying Condition

ANTI-INFLAMMATORY MEDICATIONS SYNOVECTOMY

ASPIRATIONS ARTHROTOMY ANTIBIOTICS

Treat Underlying Problem

# MEDIAL JOINT LINE PAIN

## INTRODUCTION

Medial joint pain is a common presenting complaint. It may be caused by a variety of afflictions, including patellar tracking problems, meniscus injuries, medial collateral ligament sprains, and degenerative joint disease. Sometimes no cause can be found. Careful examination is necessary to establish the presence of objective findings.

## COMMENTS

A. Obtain a careful history, one that relates the pain to specific activities such as stair climbing, running, pivoting, and squatting; determine whether symptoms are relieved by rest. In middle-aged individuals, the pain usually results from lateral patellar tracking problems, meniscus injury or degenerative joint disease of the medial compartment.

B. The physical examination should concentrate on documenting objective evidence of knee pathology. Quadriceps atrophy, effusion, lack of range of motion, and meniscus entrapment signs are reliable indicators of internal problems within the knee. Early degenerative changes may not be associated with objective findings. Patients with persistent complaints should be observed over a period of time, since underlying pathology will eventually declare itself. Routine AP and lateral x-rays are examined for degenerative disease of the medial compartment; tangential views should be checked for patellofemoral problems, including abnormal lateral tracking.

C. Careful examination will distinguish between retinacular tenderness slightly above the joint line compared with true joint line pain. Retinacular tenderness is consistent with a lateral patellar tracking syndrome, usually a consequence of misalignment of the patellofemoral tracking mechanism. This is discussed in the section entitled Treatment of Patellar Subluxation in the Adult. Diffuse joint line tenderness is more consistent with degenerative joint disease, whereas specific joint line tenderness is caused by either medial collateral ligament strain or meniscus pathology. A valgus force exerted on the knee elicits medial collateral ligament pain and meniscus entrapment maneuvers help in the evaluation of meniscal disease. Medial collateral ligament pain may arise from chronic stretching due to valgus thrust during ambulation, or from repeated injuries. In the latter situation, bone formation over the vastus tubercle may be noted radiographically (Pellegrini-Stieda disease). The medial collateral ligament-deficient knee with valgus thrust during ambulation requires orthotics or, in more severe cases, ligament reconstruction.

## REFERENCES

1. O'Donoghue DH. Reconstruction for medial instability of the knee, J Bone Joint Surg. 1973; 55–A: 941–955.
2. Insall J. Current concepts review: patellar pain. J Bone Joint Surg. 1982; 64–A:147–152.
3. Smillie IS. *Injuries of the knee joint*. 4th ed. New York: Churchill–Livingstone, 1981.

MEDIAL JOINT LINE PAIN

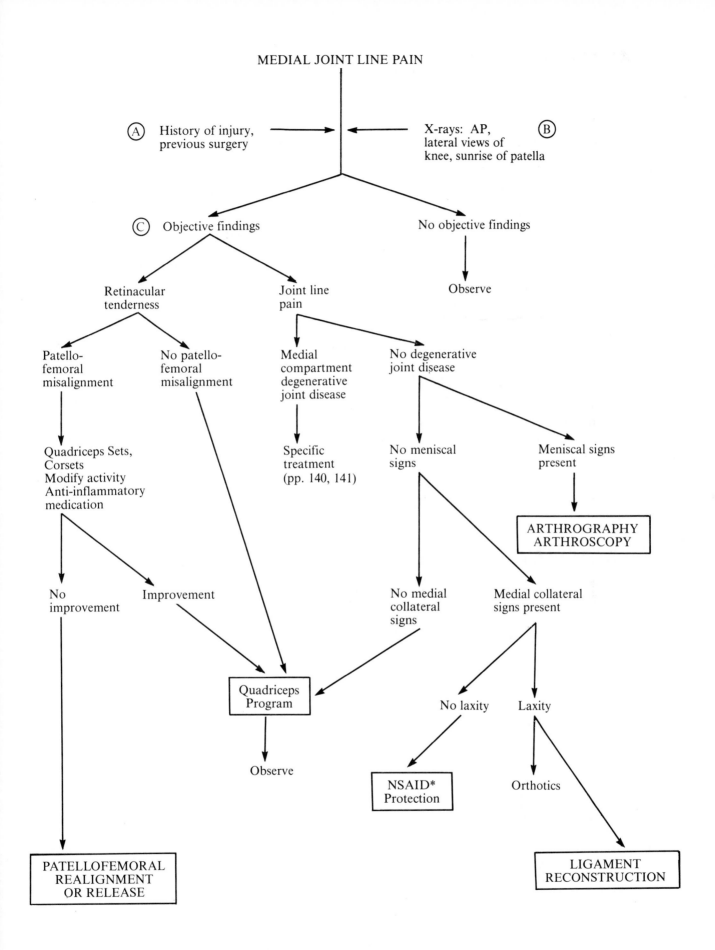

*Nonsteroidal anti-inflammatory drugs

# LATERAL JOINT LINE PAIN

## INTRODUCTION

Lateral joint line pain is less common than medial joint line pain. The most common causes include meniscus disease, degenerative joint disease of the lateral compartment, and irritation of the bursa overlying the lateral femoral epicondyle as the iliotibial band rubs back and forth during range of motion.

## COMMENTS

A.  Relate the symptoms to previous injury or to specific activities, such as stair climbing, which makes the pain worse. Locking is less likely than with medial meniscal tears. A meniscal cyst usually increases with size after activity and decreases during periods of rest.[3]

B.  Palpate the lateral femoral epicondyle during flexion and extension, searching for crepitus and tenderness suggestive of an iliotibial band syndrome. A positive flexion rotation drawer test is indicative of anterolateral rotatory instability and suggests a torn lateral meniscus.

C.  Objective findings consist of quadriceps atrophy, joint effusion, joint line cysts, positive meniscal entrapment tests and a lack of complete extension or flexion of the knee, and anterior/posterior drawer and combined instability tests.[1]

D.  The iliotibial band syndrome is caused by friction between the lateral femoral epicondyle and the iliotibial band as it moves back and forth during range of motion of the knee.[2] The syndrome appears typically after a sudden increase in activity. A long hike or increase in one's jogging routine may provoke the syndrome. Activity modification, including rest, and anti-inflammatory medication are usually sufficient to control the symptoms.

E.  Lateral compartment degenerative joint disease typically follows trauma or a long-standing valgus alignment secondary to previous injury or surgery. Avascular necrosis of the lateral femoral condyle could also produce this problem (pp. 140, 141).

F.  Other usual causes of lateral joint line pain are loose bodies and meniscus injuries. Intermittent catching with symptoms referable to the lateral side of the knee and a visible protrusion of the overlying skin suggest loose body symptoms. An x-ray examination frequently confirms the diagnosis.

G.  Cysts of the lateral meniscus usually follow trauma to the meniscus.[3] No specific injury may be recalled, but a gradual swelling at the lateral joint line, typically disappearing on full flexion and extension, is pathognomonic. If left to enlarge, erosion of the condyle may occur. Lateral meniscectomy is the treatment of choice.

## REFERENCES

1.  Grood ES, Noyes FR, Butler DL, Suntay WJ. Ligamentous and capsular restraints preventing straight, medial and lateral laxity in intact human cadaver knees. J Bone Joint Surg. 1981; 63–A: 1257–1269.
2.  Ruene JW. The iliotibial band function syndrome. J Bone Joint Surg. 1975;57–A: 1110–1111.
3.  Smillie IS. Injuries about the knee joint. New York: Churchill–Livingstone. 1970, p.52.

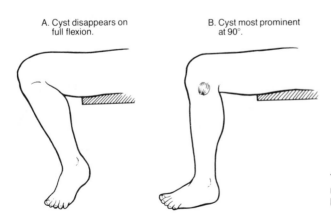

A. Cyst disappears on full flexion.

B. Cyst most prominent at 90°.

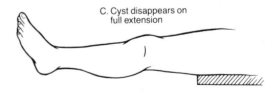

C. Cyst disappears on full extension

The cystic meniscus is less prominent at the extremes of motion due to movement of the meniscus and the iliotibial band.

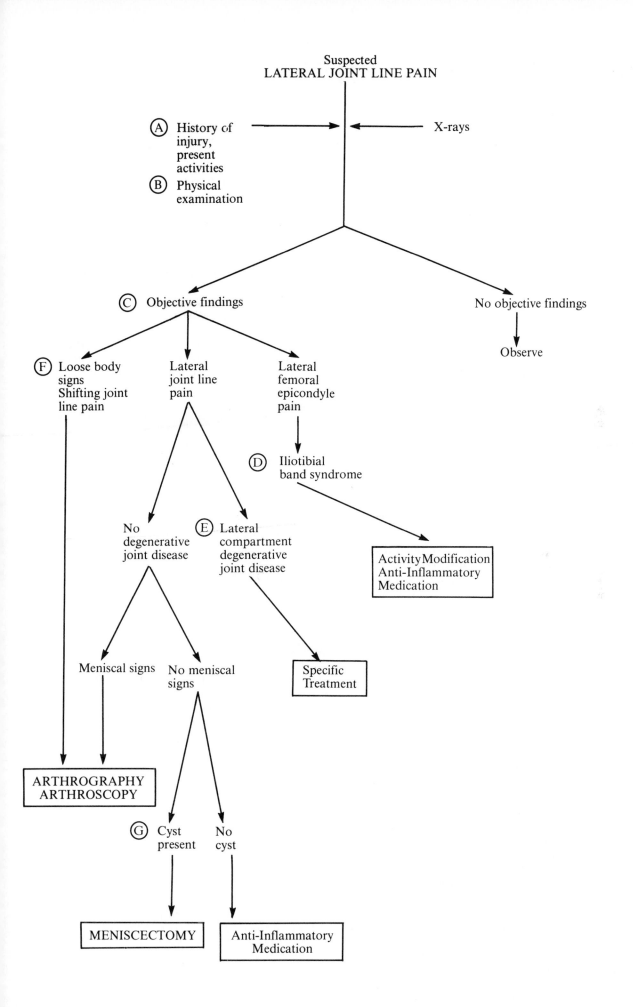

# ANTERIOR KNEE JOINT PAIN

## INTRODUCTION

Anterior knee joint pain is usually caused by abnormalities of patellar tracking, anterior meniscus, and overlying bursae. The patellar tracking system is in delicate balance and is susceptible to changes in activity type and level. An increase in one's jogging routine or a change in job locations, where more stair climbing is required, are good examples. Continuous trauma to the anterior aspect of the knee may produce prepatellar bursitis and other local irritations.

## COMMENTS

A. Attempt to relate the onset of symptoms with a specific injury or activity. Determine whether the knee locks, pops, snaps, grinds, or gives way: determine the relationship of the sensations to the location within the knee.

B. Begin by examining the gait and overall alignment of the lower extremity. An increase in the quadriceps angle suggests a possible tracking disorder. Assess the overall firmness of the quadriceps mechanism. Range the knee and palpate along each joint line for crepitus. Note the location of pain. Meniscal entrapment maneuvers should be used. Have the patient jump up and down on the involved extremity and then walk in a duck waddle position for several steps, rising at least once on the involved side to the fully extended position. If the patient can perform these maneuvers without difficulty, serious internal derangement is unlikely.

C. Anterior joint line tenderness suggests anterior meniscal horn or patellar tendon pathology. Hyperextension of the knee and meniscal entrapment maneuvers help to distinguish these entities from patellar tendinitis. Point tenderness at the inferior pole of the patella is more consistent with patellar tendinitis.

D. "Jumper's knee" is suggested by a history of increased activity with high impact loading. It is diagnosed by the presence of point tenderness, usually at the attachment of the patellar tendon to the patella.

E. Prepatellar bursitis must be distinguished from an overlying cellulitis or a knee effusion. A knee effusion produces general swelling and obliteration of landmarks about the knee; the prepatellar bursa, when swollen, presents as a well-circumscribed area anterior to the patella without distortion of other landmarks. Cellulitis is accompanied by overlying erythema spreading beyond the boundaries of the prepatellar and knee joint capsule. Ballottement of the patella and transillumination provide further help in establishing the diagnosis.

F. Stress fractures of the patella typically present with pain on running and at sport, ceasing with rest. Tangential x-ray films of the patella may show irregularity of the joint surface and partial avulsion of a small fragment. The patella is seldom badly displaced and rarely requires operative treatment.

G. Chrondromalacia usually refers to the clinical syndrome characterized by retropatellar pain with isotonic–type activities such as running, stair climbing and hiking. Initially the patellofemoral joint may be smooth to examination and normal appearing to arthroscopy. Eventually the articular surface becomes frayed and disrupted. The source of the pain is unclear. The common underlying condition is lateral patellar tracking secondary to either a static or dynamic alignment deficiency. Key physical findings include an increase in the quadriceps angle, a positive patellar apprehension sign (the patient demonstrates anxiety by attempting to restrain the physician's hands when he laterally subluxes the patella), patellofemoral compression pain, and patellofemoral crepitus on range of motion. Individuals who have undergone surgery of the knee or have been inactive with loss of quadriceps tone develop a transitory component of this syndrome during return to normal activity. Treatment includes activity modification, reduction of isotonic maneuvers, quadriceps rehabilitation, patellar shaving, and various forms of realignment of the patellar tracking mechanism.

## REFERENCES

1. Devas MB. Stress fractures of the patella. J Bone Joint Surg. 1960; 42–B:71–74.
2. Insall J. Current concepts review: patellar pain. J Bone Joint Surg. 1982;64–A:147–152.

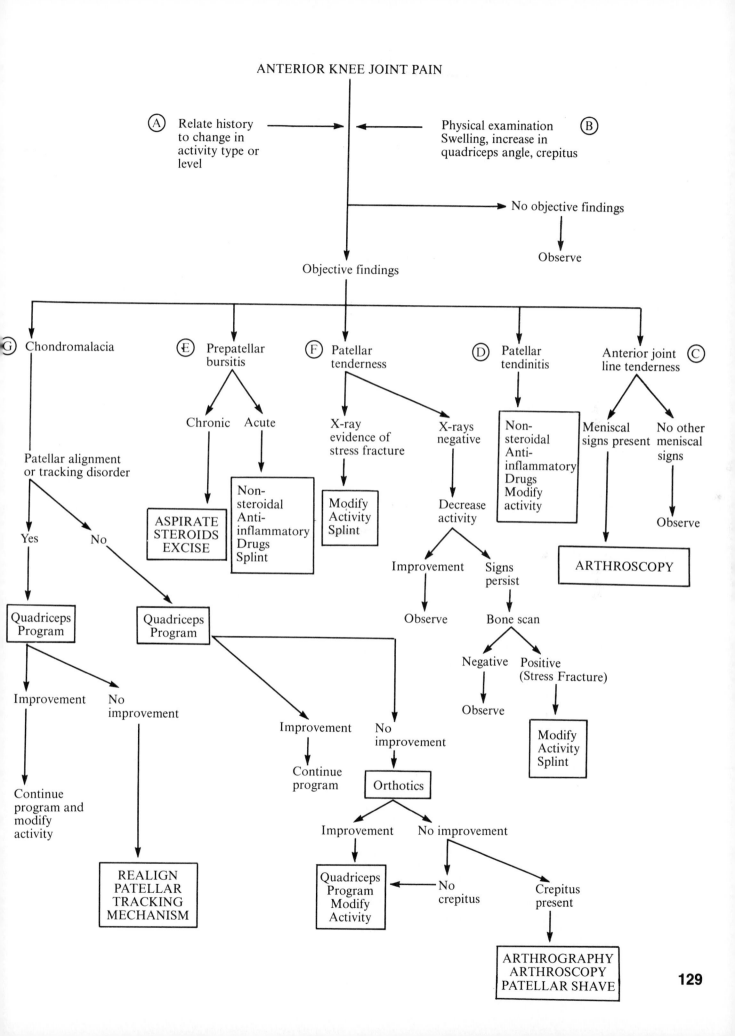

ANTERIOR KNEE JOINT PAIN

Ⓐ Relate history to change in activity type or level

Ⓑ Physical examination Swelling, increase in quadriceps angle, crepitus

No objective findings

Observe

Objective findings

Ⓖ Chondromalacia

Ⓔ Prepatellar bursitis

Ⓕ Patellar tenderness

Ⓓ Patellar tendinitis

Ⓒ Anterior joint line tenderness

Patellar alignment or tracking disorder

Chronic          Acute

X-ray evidence of stress fracture

X-rays negative

Non-steroidal Anti-inflammatory Drugs Modify activity

Meniscal signs present

No other meniscal signs

Yes          No

ASPIRATE STEROIDS EXCISE

Non-steroidal Anti-inflammatory Drugs Splint

Modify Activity Splint

Decrease activity

Observe

Quadriceps Program

Quadriceps Program

Improvement          Signs persist

ARTHROSCOPY

Improvement          No improvement

Observe          Bone scan

Improvement          No improvement

Negative          Positive (Stress Fracture)

Continue program and modify activity

Continue program

Orthotics

Observe

Modify Activity Splint

REALIGN PATELLAR TRACKING MECHANISM

Improvement          No improvement

Quadriceps Program Modify Activity

No crepitus          Crepitus present

ARTHROGRAPHY ARTHROSCOPY PATELLAR SHAVE

**129**

# POSTERIOR KNEE JOINT PAIN

## INTRODUCTION

Posterior knee joint pain is less common than pain in other sites about the knee. It is most often caused by hamstring spasm, a protective reflex indicative of internal derangement or other extra-articular conditions that cause pain.

## COMMENTS

A. Determine whether the pain is recent or long-standing and whether it is associated with swelling, disability, and previous trauma. Palpate the knee for signs of inflammation, such as increased warmth, swelling, and quadriceps atrophy. Palpate the politeal fossa for the presence of a cyst. If a flexion contracture is present, determine whether it is caused by hamstring spasm or soft tissue contracture. A firm end point is more typical of soft tissue contracture. Local tenderness along the posterior joint line is suggestive of meniscus pathology. Perform the meniscus entrapment maneuvers: flexion and extension while rotating the tibia. Pain and clicking at the posterior joint line represent a positive test. With the knee at 90° of flexion, perform a posterior drawer and view the knee from the side. Compare with the opposite knee to determine whether a posterior sag is present; posterior cruciate deficiency allows the tibia to sag posteriorly.

B. X-rays during anterior and posterior drawer stress may demonstrate the amount of posterior subluxation present.

C. Popliteal cysts are classified as congenital or acquired. A congenital cyst does not communicate with the joint and is usually caused by enlargement of the gastrocnemius/semimembranous bursa. An acquired cyst is caused by prolonged knee effusion from either an internal derangement or a chronic inflammatory arthritis. Chronic synovitis may lead eventually to herniation through the posterior capsule and form a popliteal cyst. An arthrogram will demonstrate whether the cyst communicates with the joint and will help to diagnose the presence of an internal derangement. Further definition of the pathology, definitive management, or biopsy of synovial tissues can then be accomplished through arthroscopy. Cyst excision is indicated with severe symptoms or steadily increasing size, except in rheumatoid arthritis, for which anterior synovectomy is the procedure of choice.

D. Posterior tibial sag and a positive posterior drawer are indicative of posterior cruciate deficiency. Typically this follows trauma to the anterior aspect of the tibia, such as falling off a motorcycle. One should question and observe the patient closely to determine whether this represents a functional problem. Vigorous quadriceps rehabilitation and some activity modification may be all that is necessary. If instability is marked or causing functional disability, posterior cruciate reconstruction is indicated.

E. Hamstring spasm is an involuntary protective mechanism for a painful condition in and about the knee. It is a physical finding, not a diagnosis. While a chronic inflammatory condition such as rheumatoid arthritis is the usual cause, meniscus entrapment can also cause spasm. Sometimes no obvious source can be found. A period of observation is appropriate, but if improvement does not occur, arthrography and arthroscopy may be necessary to rule out the presence of intra-articular pathology.

## REFERENCES

1. Binder IM. Treatment of popliteal cyst in the rheumatoid knee. J Bone Joint Surg. 1973; 55–B:119–125.
2. Hughston JC. Degenhardt TC. Reconstruction of the posterior cruciate ligament. Clin Orthop. 1982; 164;59–77.

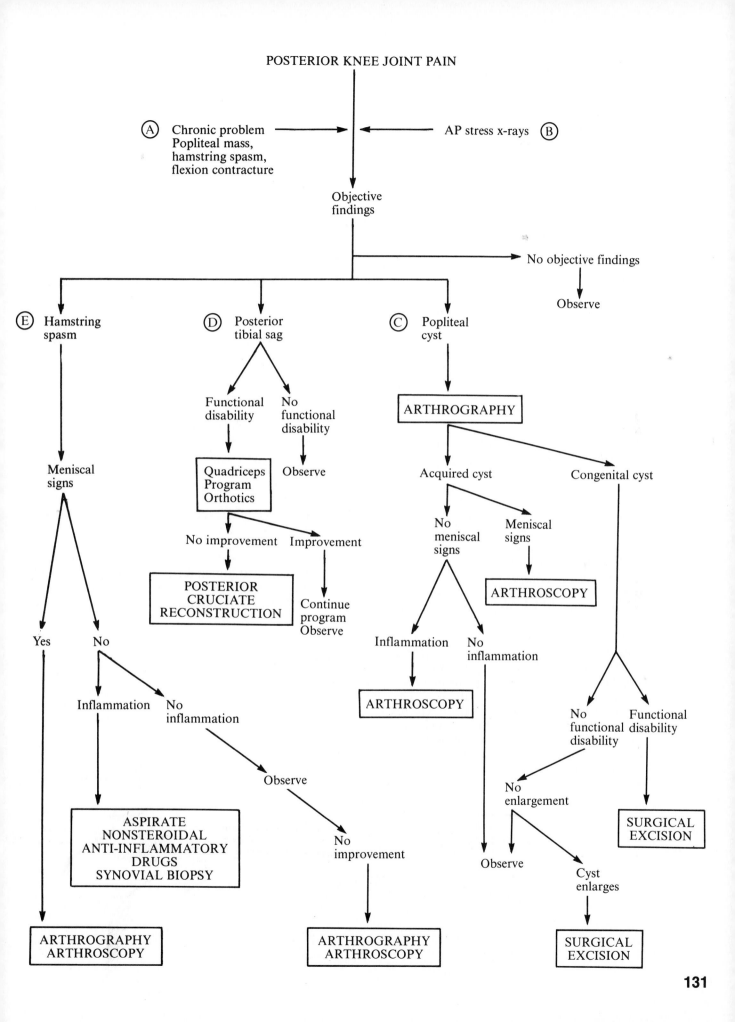

POSTERIOR KNEE JOINT PAIN

Ⓐ Chronic problem
Popliteal mass,
hamstring spasm,
flexion contracture

Ⓑ AP stress x-rays

Objective findings

No objective findings

Observe

Ⓔ Hamstring spasm

Ⓓ Posterior tibial sag

Ⓒ Popliteal cyst

Functional disability

No functional disability

ARTHROGRAPHY

Meniscal signs

Quadriceps Program Orthotics

Observe

Acquired cyst

Congenital cyst

No improvement

Improvement

No meniscal signs

Meniscal signs

POSTERIOR CRUCIATE RECONSTRUCTION

Continue program Observe

ARTHROSCOPY

Yes

No

Inflammation

No inflammation

Inflammation

No inflammation

Observe

ARTHROSCOPY

No functional disability

Functional disability

ASPIRATE NONSTEROIDAL ANTI-INFLAMMATORY DRUGS SYNOVIAL BIOPSY

No improvement

No enlargement

SURGICAL EXCISION

Observe

Cyst enlarges

ARTHROGRAPHY ARTHROSCOPY

ARTHROGRAPHY ARTHROSCOPY

SURGICAL EXCISION

**131**

# THE STIFF KNEE

## INTRODUCTION

A knee may be stiff because of mechanical reasons such as internal derangement or capsular contractures. Stiffness from inflammatory response is caused by muscle spasm, particularly of the hamstrings. Since 70° of flexion is needed for normal ambulation, 90° for stairs, and 95 to 100° for sitting, restoration of motion is important for normal function.

## COMMENTS

A. Previous injury or surgery may have produced either scarring of the quadriceps mechanism or intra-articular adhesions. Determine the amount of functional deficit in the patient's routine activities, and whether the loss is progressive. Chronic inflammatory states cause hamstring spasm and incomplete knee extension. Over a long period of time, posterior subluxation of the tibia takes place.

B. Watch the patient ambulate to determine how the stiffness affects the gait pattern. Palpate the soft tissues for scarring and range the knee to determine the type of motion end point. Hamstring spasm and internal derangement of the meniscus produce a springy end point associated with localized discomfort. Interarticular adhesions and muscle contractures cause a definite and unyielding end point.

C. An extension contracture may be acute or chronic and is usually caused by adhesions within the quadriceps mechanism. An acute contracture typically occurs following immobilization in plaster or splinting following knee surgery. For these contractures physical therapy usually suffices. If range of motion does not improve after 2 to 3 weeks, gentle manipulation under anesthesia is usually sufficient. Delayed contractures result when the quadriceps mechanism has been traumatized resulting in scarring and adhesions. Physical therapy will probably not be effective, making quadricepsplasty necessary. This procedure releases adhesions and in some cases elongates the quadriceps mechanism.

D. Acute flexion contractures typically follow plaster immobilization and arthrotomy where the knee is kept in flexion postoperatively. These usually respond to physical therapy such as quadriceps rehabilitation and active-assisted extension exercises. Chronic flexion contractures are those that have persisted for some time and typically are caused by intra-articular adhesions following severe trauma or chronic inflammatory disease with hamstring spasm, contracture of the posterior capsular structures, and posterior subluxation of the tibia. When correcting such contractures, the tibia must be pulled anteriorly while the knee is being extended; otherwise impaction of the joint surfaces will occur. Physical therapy is sometimes effective, but frequently serial casts and splints are necessary. With any form of casting the knee is brought out gradually into extension while the tibia is pulled anteriorly. This form of treatment is most specific for rheumatoid arthritis. Flexion contracture following old trauma with mature intra-and extra-articular adhesions require surgical release. All adhesions within the knee joint must be released, including both cruciate ligaments if necessary. When these adhesions have been released, attention is turned to extracapsular structures such as the hamstrings. The extent of release necessary for both flexion and extension contractures is usually greater than anticipated. A prolonged physical therapy program and sometimes orthotics will be necessary to maintain the gains achieved by surgery.

## REFERENCES

1. Engleman EP. Conservative treatment of rheumatoid arthritis. In arthritis and allied conditions. Edited by J. Hollander. Philadelphia: Lea & Febiger 1972, 441–447.
2. Nicole EA. Quadricepsplasty. J Bone Joint Surg. 1963;45-B:483–490.
3. Thompson TC. Quadricepsplasty to improve knee function. J Bone Joint Surg. 1944;24: 366–379.

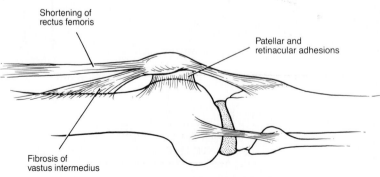

Causes of knee extension contracture.

KNEE JOINT STIFFNESS

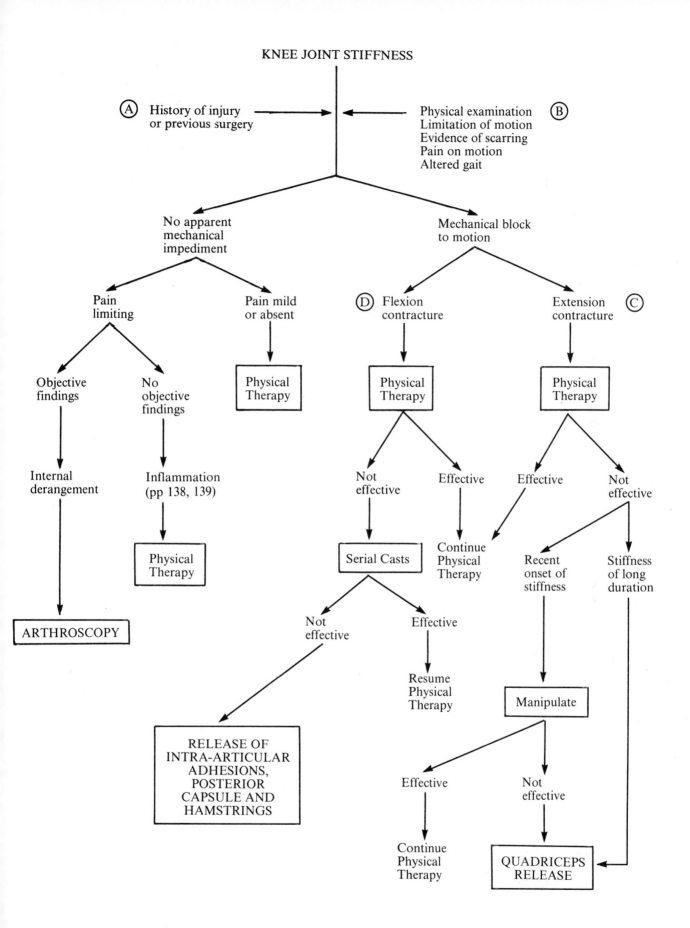

# PATELLAR SUBLUXATION

## INTRODUCTION

Patellar subluxation is caused by lateral tracking of the patella. The resulting patellofemoral incongruence causes abnormal pressures and pain. The knee is unstable and gives way during running and pivoting maneuvers. The condition is usually more common in females than in males. The tracking pathway of the patella is a function of the anatomic configuration of the lateral femoral condyle, the quadriceps angle, and the balance of pull by the quadriceps mechanism. Because the quadriceps angle is usually in some valgus, there is a laterally directed force which must be resisted by the lateral femoral condyle. A hypoplastic lateral femoral condyle or deficient vastus medialis results in lateral tracking of the patella.[1]

## COMMENTS

A.   The patient gives a history of clicking, popping, and giving way of the knee on going up and down stairs and with running and twisting activities. There is often a sensation that the knee is shifting laterally.

B.   On physical examination of the knee during range of motion, one can observe lateral tracking of the patella. This may also be elicited by having the patient flex and extend both knees simultaneously. Note the quadriceps angle.[5] Increased femoral anteversion with compensatory external tibial torsion, increased knee valgus, and lateral positioning of the tibial tubercle increase the quadriceps angle. Manually assess the medial lateral mobility of the patella, which may be reduced by lateral retinacular contractures. Obtain AP, lateral, and tangential x-ray views. Patella alta is present when the patellar length is less than the length of the patellar tendon.[3,4] A deficient lateral-femoral condyle and tilting of the patella laterally, as seen on the tangential view, are characteristic of the lateral tracking problem.

C.   Conservative treatment is always tried first. Quadriceps rehabilitation, the mainstay of conservative treatment, consists of 100 isometric quad sets per day followed by short-arc isotonic exercises. Weight loss is helpful in the obese. Daily activities that place a great demand on the quads may make a susceptible knee symptomatic. Reducing the amount of stair climbing is helpful. Knee orthotics include various corsets which attempt to constrain the patella by means of padding and tethering straps. Although significant control of patellar tracking probably is not possible, knee orthotics do help symptomatically.[2]

D.   Deficient vastus medialis bulk, function, or proximal attachment results in an imbalance in the forces controlling patellar tracking. Previous injury to the quadriceps would produce a similar result.

E.   A proximal realignment alters the direction of the quadriceps forces acting on the patella. It does not change the quadriceps angle. Proximal realignment usually involves an extensive lateral release and advancement of the vastus medialis.[2,6]

F.   Patella alta is a condition in which there is a relatively longer patellar tendon, thereby altering the relationship of the patella to the femoral condyles. In extension there may be no patellofemoral contact. The lack of condylar containment of the patella predisposes to subluxation.[4]

G.   Knee orthotics has been described in the discussion of conservative treatment, paragraph C.

H.   Abnormal knee alignment refers either to axially increased quadriceps angle, caused by such rotational problems as increased femoral anteversion, or to an increased tibiofemoral angle, caused by previous trauma or anatomic development. An increased quadriceps angle may be associated with lateral retinacular contractures, which restrain the patella laterally during tracking.[5,6]

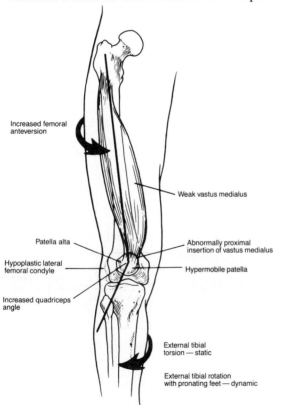

Increased femoral anteversion

Weak vastus medialus

Patella alta

Hypoplastic lateral femoral condyle

Increased quadriceps angle

Abnormally proximal insertion of vastus medialus

Hypermobile patella

External tibial torsion — static

External tibial rotation with pronating feet — dynamic

**134**    Factors contributing to patellar subluxation.

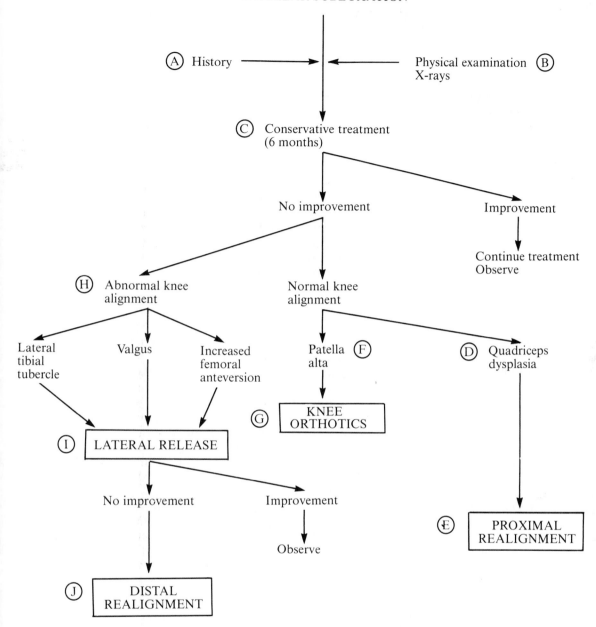

PATELLAR SUBLUXATION

(A) History → ← Physical examination (B)
X-rays

(C) Conservative treatment
(6 months)

No improvement → Improvement

Continue treatment
Observe

(H) Abnormal knee          Normal knee
alignment                alignment

Lateral        Valgus    Increased      Patella (F)        (D) Quadriceps
tibial                   femoral        alta                   dysplasia
tubercle                 anteversion

(G) KNEE
ORTHOTICS

(I) LATERAL RELEASE

No improvement    Improvement

Observe

(E) PROXIMAL
REALIGNMENT

(J) DISTAL
REALIGNMENT

## REFERENCES

I.  The objective of a lateral release is to eliminate the tethering influence of the lateral retinaculum on patellar tracking. This can be done under arthroscopic control through a small incision made just above the patella on the lateral aspect. The release should go through the full thickness of the retinaculum from several centimeters above the patella down to the joint line.[6]

J.  The purpose of a distal realignment is to diminish the quadriceps angle. This is accomplished by transplanting the tibial tubercle medially. There are many ways of accomplishing this transfer, but the technique selected should avoid posterior positioning of the tubercle. The effect of such a location is to increase patellofemoral force.[2,7]

1.  Fox TA. Dysplasia of the quadriceps mechanism, hypoplasia of the vastus medialis muscle as related to the hypermobile patellar syndrome. S Clin N Amer. 1975; 55:199–266.
2.  Insall J. Current concepts review of patellar pain. J Bone Joint Surg. 1982; 64–A:147–152.
3.  Insall J, Salvati E. Patellar position in the normal knee joint. Radiology. 1971; 101:101–104.
4.  Lancourt JE, Cristini JA. Patella alta and patella baja. J. Bone Joint Surg. 1975; 57–A;1112–1115.
5.  Laurin CA, et al. The abnormal lateral patellofemoral angel. J Bone Joint Surg. 1978; 60–A:55–60.
6.  Merchant AC, Mercer RL. Lateral subluxation of the patella. Clin Orthop Rel Res. 1974; 40–45:103.
7.  Merchant AC, isolated Patellofemoral arthritis—significance and treatment. Contemp Orthop. 1981; 11:1015.

**135**

# LIGAMENTOUS INSTABILITY OF THE KNEE

## INTRODUCTION

Disruption or stretching of the collateral and cruciate ligaments results in laxity of primary knee restraints and loading of secondary restraints including contours of the joint surfaces, menisci, and joint capsule. Secondary restraint failure is associated with meniscal tears, loose bodies, and degenerative joint disease. Laxity causing functional deficits tends to be multidirectional. Isolated anterior instability is rare.

## COMMENTS

A. Establishing the injury mechanism will help explain the observed instability. Determine whether the presenting complaint is actually causing a functional deficit, as evidenced by episodes of giving way followed by swelling, and whether symptoms are progressive. Establish whether symptoms are present only with heavy activity, such as contact sports, or whether they occur on level ground. Instability may be important to the professional athlete, but not to the sedentary desk worker.[4]

B. Examination of ligamentous laxity in the knee can be complicated. Ligament tension is highly variable. Apprehensive patients do not relax; they stabilize their knee with voluntary muscle contractions. Pain may prevent the patient from completely relaxing. Examination under anesthesia is often necessary before deciding on surgery. The knee should be examined while fully extended, while in 30° of flexion, and while in 90° of flexion. Results should be compared with the opposite knee. Pure anterior-posterior and medial-lateral stress testing and rotatory maneuvers are used to elicit combined instabilities. The jerk test, pivot shift, and flexion rotation drawer are highly specific for combined instabilities. The examination should be repeated to confirm the presence of instability.

C. Conservative treatment for a ligamentous instability with a functional deficit requires development of strong hamstrings and quadriceps. The patient should avoid running and cutting maneuvers during rehabilitation. Urge that the patient's activities be accomplished with his center of gravity over the center of support so the knee will be less apt to buckle and give way. A variety of orthotics is available to control anterior rotatory instability (e.g., Lenox Hill Derotation Brace, Poliaxial Knee Cage). Control of posterior instability by bracing is less effective.[1,2,4]

D. Anterolateral rotatory instability is demonstrated by the flexion rotation drawer test. If giving way occurs frequently during routine activites, laxity will increase leading to meniscus damage. Surgical management includes both intra- and extra-articular reconstruction.[4]

E. Anteromedial instability is demonstrated by a positive drawer with the foot externally rotated and the knee at 90° of flexion. Pes plasty increases the internal rotating forces generated during activity and provides a dynamic sling. Both intra-articular cruciate reconstruction and pes plasty may be indicated.[3]

F. The clinical significance of posterior instability is controversial. The presence of posterolateral and posteromedial instability is less common and more difficult to elicit. Positive posterior drawer and posterior Lachman's maneuver, associated with visible posterior sag of the tibia, are the hallmarks of posterior laxity. When posterior laxity affects function, the ligament may be reconstructed by various means, but long-term results remain to be demonstrated.

Anterior Drawer — Lachmann

Pivot shift
Flexion-Rotation Drawer

AM  AL

PM  PL

Fibula

Posterior Drawer

Summary of axis and rotational laxities.

## REFERENCES

1. Giove TP, Sayer JM, Kent BE, Sanford TL, Garrick JG. Non-operative treatment of the torn anterior cruciate ligament. J Bone Joint Surg. 1983; 65–A:184.
2. Nicholas JA. Bracing the anterior cruciate ligamentous deficient knee using the Lenox Hill derotation brace. Clin Orthop. 1983; 172:173.
3. Noyes FR, Sonstegard PA. Biomechanical function of

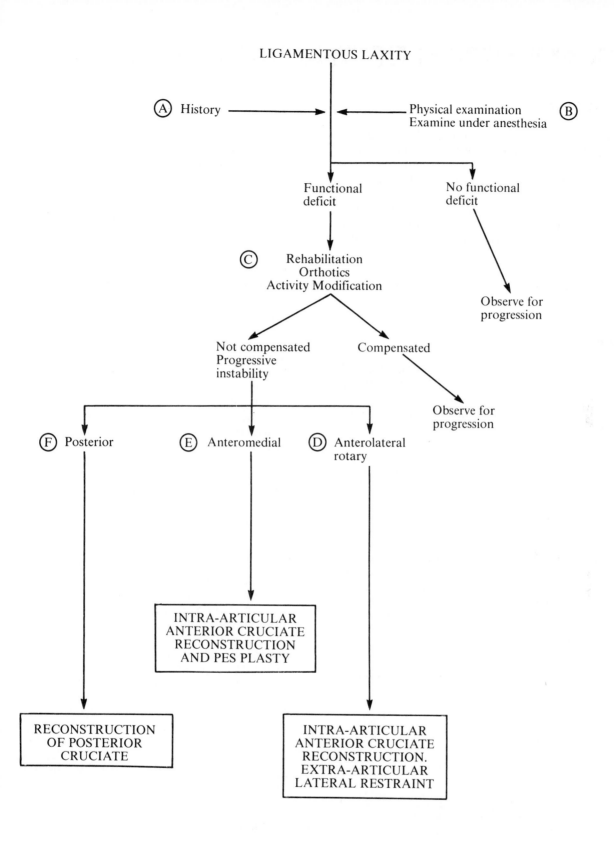

LIGAMENTOUS LAXITY

(A) History — → ← — Physical examination
Examine under anesthesia (B)

Functional deficit        No functional deficit

(C) Rehabilitation
Orthotics
Activity Modification

Not compensated
Progressive instability        Compensated

Observe for progression        Observe for progression

(F) Posterior        (E) Anteromedial        (D) Anterolateral rotary

INTRA-ARTICULAR
ANTERIOR CRUCIATE
RECONSTRUCTION
AND PES PLASTY

RECONSTRUCTION
OF POSTERIOR
CRUCIATE

INTRA-ARTICULAR
ANTERIOR CRUCIATE
RECONSTRUCTION.
EXTRA-ARTICULAR
LATERAL RESTRAINT

the pes anserinus at the knee and the effect of a transplantation. J Bone Joint Surg. 1973; 55-A:1225.
4. Noyes SL, Mooar PA, Matthews DS, Butler BL. The symptomatic anterior cruciate deficient knee–Part I, the long term functional disability in athletically active individuals. Part II, results of rehabilitation, activity modification and counseling on functional disability. J Bone Joint Surg. 1983; 65–A:155–175.

# INFLAMMATION OF THE KNEE JOINT

## INTRODUCTION

The diagnosis of inflammatory joint disease of the knee is established by clinical criteria and joint fluid analysis. The differential diagnosis of inflammatory joint disease includes hemorrhagic arthritis (e.g., pigmented villonodular synovitis), septic arthritis including bacterial infections, and noninflammatory arthritis, such as trauma and degenerative joint disease. Inflammatory arthritis of the knee can be divided into three main categories for treatment purposes:[1] Rheumatoid arthritis,[2] acute crystal-induced synovitis (gout and pseudo-gout), and[3] all other inflammatory arthritides.

## COMMENTS

A. The objectives in the treatment of rheumatoid arthritis are to control the synovitis and, at the same time, to minimize any effects of the synovitis on joint structures. The best approach to acute crystalline-induced synovitis consists of diminishing the inflammatory response of the joint to the crystals and, in the case of gout, lowering the blood uric-acid level on a long-term basis. The remainder of the inflammatory arthritides that produce arthritis of the knee are treated symptomatically, usually with anti-inflammatory drugs. The main treatment is that of the underlying disease process. When the inflammatory arthritides lead to destruction of the knee joint, either knee fusion or total joint replacement is performed. Physical examination of the inflamed knee should concentrate on the effects of the inflammatory process in terms of alignment, muscle function, range of motion, joint contracture, and ligament laxity. Knee flexion contractures are usually associated with some degree of posterior tibial subluxation.

With gout, the presence of tophi should be established, as involvement of ligaments and the quadriceps mechanism may lead to eventual failure of those structures. Medical management of inflammatory knee joint disease in general involves the use of anti-inflammatory medication, analgesics, protection of the joint through rest and splinting, quadriceps maintenance for control of the joint, and prevention of knee flexion contracture.

B. When medical therapy for rheumatoid arthritis has not been effective for at least 3 to 6 months, a synovectomy will help decrease pain and protect the joint. Once destruction has occurred, the main role of synovectomy is pain relief. The natural history of the disease is such that it may last a brief period of time, be subject to intermittent attacks, or eventually burn out, leaving a residual degenerative joint disease. When synovitis persists and results in progressive joint destruction and loss of stability, synovectomy and total knee replacement is the procedure of choice. To obtain a more durable limb, young working patients should probably undergo a knee fusion rather than total knee replacement.

C. Acute crystal-induced synovitis refers either to gout or pseudo-gout. Pseudo-gout can be managed by nonsteroidal anti-inflammatory drugs. Gout is divided into acute and intercritical phases. The management of acute gout consists of either colchicine, which helps to establish the diagnosis as well as control the initial symptoms, or a nonsteriodal anti-inflammatory medication. Once the acute phase has been managed, the patient enters the intercritical phase of treatment, which involves control of hyperuricemia by proper medication and diet. Frequently this regimen will contain the disease. If progression occurs, with gradual destruction of the joint from acute flare-ups, total knee replacement will be required. If tophi involve the tendons and ligaments, these deposits should be excised in order to prevent rupture of the quadriceps tendon and other ligaments about the knee.

## REFERENCES

1. Primer on the rheumatic diseases. Prepared by the Committee on the American Rheumatism Association Section of the Arthritis Foundation. 7th Ed. The Arthritis Foundation, New York, NY.

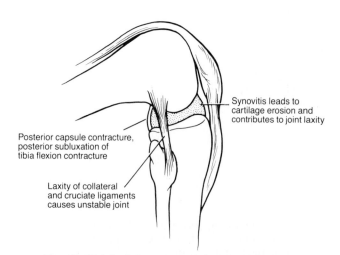

Synovitis leads to cartilage erosion and contributes to joint laxity

Posterior capsule contracture, posterior subluxation of tibia flexion contracture

Laxity of collateral and cruciate ligaments causes unstable joint

The effect of the inflammatory process on key structures within the knee.

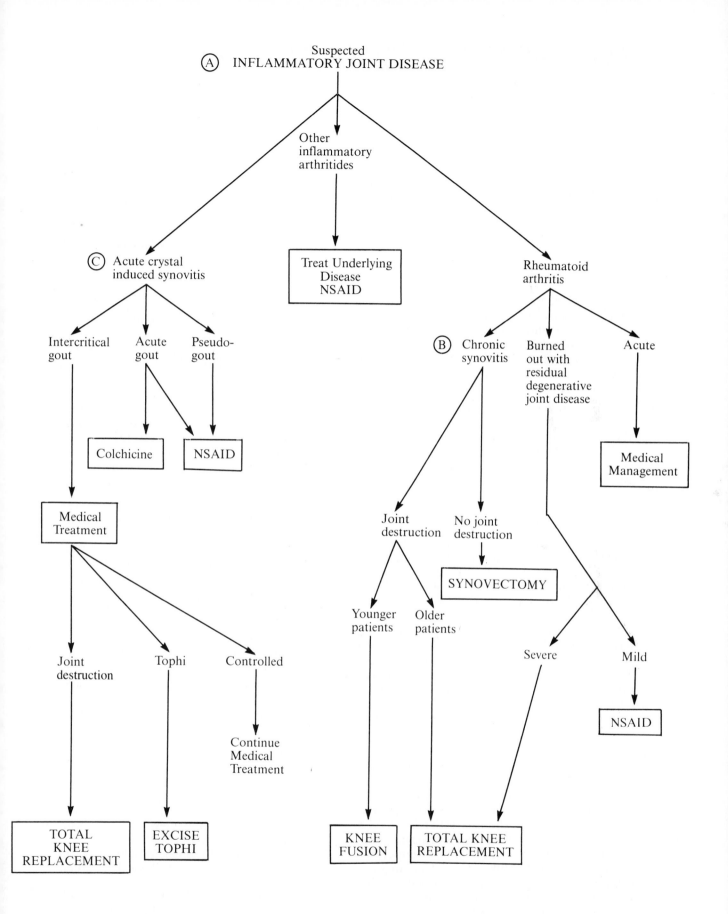

# DEGENERATIVE JOINT DISEASE OF THE KNEE

## INTRODUCTION

Degenerative joint disease of the knee (osteoarthritis) results in bony structural changes and loss of articular cartilage, which produce mechanical symptoms of impingement or restricted range of motion and gradually progressive deformity.

## COMMENTS

A. Whereas osteoarthritic pain tends to be aching in quality, aggravated by activity and relieved by rest, a neuropathic joint (Charcot) may not be particularly symptomatic in the face of severe instability and destruction. The presence of infection should be sought in the event that total knee replacement is a treatment alternative.

B. Check the overall alignment in order to determine the relationship of the mechanical axis to the knee joint. The mechanical axis passes from the center of the femoral head through the middle of the knee to the center of the talus. Observe the gait for varus or valgus thrust indicative of medial or lateral compartment joint surface loss. Osteoarthritic joints do not usually have an effusion, unlike inflammatory joints.

C. Conservative treatment for degenerative joint disease includes nonsteroidal anti-inflammatory drugs, weight reduction, rest, and isometric exercises. Shoe wedges may be effective if the mechanical axis is not far from the center of the knee joint. For instance, a progressive varus deformity could be treated by a lateral shoe wedge, which thrusts the knee dynamically into valgus and shifts the mechanical axis more laterally. Orthotics are more helpful for valgus than for varus knees. A job change may be indicated, particularly if the patient is a heavy construction worker. Conservative treatment usually is effective early and may retard the progression of the disease.

D. Medial compartment degenerative joint disease frequently follows a previous medial meniscectomy or excessive tibia vara. A high valgus tibial osteotomy shifts the mechanical axis into the lateral compartment and is effective in 85% of cases.[5] It has the advantage of not being an intra-articular procedure, which might jeopardize a future total joint replacement. Unicompartmental knee replacement is an alternative with variable results.[4] The main problem occurs at revision to a total knee, when removal of the components can cause loss of bone stock. This makes the total knee technically more difficult.

E. Lateral compartment degenerative joint disease typically results from lateral tibial or femoral condyle fractures, avascular necrosis of the lateral femoral condyle, or an excessive amount of knee valgus. The treatment is a choice between a femoral distal osteotomy and a hemiarthroplasty. The end result must decrease the tibiofemoral angle toward neutral.[3]

F. Severe patellofemoral degenerative joint disease commonly follows a comminuted patellar fracture, but may occur without obvious cause. In young individuals the treatment of choice is patellectomy. Older individuals may be temporarily relieved by patellofemoral resurfacing, but if other compartments are also involved, a total joint replacement is more predictable. Elevating the tibial tubercle decreases the patellofemoral force and may decrease the symptoms to a tolerable degree. When patellectomy is necessary, the tubercle elevation provides a better mechanical advantage for the quadriceps mechanism.[2]

G. Bi- or tri-compartment disease is best managed by total joint replacement.

H. Previous infection always carries with it the risk of reactivation with any subsequent procedure. Therefore, total knee arthroplasty is not usually performed with a history of sepsis. In young individuals, a knee fusion is the treatment of choice. When the responsible organism is Staphylococcus epidermidis a staged arthroplasty using antibiotic impregnated cement may be attempted. The long-term durability of this approach has yet to be determined.[1]

I. A neuropathic (Charcot) joint will not fuse and will destroy a total knee replacement because the patient has no proprioceptive feedback and cannot protect his own knee. Bracing for instability is the best approach.

## REFERENCES

1. Gristina AG, Kolkin J. Current concepts review. Total joint replacement and sepsis. J Bone Joint Surg. 1983; 65-A:128.
2. Insall J. Current concepts review. Patellar pain. J Bone Joint Surg. 1982; 64-A:147–152.
3. Rozing PM, Insall J, Bohne WH. Spontaneous osteonecrosis of the knee. J Bone Joint Surg. 1980; 62–A:2–7.
4. Shurley TH, O'Donoghue OH, Smith WD, Paine PE, Granna WA. Unicompartmental arthroplasty of the knee. Clin Orthop. 1982; 164:236–240.
5. Torgerson WR, Kettelkamp DB, Igou RA, Leach RE. Tibial osteotomy for the treatment of degenerative arthritis of the knee. Clin Orthop. 1974; 101:46.

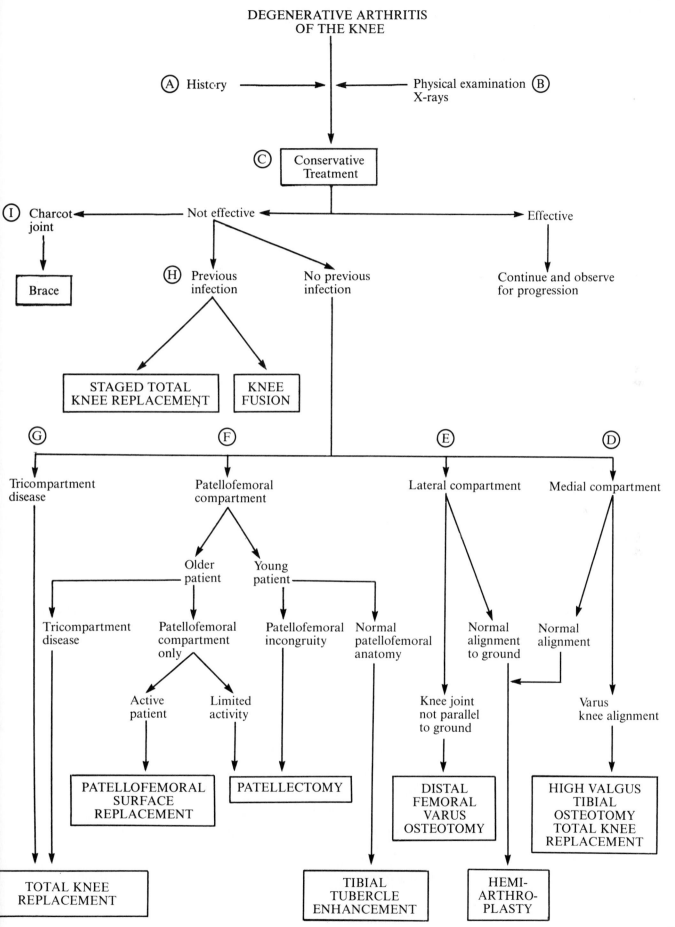

DEGENERATIVE ARTHRITIS
OF THE KNEE

Ⓐ History          Physical examination Ⓑ
                   X-rays

Ⓒ Conservative
   Treatment

Ⓘ Charcot joint ← Not effective ←          Effective

Brace

Ⓗ Previous          No previous          Continue and observe
   infection           infection          for progression

STAGED TOTAL          KNEE
KNEE REPLACEMENT      FUSION

Ⓖ                Ⓕ                Ⓔ                Ⓓ

Tricompartment       Patellofemoral       Lateral compartment    Medial compartment
disease              compartment

                     Older          Young
                     patient        patient

Tricompartment       Patellofemoral    Patellofemoral    Normal            Normal           Normal
disease              compartment       incongruity       patellofemoral    alignment        alignment
                     only                                anatomy           to ground

Active          Limited                              Knee joint                        Varus
patient         activity                             not parallel                      knee alignment
                                                     to ground

PATELLOFEMORAL       PATELLECTOMY                    DISTAL            HIGH VALGUS
SURFACE                                              FEMORAL           TIBIAL
REPLACEMENT                                          VARUS             OSTEOTOMY
                                                     OSTEOTOMY         TOTAL KNEE
                                                                       REPLACEMENT

TOTAL KNEE                          TIBIAL            HEMI-
REPLACEMENT                         TUBERCLE          ARTHRO-
                                    ENHANCEMENT       PLASTY

141

# TREATMENT OF MENISCAL DERANGEMENT

## INTRODUCTION

Meniscal derangements interfere with normal motion of the knee and cause articular erosions that lead to degenerative joint disease. On the other hand, complete removal of the meniscus produces long term degenerative changes. Management of meniscus pathology requires careful identification of the lesion and judgment regarding effects of the lesion on the knee joint and the patient's goals and activities. The trend is toward more conservatism.[1,3,4] If knee function is not seriously affected, particularly in older individuals, at least part of the meniscus is retained. The weight bearing function of the menisci dictate that these structures should be preserved whenever possible.[7] Thus, peripheral tears are encouraged to heal with simple suturing.[5,6] In bucket handle tears only the bucket handle portion is excised.[1] Other tears are simply trimmed and balanced to eliminate mechanical interference yet preserve some weight-bearing function of the residual meniscus. Management of meniscal derangements has changed with the development of diagnostic and operative arthroscopy. The lack of tissue plane dissection significantly decreases postoperative morbidity. An athlete whose meniscus derangement is managed arthroscopically may return to his sport as soon as 13 days postoperatively.

## COMMENTS

A. The history establishes the injury mechanism, site of the meniscus injury and functional disability produced by the lesion. Physical examination elicits objective findings indicative of an internal derangement and further helps to establish the location of the meniscus injury. Look for the presence of effusion, quadriceps atrophy, restriction of range of motion, point/joint line tenderness which does not change with range of motion and positive meniscal entrapment tests.

B. Arthrography is most helpful in identifying meniscal lesions in the posteromedial corner and least helpful for lateral lesions where other structures make interpretation difficult. Arthroscopy is easily performed in the lateral compartment but is very difficult to perform in the posterior compartment without additional equipment and entry portals. Arthroscopy and arthrography together increase the diagnostic capability of finding the lesion. Clinical experience and judgment are required to determine how to deal with the lesion. In some instances this may require conservatism, given the individual patient, and in others only limited excision. Where possible as much of the meniscus is retained as is consistent with normal function of the knee.

C. Marginal tears in the lateral compartment have the best chance of healing. As seen through the arthroscope, these tears can be divided into red–red, red–white, and white–white, depending on whether the tissue on either side of the tear is connective tissue which heals or meniscal tissue which does not heal.[5] Thus, a red–red marginal tear is one primarily through connective tissue and has a high likelihood of healing while the white–white tear is through meniscus tissue and will not heal.

D. Bucket handle tears produce a mechanical derangement caused by intercondylar displacement of the handle portion of the lesion. Simple excision of the handle is the treatment of choice and can usually be done arthroscopically.[1,4]

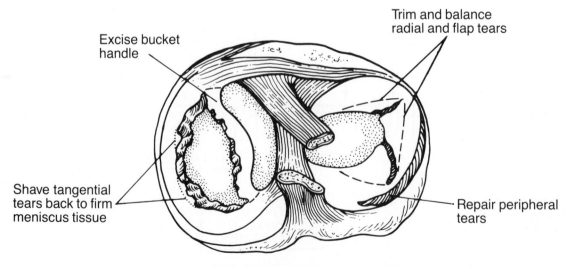

Arthroscopic management of meniscus lesions.

Excise bucket handle

Trim and balance radial and flap tears

Shave tangential tears back to firm meniscus tissue

Repair peripheral tears

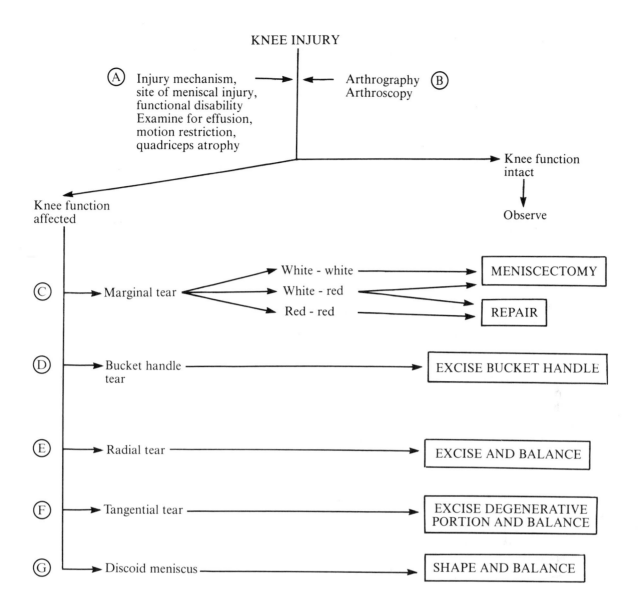

KNEE INJURY

(A) Injury mechanism, site of meniscal injury, functional disability Examine for effusion, motion restriction, quadriceps atrophy

Arthrography Arthroscopy (B)

Knee function intact → Observe

Knee function affected

(C) → Marginal tear → White - white → MENISCECTOMY
White - red
Red - red → REPAIR

(D) → Bucket handle tear → EXCISE BUCKET HANDLE

(E) → Radial tear → EXCISE AND BALANCE

(F) → Tangential tear → EXCISE DEGENERATIVE PORTION AND BALANCE

(G) → Discoid meniscus → SHAPE AND BALANCE

E. Radial tears which do not extend completely through to the periphery may be trimmed and balanced, removing only those portions of the meniscus adjacent to the tear and leaving a gently contoured area of excision.

F. Tangential tears, usually the result of degenerative changes within the meniscus, do not necessarily require treatment unless they are producing functional disability. Considerable tangential pathology may be present in patients who have no functional disturbance. Rotary shaving instruments can sculpt these menisci so that the medial margins are contoured back to healthier tissue.

G. Congenital discoid menisci cause a characteristic loud snapping accompanied by an audible click when the knee is flexed or extended. A palpable tender mass felt along the joint line is exaggerated as the knee is brought from a flexed position to extension. The lesions may be a complete disc or discoid in shape. Operative arthroscopy allows limited excision and contouring of the meniscus so that in some cases a remnant can be retained.

## REFERENCES

1. Carghill A, Jackson TP. Bucket handle tears of the medial meniscus. J Bone Joint Surg. 1976; 58–A:248–251.
2. Gillies H, Siligson D. Precision in the diagnosis of meniscal lesions. a comparison of clinical evaluation arthrography and arthroscopy. J Bone Joint Surg. 1979; 61–A:343–346.
3. Jackson RW, Rouse DW. Results of partial arthroscopic meniscectomy in patients over forty. Scientific Exhibit, 49th Annual Meeting Acad Orthopaedic Surg. New Orleans, 1982.
4. McGinty JB, Guen LF, Marvin RA. Partial or total meniscectomy: a comparative analysis. J Bone Joint Surg. 1977; 59–A:763–766.
5. Mulhollan JS. Peripheral detachment of meniscus. In *Advanced Techniques in operative arthroscopy.* Williamsburg, Virginia; 1982.
6. Price CT, Allen WC. Ligament reapir in the knee with preservation of the meniscus. J Bone Joint Surg. 1978; 60–A:61–67.
7. Walker P, Echman M. The role of the menisci in force transmission across the knee. Clin Ortho. 1975; 109:184–192.

# OSTEOCHONDRITIS DISSECANS OF THE KNEE

## INTRODUCTION

Osteochondritis dissecans refers to the process by which an area of subchondral bone in the knee becomes avascular, later undergoes degenerative changes of the overlying cartilage, and eventually separates to become a loose body within the knee. Trauma is believed to be the precipitating event. Treatment has become more conservative and depends on the stage of the disease.

## COMMENTS

A. Symptoms are usually less severe than those caused by tears of the menisci. A dull aching pain within the center of the joint is typical. If separation of the fragment has occured, loose body symptoms with intermittent locking can be elicited. When questioned, the patient may report that he can palpate the loose body himself.

B. Physical examination consists of palpation of medial femoral condylar area with the knee flexed in an attempt to feel the defect. This is often possible once the avascular fragment has become separated. X-ray examination should include AP, lateral, and notch view. The most common location is the articular margin of the medial condyle. One or more loose bodies may be seen within the joint. The status of the fragment may sometimes be determined with an arthrogram. Dye that is seen to surround the fragment would suggest imminent separation.

During arthroscopy, the area can be viewed directly and probed for further definition of the status of the lesion.

C. Treatment of osteochondritis dissecans in adults has become nonsurgical except when symptoms are definite. Compared to children, the prognosis in adults with this condition is poor. Three-fourths of Linden's patients with adult onset had osteoarthritis of all three compartments of the knee joint. The two main decisions that must be made are whether or not the fragment is detached and whether or not it is located on a major weight-bearing surface. Undetached fragments on weight-bearing surfaces should be drilled in an effort to prevent future detachment. Lesions not on a weight-bearing surface can be simply removed. If detachment of a large piece has already taken place from a weight-bearing surface, reattachment is indicated. When not on a weight-bearing surface, simple removal of a loose body is all that is required.

## REFERENCES

1. Green JP. Osteochondritis dissecans of the knee. J Bone Joint Surg. 1966; 48-B:82–91.
2. Linden B. Osteochondritis dissecans of the medial femoral condyle. J Bone Joint Surg. 1977; 59-A:769.
3. Smillie IS. Diseases of the Knee Joint. New York Churchill Livingstone, 1974. 369 .

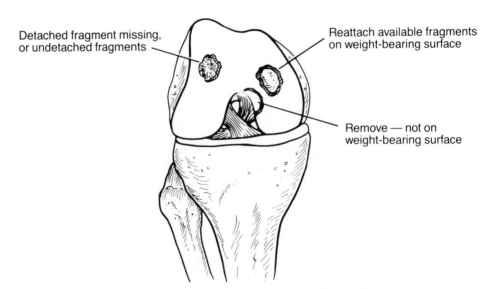

Detached fragment missing, or undetached fragments

Reattach available fragments on weight-bearing surface

Remove — not on weight-bearing surface

Disposition of osteochondritis dissecans fragments within the knee.

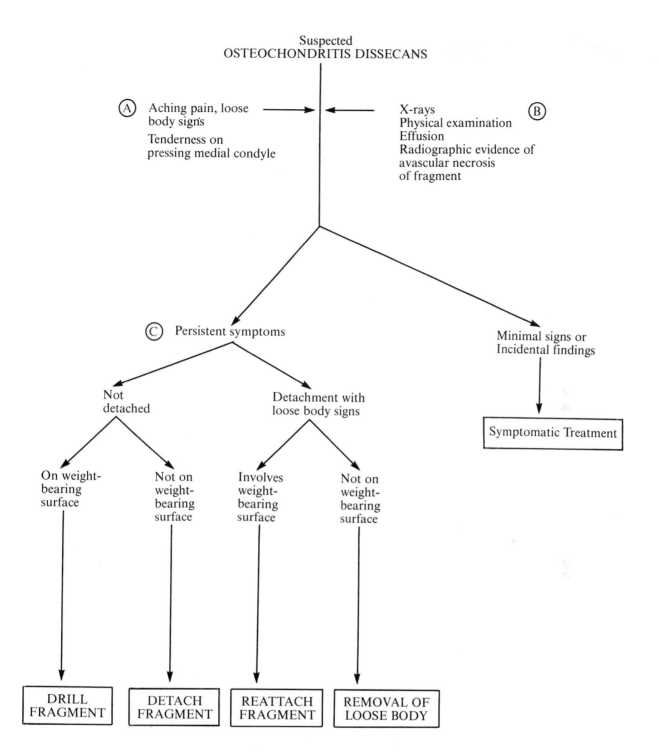

Suspected
OSTEOCHONDRITIS DISSECANS

(A) Aching pain, loose
body signs

Tenderness on
pressing medial condyle

(B) X-rays
Physical examination
Effusion
Radiographic evidence of
avascular necrosis
of fragment

(C) Persistent symptoms

Minimal signs or
Incidental findings

Not
detached

Detachment with
loose body signs

Symptomatic Treatment

On weight-
bearing
surface

Not on
weight-
bearing
surface

Involves
weight-
bearing
surface

Not on
weight-
bearing
surface

DRILL
FRAGMENT

DETACH
FRAGMENT

REATTACH
FRAGMENT

REMOVAL OF
LOOSE BODY

# CHRONIC ANKLE SWELLING

## INTRODUCTION

Chronic swelling of the ankle may or may not be painful and frequently is a phenomenon for which the patient has no immediate answer. The main differential is between a specific arthritic disorder and old trauma which produces chronic instability.

## COMMENTS

A. Previous trauma to the ankle, including multiple sprains, is often forgotten by the patient. Ankle instability is usually associated with frequent inversion episodes while running, pivoting, or walking on uneven ground. The unstable ankle may swell after prolonged activity with some resolution after rest. An increase in activity for even one day may cause severe pain, swelling and discoloration. The presence of underlying disease, such as rheumatoid arthritis or diabetes mellitus, should be sought. Physical examination begins with accessing alignment of the ankle and ambulation. Palpate tissues to determine the source and temperature of the swelling and access mortice stability. Palpation of the tendon sheaths that cross the ankle joint while the patient voluntarily moves his foot may reveal localized crepitus, indicative of tendinitis. Swelling of the ankle is most commonly seen around the anterior aspect of the ankle joint, unlike the diffuse localized swelling of an ankle sprain that is anterolateral. Test ankle stability in the anterioposterior and mediolateral directions and correlate with the normal side. Excessive AP drawer or mediolateral laxity (talar knock) usually indicates a previous sprain with residual ligamentous laxity.

B. X-ray studies include AP, lateral, and mortice views. Widening of the mortice and osteophytic changes reflect previous trauma. Defects in the talar dome, such as osteochondritis dissecans, are best evaluated with arthrotomography. Talar and subtalar tilt are compared with the normal side using stress x-rays. Arthroscopy of the ankle allows lesions of the talus to be visualized directly.[6]

C. Acute tendinitis often follows strenuous and unusual activity in which the foot and ankle are used excessively. Treat by splinting or immobilizing the ankle in plaster for 3 to 10 days and give anti-inflammatory medications. Steroids should not be injected into tendon sheaths as rupture might result.

D. Specific arthritic disorders may affect the ankle joint. Treatment consists of rest, splinting, and anti-inflammatory medication while treating the underlying disease.

E. Osteochondritis dissecans[1] of the ankle is thought to be caused by a twisting injury in which the talus is impacted against the mortice. A subchondral bone fragment is produced while the overlying cartilage may remain intact. If separation occurs producing a loose body within the ankle joint, destruction becomes a major concern. Arthrotomograms are helpful in establishing whether the fragment is separated. Treatment of choice is excision of the abnormal cartilage and avascular fragment, followed by drilling into the subchondral bone at the base of the defect.

F. Degenerative joint disease of the ankle frequently follows old injury. Ankle motion gradually decreases and pain becomes more or less constant, aggravated by activity and relieved partly by rest. Reduce ankle motion by a below-knee orthotic with the ankle joint locked in neutral. A rocker bottom sole then compensates for the lack of ankle motion. Sometimes wearing a firm hiking boot is sufficient. A patellar tendon-bearing brace[4] will transfer impact loads from the metatarsal heads directly to the proximal tibia, bypassing the ankle joint. For patients involved in heavy manual labor, such as logging and construction work, conservative measures may be insufficient. In this event, an ankle fusion should be done.[5] The optimal position of the fused ankle is controversial. I favor a neutral position, with shoe sole adjustments being devised to compensate for specific activity requirements. The role of total ankle replacement in degenerative joint disease is limited.

G. Loss of mortice structure will result in laxity and instability. Diabetics with early neuropathic joints who fracture their ankles frequently go on to progressive mortice destruction due to the lack of sensory feedback. The approach to this problem consists of maintaining the foot in plantar-grade alignment with casts, splints, or orthotics. Fusion is contraindicated in a Charcot joint.

H. Ligamentous instability is usually the result of previous ankle sprains. A variety of orthotics, such as ankle lacers, and corsets, may provide enough stability to partially compensate for loss of key ligaments. Usually these devices are not sufficient for heavy activity. Satisfactory restoration of stability is possible with ligament reconstruction.[2,3]

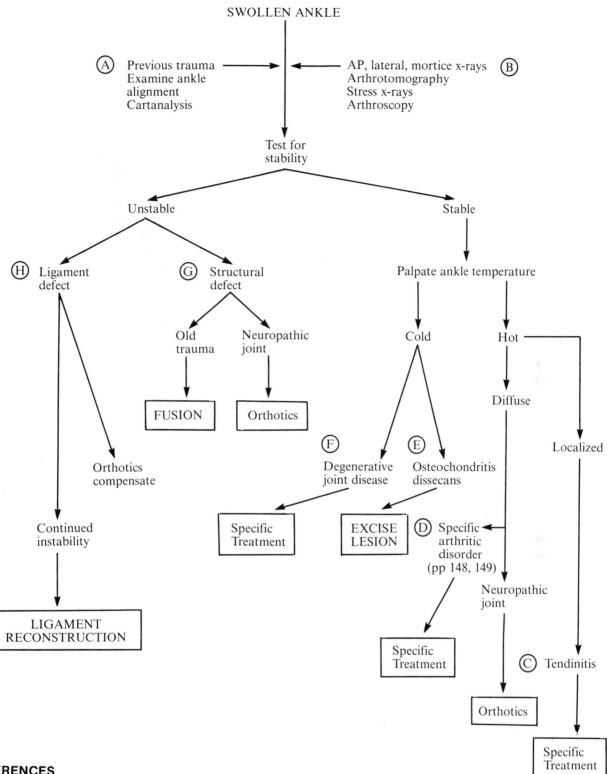

SWOLLEN ANKLE

Ⓐ Previous trauma
Examine ankle
alignment
Cartanalysis

Ⓑ AP, lateral, mortice x-rays
Arthrotomography
Stress x-rays
Arthroscopy

Test for stability

Unstable

Stable

Ⓗ Ligament defect

Ⓖ Structural defect

Palpate ankle temperature

Old trauma

Neuropathic joint

FUSION

Orthotics

Orthotics compensate

Cold

Hot

Diffuse

Localized

Ⓕ Degenerative joint disease

Ⓔ Osteochondritis dissecans

Specific Treatment

EXCISE LESION

Ⓓ Specific arthritic disorder (pp 148, 149)

Neuropathic joint

Specific Treatment

Continued instability

LIGAMENT RECONSTRUCTION

Orthotics

Ⓒ Tendinitis

Specific Treatment

## REFERENCES

1. Berndt AL, Harty M. Transchondral fractures of talus. J Bone Joint Surg. 1959; 41–A:988–1020.
2. Brantigan JW, Pedigana LR, Lippert FG. Instability of the subtalar joint. J Bone Joint Surg. 1977; 59-A:321–324.
3. **Chrisman OD, Snook GA. Reconstruction of lateral** ligament tears of the ankle: an experimental study and clinical evaluation of seven patients treated by a new modification of the Elmslie procedure. J Bone Joint Surg. 1969; 51-A:904–912.
4. Davis FJ, Fry LR, Lippert FG, Simons BC, Remington J. The patellar tendon-bearing brace (report of sixteen patients). Orthop Dig. 1974; 37–38.
5. Lance ML, et al. Arthrodesis of the ankle joint. A follow-up study. Clin Orthop Rel Res. 1979; 142:146.
6. Parisien SJ. Arthroscopy of the ankle: state of the art. Contemp Orthop. 1982; 5:21–27.
7. Primer on the Rheumatic Diseases: The Arthritis Foundation, 475 Riverside Drive, New York, NY 10027.

# CHRONIC ANKLE PAIN

## INTRODUCTION

Chronic ankle pain may be localized or diffuse and may be the result of previous trauma, inflammatory or degenerative states, and various overuse syndromes. Specific diagnosis is sometimes difficult. Specific treatment for each condition is covered in the sections *Chronic Ankle Swelling* and *The Unstable Ankle*. Local injection with Xylocaine, into specific sites such as the ankle joint or subtalar joint, will help to localize the site of pain. A short period of cast immobilization puts the ankle and foot at rest and decreases the pain. As the patient walks out of plaster for the first time, it is easier to localize the site of discomfort.

## COMMENTS

A.  A patient with previous trauma to the ankle who engages in high-impact loading activities, such as jogging and racquet sports, will aggravate the effect of a previous injury on the ankle. A history of repeated sprains suggests chronic instability as a source of pain. Even one bad sprain, inadequately treated, may result in long-term pain due to instability. The effects of neuropathic joints are alarming, but not often symptomatic. Evaluate the overall alignment of the foot during walking and standing. Tibial malalignment from previous shaft fractures may cause ankle pain. Range of motion will be decreased by impinging osteophytes. The site of impingement is usually painful. Old non-unions of medial and lateral malleoli have point tenderness, in contrast to the more diffuse tenderness of degenerative joint disease. Look for laxity of the tibiotalar and subtalar joints. Ligamentous laxity from previous injury may cause pain after prolonged walking, standing, or strenuous activities.

B.  X-ray examination should include AP, lateral, and mortice views.[2] With instability, stress roentgenograms are indicated. Arthrotomograms are helpful in identifying the presence of joint surface abnormalities and to further delineate the degree of attachment of osteochondritis dissecans. Arthroscopy of the ankle may be helpful for accessible lesions but requires experience.[3] When doubt exists about the exact source of the pain, specific injection of the area, e.g., in the subtalar joint, is helpful. This should be done under image intensifier control with an initial injection of Renografin to substantiate the presence of the needle in the joint.

C.  There may be no correlation between the severity of the x-ray findings and the clinical symptoms. Degenerative joint disease tends to improve with rest, orthotics, or casts that immobilize the involved joints.

D.  Osteochondritis dissecans may cause general and vague ankle aching, particularly after heavy activity. The extent of the lesion and the degree to which it is attached to the talus can be clarified by the use of arthrotomograms.

E.  Ankle instability is usually the result of ankle sprains. There may be both an AP drawer and talar knock, signifying mortice instability. As loose-jointed people may also appear unstable on examination, comparison with the opposide side during inversion stress x-ray examination is important. The use of an orthosis, such as an ankle corset to inhibit excessive mobility, may also be diagnostic in determining whether the instability itself is the source of the pain.

F.  Malalignment of tibial fractures—producing varus, valgus, or anterior-posterior angulation at the ankle—may cause ankle discomfort with active use. Malalignments which are not easily compensated by subtar or ankle motion should be corrected prophylactically to prevent later degenerative changes.

G.  The ankle is frequently affected by rheumatoid arthritis, crystal-induced synovitis, and other inflammatory conditions. It usually is just one of many involved joints. Synovial proliferation is much more prominent than with other painful conditions involving the ankle.[4]

## REFERENCES

1.  Chapman MW. Sprains of the Ankle. AAOS. Instructional Course Lectures. St. Louis, CV Mosby. 1983; 24:294.
2.  Brantigan JW, Pedegana LR, Lippert FG. Instability of the sub-talar joints: Diagnosis by stress tomography in three cases. J Bone Joint Surg. 1977; 59-A:321.
3.  Parisien SJ. Arthroscopy of the ankle—state of the art. Contemp Orthop. 1982; 5:21.
4.  Primer on the Rheumatic Diseases. The Arthritis Foundation, 475 Riverside Drive, New York, NY 10027.

# CHRONIC ANKLE PAIN

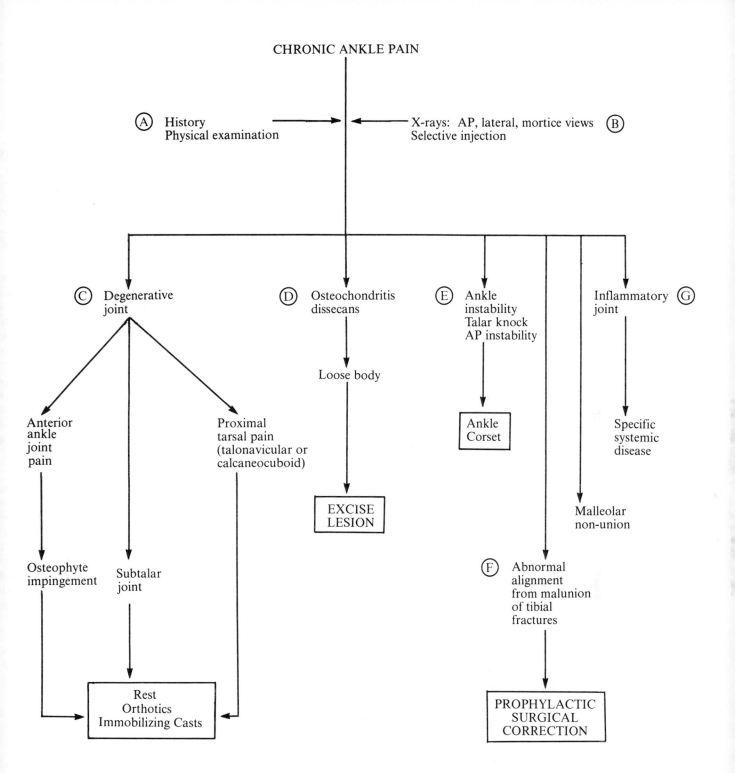

(A) History
Physical examination

(B) X-rays: AP, lateral, mortice views
Selective injection

(C) Degenerative joint

(D) Osteochondritis dissecans

(E) Ankle instability
Talar knock
AP instability

(G) Inflammatory joint

Anterior ankle joint pain

Proximal tarsal pain (talonavicular or calcaneocuboid)

Loose body

Ankle Corset

Specific systemic disease

Osteophyte impingement

Subtalar joint

EXCISE LESION

Malleolar non-union

(F) Abnormal alignment from malunion of tibial fractures

Rest
Orthotics
Immobilizing Casts

PROPHYLACTIC SURGICAL CORRECTION

# THE UNSTABLE ANKLE

## INTRODUCTION

The patient's interpretation of the term "unstable ankle" is different from that of the physician. The important distinction to be made is whether the ankle actually turns inward or outward unexpectedly, leaving residual symptoms of swelling and pain. Severe ankle sprains with demonstrable laxity should be treated appropriately to prevent chronic problems of instability. If an anterior drawer or talar knock is present, protection for 3 to 4 weeks in a cast is sometimes desirable. A loss of mortice integrity caused by injury to the syndesmosis requires surgical repair. Following any ligamentous injury, adequate muscle rehabilitation, particularly of the peroneal tendons, is essential.

## COMMENTS

A. Determine whether the instability is event-related, e.g., resulting from a sprain or fracture. If the patient has diabetes, the instability may be due to a neurotrophic joint. Any problems that affect normal functioning of the neuromuscular system should be sought, e.g., stroke, lumbar disc disease, peroneal palsies. One should check the static alignment of the lower extremity looking for heel varus and the ambulatory alignment for any heel roll-over. Inspect the patient's shoes for evidence of outward or inward heel roll. Peroneal strength should be carefully assessed. Mortice integrity is checked by stressing the talus in both the AP and mediolateral directions. Excessive displacement compared to the normal side means abnormal laxity.

B. AP, lateral, mortice, and stress roentgenograms of the ankle are important. Symmetrical stress should be applied with the foot being inverted in order to assess talar tilt.[1]

C. Ankle stability is affected by the bony integr[ity] of the mortice. Destruction of the mortice [by] trauma or by a neuropathic joint process res[ults] in loss of articulating surfaces and mechani[cal] congruence. Loose bodies, from osteochond[ritis] dissecans and previous trauma, that float in a[nd] out of the ankle cause the ankle to be unpre[dic]tably unstable.

D. Some patients have generalized joint laxity ty[pi]cally seen on examination of metatarsophal[an]geal, elbow, and knee joints. Ankle sprains [can] be prevented by orthotics that provide late[ral] stability, such as a lateral heel wedge, and [by] educating the patient about activities to [be] avoided.

E. Weakening of the peroneal muscles predispo[ses] to instability and inversion type injuries. Lu[m]bar disc disease, neurapraxia of the peron[eal] nerve, or Charcot-Marie Tooth disease may [be] responsible. An ankle corset, lateral wedges, a[nd] even bracing may be necessary to control t[he] problem.

F. Lateral ligamentous instability of the ankle [is] often caused by inadequate treatment of a p[re]viously sprained ankle. The instability may be [in] the tibiotalar joint or in the subtalar joint. Str[ess] roentgenograms and tomograms are necessa[ry] to determine which joints are involved. A tria[l of] orthotics is appropriate before surgery is con[si]dered because the combination of activity mo[di]fications and the orthotic may be sufficie[nt]. When pain and instability persist, ligame[nt] reconstruction is indicated. Good stability c[an] be achieved by a variety of procedures. I perso[n]ally prefer the modified Elmslie procedu[re] which stabilizes both tibiotalar and subta[lar] joints.

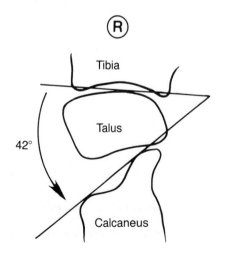

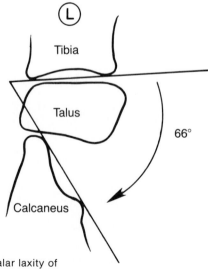

AP inversion stress tomogram showing subtalar laxity of the left ankle.

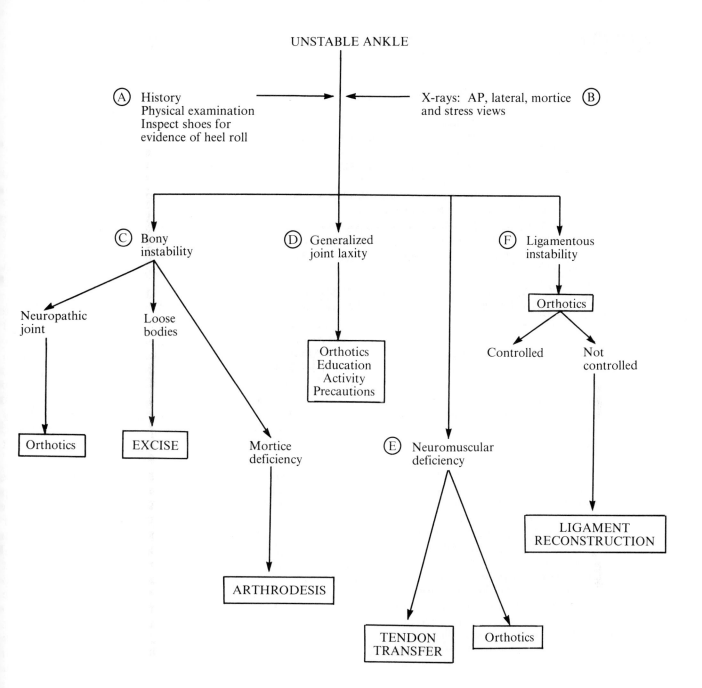

UNSTABLE ANKLE

Ⓐ History
Physical examination
Inspect shoes for
evidence of heel roll

Ⓑ X-rays: AP, lateral, mortice
and stress views

Ⓒ Bony
instability

Neuropathic
joint

Loose
bodies

Orthotics

EXCISE

Mortice
deficiency

ARTHRODESIS

Ⓓ Generalized
joint laxity

Orthotics
Education
Activity
Precautions

Ⓔ Neuromuscular
deficiency

TENDON
TRANSFER

Orthotics

Ⓕ Ligamentous
instability

Orthotics

Controlled

Not
controlled

LIGAMENT
RECONSTRUCTION

## REFERENCES

1. Brantigan JW, Pedegana LR, Lippert FG. Instability of the subtalar joint. J Bone Joint Surg. 1977; 59-A:321.
2. Chrisman OD, Snook GA. Reconstruction of lateral ligamentous tears of the ankle. An experimental study and clinical evaluation of seven patients treated by a new modification of the Elmslie procedure. J Bone Joint Surg. 1968; 51-A:904.

# MEDIAL ARCH PAIN

## INTRODUCTION

Increased participation in high-impact loading sports such as jogging, hiking, and tennis may cause medial arch pain. Feet that pronate during ambulation are especially susceptible because the medial arch structures are strained. The medial arch is formed by the skeletal architecture and supported by soft tissues such as posterior tibial tendon, plantar fascia, and long plantar and spring ligaments. The tendo Achilles may become contracted, potentiating a pronation deformity. The treatment of medial arch pain, regardless of diagnosis, is initially conservative with supportive orthotics. If symptoms persist, a variety of surgical procedures are available, depending on the underlying problem.

## COMMENTS

A. Foot symptoms are usually related to activity and type of shoes. Patients should be questioned about the relationship of activity to symptoms and shoe wear. If the individual is a jogger, a careful history must be taken to identify the type of running program, the running surface, the make of shoe, and exercise protocol. The examination of a patient with medial arch pain should include walking (sometimes running), standing, and sitting. The objective is to determine the static alignment of the foot and lower extremity as well as the effect of dynamic forces on this alignment. Careful inspection of the patient's shoe will show wear patterns that are caused by these dynamic forces. Medial arch pain is commonly associated with pronated feet. The cause of the pronation may be either local or due to some misalignment of the ipsilateral extremity more proximally. Careful range of motion examination of the hips, knees, ankles, subtalar joint, and mid-foot is essential. One of the more frequently missed findings is restricted subtalar motion due to a tarsal coalition.

B. X-ray studies include AP and lateral weight-bearing plus Harris views[4] if tarsal coalition is suspected. Osteophytes around the talonavicular joint should alert the orthopaedist to a possible tarsal coalition.

C. Medial arch pain may be due to bony protrusions such as accessory navicular. This condition makes the wearing of ski boots and other hiking footwear uncomfortable due to the local pressure. Excision of the accessory navicular must be accompanied by reattachment of the posterior tibial tendon, or collapse of the arch will result.

D. Osteochondritis of the talar head[2] (Köhler's disease) may progress to degenerative changes at the talonavicular joint. When conservative measures such as orthotics fail, a triple arthrodesis is required.

E. A flattened medial arch or pes planus can be either a hypermobile foot or rigid flatfoot.[6] The hypermobile foot subjected to repetitive high-impact loading frequently becomes symptomatic. Medial arch supports, which range from soft leather to plastic, are effective in maintaining a normal arch configuration and relieving symptoms. In severe cases with persistent symptoms, stabilization of the arch either by soft tissue support or by fusion may be necessary.

F. The most common cause of rigid flatfeet in the adult is a tarsal coalition, which has gone undiagnosed through the years and which has been relatively asymptomatic until there is an increase in activity.[4] The hallmark of this condition is reduced subtalar motion compared to the opposite side. X-rays will determine the location of the coalition. Degenerative changes usually result from the restricted motion. Medial arch supports and activity modification may control symptoms, but with persistence a triple arthrodesis is the procedure of choice. Old calcaneal fractures extending into the subtalar joint will also decrease subtalar motion and may produce similar symptoms. The treatment is the same for a tarsal coalition. The treatment of rheumatoid arthritis is well described.[3]

G. Patients who present with medial arch complaints and do not show objective findings often respond to a limited trial of anti-inflammatory medication, rest, and soft medial arch supports. Medial arch supports range from felt pads, which can be glued to the shoe, to molded plastic supports, which can be transferred to different shoes.[5,9,10] Molded arch inserts generally fit better, support better, and allow use in a variety of shoes. Insert materials range from soft foam rubber to plastic. "Posts" added to the bottom of the orthotic or heel and sole on the medial aspect can tip the foot into inversion, transferring more weight to the lateral aspect of the foot and less weight to the medial arch. The rigidity of the orthotic depends on the structural problem and the amount of activity. Thus, runners with hypermobile feet require firmer support, and plastic orthotics are required.

## REFERENCES

1. Camper T. Dissertation on the best form of shoe, the classic. Clin Orthop Rel Res. 1975; 110:2–5.
2. Carp N. Köhler's disease of the tarsal scaphoid. J Bone Joint Surg. 1937; 19:84.
3. Clayton ML. Surgical treatment of the rheumatoid foot. In *Foot Disorders: Medical and Surgical Management*, NJ Edited by Giannestras, Philadelphia:Lea & Febiger, 1967, pp. 319–340.

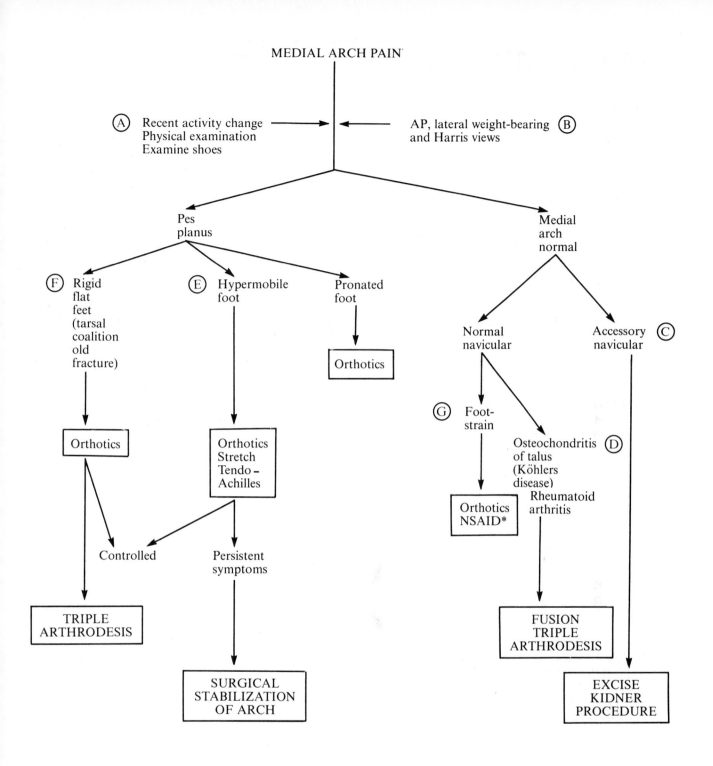

MEDIAL ARCH PAIN

(A) Recent activity change
Physical examination
Examine shoes

AP, lateral weight-bearing (B)
and Harris views

Pes planus

Medial arch normal

(F) Rigid flat feet (tarsal coalition old fracture)

(E) Hypermobile foot

Pronated foot

Normal navicular

Accessory navicular (C)

Orthotics

Orthotics

(G) Foot-strain

Osteochondritis of talus (Köhlers disease) (D)

Orthotics
Stretch Tendo-Achilles

Rheumatoid arthritis

Orthotics
NSAID*

Controlled

Persistent symptoms

TRIPLE ARTHRODESIS

FUSION TRIPLE ARTHRODESIS

SURGICAL STABILIZATION OF ARCH

EXCISE KIDNER PROCEDURE

*Nonsteroidal anti-inflammatory drug

4. Harris RL, Beath TJ. Rigid spastic flatfeet. J Bone Joint Surg. 1950; 32-B:203.
5. Hauser ED. Office management of painful feet. Orthop Clin N Am. 1957; 75–89.
6. Inman VT, Mann RA. Biomechanics of the foot and ankle. In Surgery of the Foot. Edited by VT Inman and HL DuVries. St. Louis: CV Mosby, 1973, pp. 3–22. pp. 3–22.
7. James S. Injuries to Runners. Presented at the American Academy of Orthopaedic Surgeons Annual Meeting, Las Vegas, Nevada, 1977.
8. Kidner FC. The pre-hallux (accessory scaphoid) and its relation to flatfoot. J Bone Joint Surg. 1929; 11:831.
9. Milgram JE, Jacobson MA. Foot gear—therapeutic modifications of the sole and heel. Orthop Rev. 1978; 11:57–62.
10. Newell S. The conservative treatment of plantar fasciitis. Physician in Sports Medicine, October, 1977.

# PLANTAR FASCIITIS

## INTRODUCTION[1]

Plantar fasciitis is characterized by pain at the attachment of the plantar fascia to the os calcis. It is related to factors that produce stretch on the plantar fascia such as a pronating foot, overuse, increased weight, and poor shoe support. Plantar fasciitis is a frequent problem of runners. It must be distinguished from a tarsal tunnel syndrome, usually characterized by parasthesias radiating into the foot and a positive Tinel's test; Reiter's disease, a spondyloarthropathy in which the pain is usually more posteriorly located and the HLA B-27 is positive; a cyst of the os calcis can be seen by x-ray. Plantar fasciitis can become chronic and takes a long time to heal. Patients tend to be discouraged and frustrated with the lack of response to treatment. The patient needs to be informed that a protracted time for healing is not uncommon.

## COMMENTS

A.  Plantar fasciitis may be precipitated by a sudden increase in weight, change in activity profile, or return to activity suddenly after a long period of rest, as in a cast. Symptoms tend to be worse in the morning, after standing or walking, and on the first few steps after a period of sitting. Patients are commonly referred with a diagnosis of bone bruise or heel spur. Physical examination begins with the patient standing and walking barefoot to show pronation tendencies, valgus heels, and tight Achilles tendons. Inspection of the sole often reveals swelling over the plantar fascia attachment to the os calcis. Palpation reveals increased warmth and localized tenderness.

B.  A lateral radiograph of the foot may show a small spur at the origin of attachment of the plantar fascia which represents an inflammatory response. The spur is not the cause of the pain.

C.  Patients often tolerate the pain for a period of time until they can no longer endure either the annoyance or the discomfort. Prompt relief is expected from the physician. One of the first tasks is to make the patient understand that improvement may take longer than expected. When the condition is of recent origin, anti-inflammatory medications along with a medial heel wedge or a molded insert to prevent pronation of the foot may be all that is necessary. Various methods for taping the foot into inversion are effective when used by physicians experienced in this technique. Loss of excess weight, good shoes and sedentary activities aid treatment. If no response has occurred after 2 to 3 weeks, a cortisone injection from the medial aspect of the heel often brings prompt relief. If that fails, I suggest a month in a short-leg walking cast. The patient should use his orthotics until asymptomatic. When the plantar fascia is no longer tender to palpation, gradual resumption of normal activity may begin. Patients with pronation tendencies should retain the use of the orthotics for running activities. In individuals with normal alignment, a gradual weaning from orthotics is usually successful.

D.  When all forms of conservative treatment fail and the patient is still symptomatic and incapacitated after 6 months, surgical release of the plantar fascia may provide relief. In my experience, surgical release of the plantar fascia has rarely been necessary. Release is accomplished through a medial incision under tourniquet control. The plantar fascia is easily visualized and sectioned under direct vision. Completeness of release can be tested by tensing the plantar fascia while palpating for remaining strands attached to the os calcis.

## REFERENCE

1.  Clancy WG. Tendinitis and the plantar fascia in runners. Orthop 1983; 6:230–233.

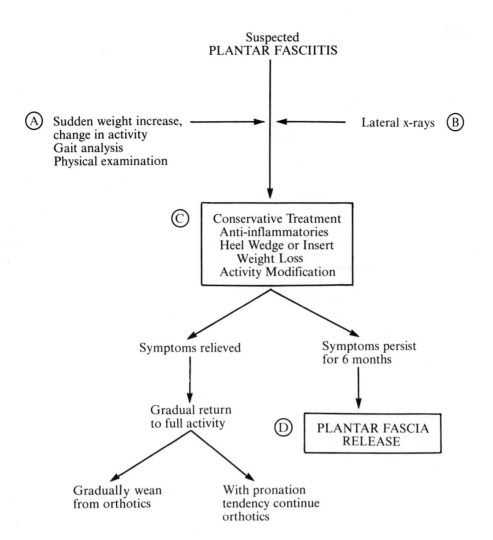

Suspected
PLANTAR FASCIITIS

Ⓐ Sudden weight increase,
change in activity
Gait analysis
Physical examination

Lateral x-rays Ⓑ

Ⓒ Conservative Treatment
Anti-inflammatories
Heel Wedge or Insert
Weight Loss
Activity Modification

Symptoms relieved

Symptoms persist
for 6 months

Gradual return
to full activity

Ⓓ PLANTAR FASCIA
RELEASE

Gradually wean
from orthotics

With pronation
tendency continue
orthotics

# ACHILLES TENDINITIS

## INTRODUCTION

Achilles tendinitis is a primary inflammation of the tendon with secondary involvement of the tendon sheath. This condition must be distinguished from retrocalcaneal bursitis or tenosynovitis caused by local irritation from boots, and other causes of overlying friction. Achilles tendinitis can be divided into two broad categories. The first is related to underlying systemic disease such as the inflammatory arthritides. The second is due to overuse. In the former condition, involvement of the tendon occurs from the inflammatory process of the tenosynovium, while the second category results from repeated microtrauma. Areas of degeneration with central necrosis form and rupture may result. Tight heel cords, valgus heels, and pronated feet predispose to Achilles tendinitis. A poor understanding of proper exercise routine, shoe wear, and running surfaces also contributes. The treatment depends to some extent on the goals and expectations of the patient. A sedentary office worker with an acute Achilles tendinitis has different goals from those of the serious athlete who wishes to perform on a daily basis. For Achilles tendinitis secondary to systemic disease, treat the specific disease and use local measures for the tendinitis. The overuse syndrome responds to rest, anti-inflammatories, and tendon stretching. Occasionally surgery may be necessary to remove a large degenerative focus. Achilles tendinitis can be broadly classified into acute, (less than 3 weeks duration), subacute (less than 6 months), and chronic (longer than 6 months).[2,3]

## COMMENTS

A. A careful history should be taken regarding the patient's ambulatory activity, particularly with regard to running sports. A change in the extent or nature of the exercise routine, particularly if there has been a period of intervening rest, frequently contributes to this condition. Evidence for underlying systemic disease should be sought. Carefully inspect the patient's shoes, particularly the athletic shoes, for evidence of wear, support, and heel protection. Patients with tight tendo Achilles, valgus heels, and pronated feet are susceptible to Achilles tendinitis. Inspect the calcaneal region for evidence of retrocalcaneal bursitis sometimes confused with Achilles tendinitis. This condition is localized to the tendinous insertion along the posterior aspect of the calcaneus and is frequently associated with a bony prominence, which may need to be removed. Inspection of the Achilles tendon is best performed with the patient prone on the examining table. Look for swelling, nodularity of the tendon, and tenderness. The patient should move his foot up and down while the examiner palpates the tendon sheath for crepitus. A warm boggy tenosynovium is more consistent with underlying systemic disease than an overuse syndrome.

B. Chronically inflamed tenosynovium with a previous history of tendon rupture may reflect rheumatoid arthritis, tuberculous synovitis, or SLE. Treat the underlying disease and institute local measures to protect the tendon. These will be described under "conservative treatment."

C. Overuse Achilles tendinitis can be divided into acute, subacute, and chronic, depending upon the duration of symptoms. Conservative treatment is indicated for all cases seen initially. The longer the presence of symptoms, the longer will be the period before response to treatment.

D. Conservative treatment[2] consists of local measures related to the tendinitis, shoe modification, and activity modification. Local measures consist of hot and cold contrast baths, plus non-steroidal anti-inflammatory medications. Cortisone injected into the tendon sheath is not advisable because it may mask an underlying inflammation and render the tendon susceptible to rupture. A three-eighths inch heel lift or higher heels as in cowboy-type boots will eliminate some tension in the tendon and provide immediate symptomatic relief during ambulation. As symptoms subside, tendo Achilles heel stretching exercises are added, particularly when tight heel cords are contributing to the condition. The best clinical guide to the success of treatment is the disappearance of pain on palpation of the Achilles tendon itself. When all tenderness has subsided, the patient may begin a graduated return to full competitive activity. An abrupt return to full activity is a frequent cause of recurrence.

E. In chronic cases where treatment has not brought about a response after 6 months, exploration of the tendon should be considered. At surgery the tendon is visualized and palpated. Areas of nodularity are sought. Large degenerative lesions with central necrosis should be excised and the tendon reconstructed by a Bosworth-type turndown and plantaris reinforcement.[1] Small lesions are merely closed and the patient placed back on a conservative treatment program.

## REFERENCES

1. Bosworth DM. Repair of defects in the tendo Achilles. J Bone Joint Surg. 1956; 38A:111.
2. Clancy WG. Tendinitis and plantar fasciitis in runners. Sports Med Orthop. 1983; 6:217–233.
3. Puddu G, Ippolito E, Postacchini F. A classification of Achilles tendon disease. Am J Sports Med. 1976; 4:145–150.

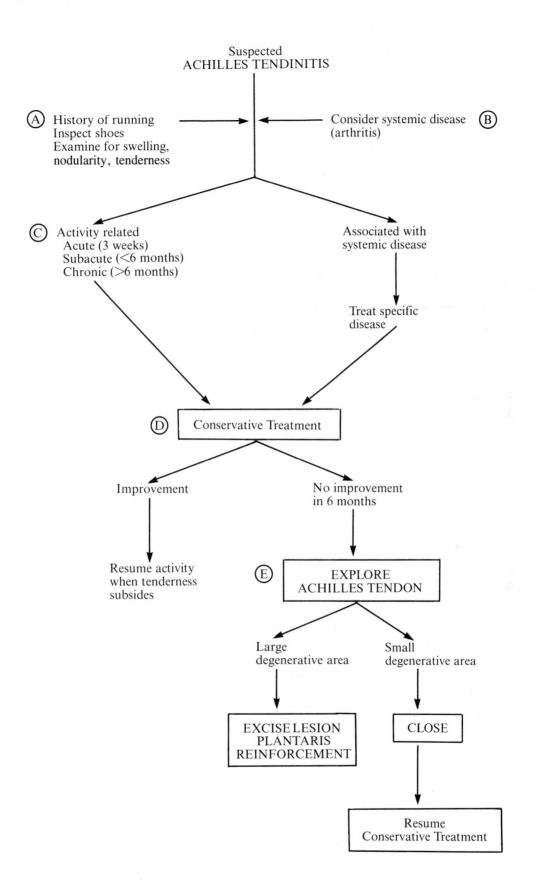

Suspected
ACHILLES TENDINITIS

Ⓐ History of running          →     ←          Consider systemic disease Ⓑ
Inspect shoes                                     (arthritis)
Examine for swelling,
nodularity, tenderness

Ⓒ Activity related                              Associated with
Acute (3 weeks)                                 systemic disease
Subacute (<6 months)
Chronic (>6 months)

                                                Treat specific
                                                disease

Ⓓ  Conservative Treatment

Improvement                          No improvement
                                     in 6 months

Resume activity                          Ⓔ  EXPLORE
when tenderness                              ACHILLES TENDON
subsides

                        Large                    Small
                        degenerative area        degenerative area

                    EXCISE LESION              CLOSE
                    PLANTARIS
                    REINFORCEMENT

                                             Resume
                                             Conservative Treatment

**157**

# METATARSALGIA

## INTRODUCTION

Metatarsalgia is pain underneath the metatarsal heads. The pain may be localized to one or more metatarsal heads. A variety of causes contribute to metatarsalgia and require that a careful analysis of the foot be accomplished before selecting treatment.[6] In the normal foot, weight bearing is distributed so that 1/3 of the body weight is carried by the first ray and 1/6 by the remaining metatarsal heads. Claw toes cannot provide this function and predispose to metatarsalgia. Individuals with a cavus-type foot concentrate weight on the metatarsal heads. The treatment of metatarsalgia attempts to redistribute or equalize weight by a variety of pads placed in the shoe or on the sole. When conservative measures fail, surgical treament is specific, depending on the etiology.

## COMMENTS

A.  The location and characteristics of the pain help to establish the diagnosis. Pain radiating into a toe is suggestive of Morton's neuroma.[3,4] The relationship of pain to activity and shoe wear is important in determining whether a patient's activity style is the main problem. Physical examination should always include inspection of stance, ambulation, and sitting alignment of the foot. The cavus and hallux valgus foot is predisposed to metatarsalgia. Clawing of the toes causes more weight to be concentrated at the metatarsal heads. Inspection of the shoes will indicate whether the wear is primarily lateral or medial, such as the medial counter bulge with pes planus. Normal shoe wear is slightly lateral to the midline of the heel. Check range of motion of the toes. Hallux rigidus causes decreased dorsiflexion of the first MTP joint and consequently a long toe lever arm. The plantar pads should be carefully palpated as a deficiency in thickness leads to metatarsalgia. Rheumatoid patients tend to have deficient plantar pads. The callous pattern will show where the weight is being concentrated. A hypermobile first ray causes a transfer of weight to the lateral metatarsal heads. Palpation of dorsalis pedis and posterior tibial pulses along with the cutaneous signs of adequate circulation (hair, nail changes, warmth) determine whether there are any vascular contraindications to surgery.

B.  Weight-bearing x-rays should be taken showing the foot in the lateral and AP positions.[6] In the lateral view of a normal foot, the talar head, cuneiforms, and metatarsals should be in a straight line. Deviation above or below will indicate planus or cavus feet. Splaying of the metatarsals will be seen in the standing AP. If the first and second intermetatarsal angle is greater than 13°, metatarsal primus varus is present, a precursor to hallux valgus. Tangential views of the hallus show the relative position of the sesamoids. A variety of pressure-measuring devices are available which demonstrate the amount of load carried by each metatarsal head.[5]

C.  Morton's neuroma is a painful affliction of the interdigital nerve, usually to toes 3 and 4.[3,4] The etiology of this condition is still not clear but is probably related to compression of the nerve. Pain shooting down into the third and fourth toe on manual compression *against* the medial and lateral aspect of the foot as well as on axial pressure exerted between the third and fourth head is characteristic. Frequently, a movable soft tissue mass can be felt between the metatarsal heads. Acute symptoms are treated by rest and metatarsal pads. A cortisone injection in the affected web space is also effective. Once the neuroma becomes enlarged with chronic symptoms, excision is the treatment of choice.

D.  Rheumatoid arthritis of the foot usually results in a fixed hallux valgus alignment and prominent metatarsal heads.[1] The synovitis of those joints usually is quite painful. Dorsal subluxation of the toes aggravates the condition. When conservative treatment fails, resection of the metatarsal heads is indicated.

E.  Freiberg's infraction, thought to be avascular necrosis of the second metatarsal head, typically occurs at the second MTP joint and is eventually characterized by sclerosis and flattening of the second metatarsal head.[2] There is concomitant enlargement of the second metatarsal shaft, joint pain and swelling. When conservative measures fail, resection of the base of the proximal phalanx is the treatment of choice.

F.  Stress fractures are common in the second metatarsal neck and shaft and may present as metatarsalgia of the second metatarsal head. Tenderness is usually present dorsally and

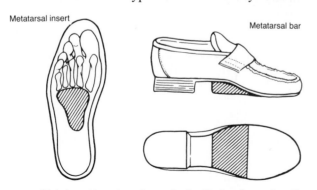

Metatarsal insert

Metatarsal bar

Metatarsal inserts or bars attached to the shoe sole relieve weight-bearing pressure on the metatarsal heads.

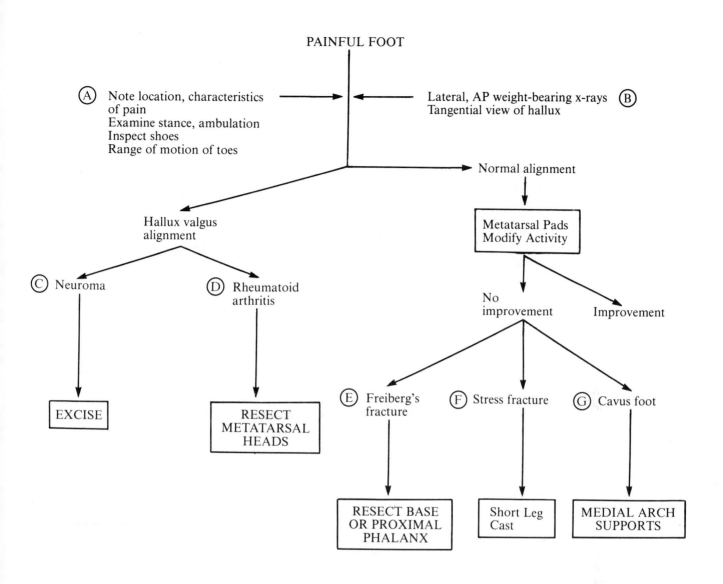

PAINFUL FOOT

(A) Note location, characteristics
of pain
Examine stance, ambulation
Inspect shoes
Range of motion of toes

(B) Lateral, AP weight-bearing x-rays
Tangential view of hallux

Normal alignment

Hallux valgus
alignment

Metatarsal Pads
Modify Activity

(C) Neuroma

(D) Rheumatoid
arthritis

No
improvement

Improvement

EXCISE

RESECT
METATARSAL
HEADS

(E) Freiberg's
fracture

(F) Stress fracture

(G) Cavus foot

RESECT BASE
OR PROXIMAL
PHALANX

Short Leg
Cast

MEDIAL ARCH
SUPPORTS

around the site of the stress fracture. X-rays may show nothing early in the process, but eventually show a small wisp of callus at the fracture site. A bone scan will detect the fracture earlier. A change in activity level is usually the cause. Treatment consists of rest, firm shoe, and crutches or a short leg walking cast for 3 to 4 weeks.

G.  This foot has a high medial arch and concentrates weight bearing on the metatarsal heads. Most metatarsalgia from this cause is relieved by molded inserts, which distribute weight bearing forces to the rest of the foot.

## REFERENCES

1.  Clayton ML. Surgery in rheumatoid arthritis. J Bone Joint Surg. 1963; 45–A:1519.
2.  Freiberg AH. The so-called infraction of the second metatarsal bone. J Bone Joint Surg. 1926; 8:257.
3.  Lassman G. Morton's toe. Clinical light and electron microscopic investigations in one hundred thirty-three cases. Clin Orthop. 1979; 142:73–84.
4.  Litchman M, et al. Morton's metatarsalgia. J Internat Coll Surg. 1964; 41:647–653.
5.  Silvino N, Evanski PN, Waugh TR. The Harris and Beath foot printing map: diagnostic validity in clinical use. Clin Orthop Rel Res. 1980; 151:265–269.

# THE DIABETIC FOOT

## INTRODUCTION

The diabetic foot presents a challenging problem to the orthopaedic surgeon. Approximately 5% of the population suffers from diabetes and about 50% of all major lower extremity amputations are in the diabetic. The foot problems arise because of microangiopathy and peripheral neuropathy. Together, the two result in changes not only of foot configuration, but also of skin susceptibility to trauma. Superficial ulcers form, but cannot be seen or felt by the patient. These ulcers progress and may involve the bone with osteomyelitis. When extensive ulceration has occurred, amputation is the only solution. The orthopaedic surgeon ensures that the diabetic patient is properly instructed in care of the feet and the wearing of proper shoes. Foot deformities which cause prominences are treated by prophylactic surgery. Doppler blood pressures, which compare blood pressure in the foot to that in the arm, provide a useful guide known as the ischemic index. When this index falls below 0.45, healing after surgery is doubtful.[4]

## COMMENTS

A.  Diabetic patients experience dysesthesias in their feet to such an extent that narcotics may be required. Paradoxically, they have diminished sensation of pain and temperature. In taking the history, one should determine the patient's knowledge about diabetic foot care and what problems have been experienced in the past. Good medical control of hyperglycemia seems to diminish the severity of symptoms.[1] Physical examination should include measurement of deep tendon reflexes, which are often reduced. Note bone vibration and position sense, as well as the skin, nails, and hair growth of the feet. Because of the microangiopathy, skin ulceration can occur despite strong pulses and a warm foot. Intrinsic atrophy and muscle imbalance often cause clawing of the toes. These cock-up deformities pull the plantar tissues distally, uncovering the metatarsal heads and rendering them more susceptible to pressure ulceration. The diabetic tends to form thick corns and calluses, which themselves lead to ulceration because the patient cannot feel the pressure exerted by these lesions on the bottom of the foot.

B.  X-rays of the diabetic foot show a spectrum of demineralization, osteolysis, and Charcot joint changes.

C.  Conservative care begins with the education of the patient and the need for a daily foot inspection.[2] Frequent sock changes and inspection of the skin for pressure areas will alert the patient to impending trouble. Meticulous care of corns, calluses, and nails requires skill by the patient because trimming corns too deeply may precipitate an ulcer. Improper trimming of nails produces ingrowing and subsequent infection of the nail bed. Shoes must have adequate depth and total contact inner soles in more advanced problems.

D.  Diabetic patients with bony prominences about the feet can benefit from prophylactic surgery in which these prominences are eliminated.[4] Clawed toes can be managed by a resection of the base of the proximal phalanges and IP fusions. Hallux valgus deformities with prominent bunions can be corrected with Keller-type procedures.

E.  Diabetic osteopathy results from continued trauma to the bony structures of an insensitive foot.[4] The warm, swollen foot may be incorrectly diagnosed as osteomyelitis. Intact skin and the lack of other septic parameters, including systemic signs, help one to make the distinction. Treatment of diabetic osteopathy is rest and protection in a walking cast. Further deformity of the foot is avoided while tissue stability in a plantigrade position develops.

F.  Superficial skin ulcers develop from shoe pressure or from corns on the bottom of the foot.[4] Ultimately an ulceration penetrates the dermis and drains. At this point, extra-depth shoes with polyethylene inserts provide total contact, reducing pressure over the ulcer. A short-leg cast with a polypropylene insert provides maximal protection. The ulcer itself is treated by local debridement and skin grafting if necessary. Remove bony prominences when skin healing is complete.

G.  For skin ulcerations that extend down to tendon, bone, and joint, first excise all necrotic tissue, then close as soon as possible with skin grafting as necessary.[4] Remove bony prominences when wounds have healed.

H.  Ulcerations that extend down into and include bone present a difficult problem.[4] If the ischemic index determined by Doppler examination is less

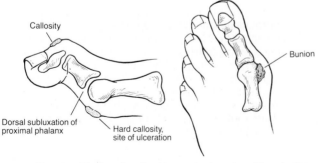

Callosity

Bunion

Dorsal subluxation of proximal phalanx

Hard callosity, site of ulceration

Structural factors involved in producing ulcerations in the diabetic foot.

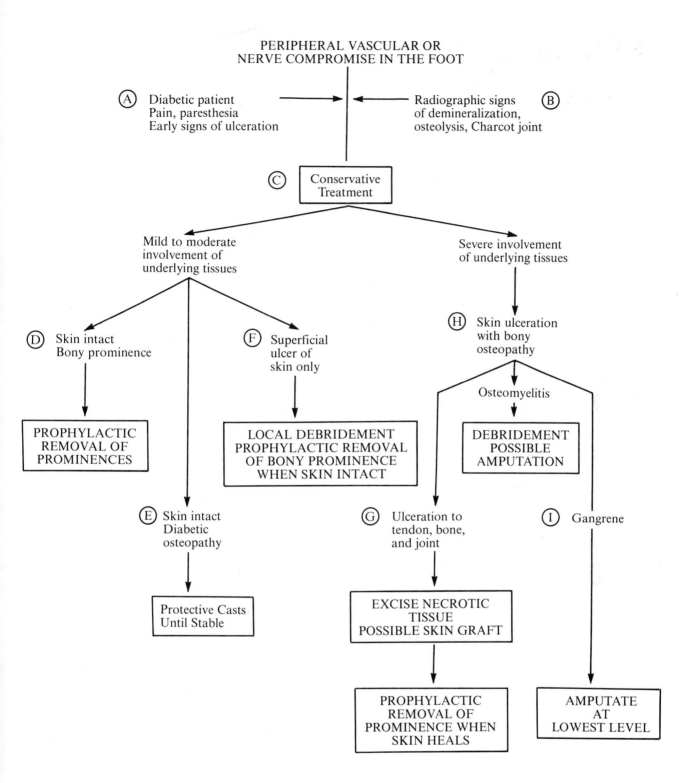

PERIPHERAL VASCULAR OR
NERVE COMPROMISE IN THE FOOT

(A) Diabetic patient
Pain, paresthesia
Early signs of ulceration

(B) Radiographic signs
of demineralization,
osteolysis, Charcot joint

(C) Conservative
Treatment

Mild to moderate
involvement of
underlying tissues

Severe involvement
of underlying tissues

(D) Skin intact
Bony prominence

(F) Superficial
ulcer of
skin only

(H) Skin ulceration
with bony
osteopathy

PROPHYLACTIC
REMOVAL OF
PROMINENCES

LOCAL DEBRIDEMENT
PROPHYLACTIC REMOVAL
OF BONY PROMINENCE
WHEN SKIN INTACT

Osteomyelitis

DEBRIDEMENT
POSSIBLE
AMPUTATION

(E) Skin intact
Diabetic
osteopathy

(G) Ulceration to
tendon, bone,
and joint

(I) Gangrene

Protective Casts
Until Stable

EXCISE NECROTIC
TISSUE
POSSIBLE SKIN GRAFT

PROPHYLACTIC
REMOVAL OF
PROMINENCE WHEN
SKIN HEALS

AMPUTATE
AT
LOWEST LEVEL

than 0.45, healing may not be possible even after surgical debridement. In this event, an amputation may be the best alternative.

I.  Gangrenous toes can become septic and should be amputated at the lowest possible level in accordance with the Doppler ischemic index.

**REFERENCES**

1.  Cahill GF, Etzwiler DD. Freinkeln  "control" and diabetes. N Engl J Med. 1976; 1004.

2.  Jacobs RL, Karmody A. The diabetic foot. In *Disorders of the Foot*. Edited by Jahss, Philadelphia: WB Saunders. 1982, pp. 1377–1397.

3.  Levin MD. Medical evaluation in treatment of the diabetic foot. In *The Diabetic Foot*. 2nd Ed. Edited by Levin and O'Neil, St. Louis: CV Mosby, 1977, pp. 1–45.

4.  Wagner WF. Transcutaneous Doppler ultrasound in the prediction of healing and the selection of surgical level for dysvascular lesions of the toes and forefoot. Clin Orthop. 1979; 102:110.

# TREATMENT OF BUNIONS

## INTRODUCTION

A bunion can be defined as medial prominence of the first MTP joint with an overlying bursa. Many etiologic theories exist, but the exact relationship of genetics, shoe wear, and activity level to bunion development has not been fully established.[1]

## COMMENTS

A. In taking the history, one should determine the impact of the bunion on the patient's life style. Occupational and recreational requirements should be evaluated. Physical examination should focus on the appearance of the foot while the patient is standing, walking, and sitting. Of particular importance is the competence of the first ray as a weight-bearing structure. This can be ascertained by examining for calluses and the mobility of the first ray. Short, mobile first rays do not assume their full share of the load and tend to cause transfer lesions laterally. Assessing mobility of the MTP joint is also helpful because lack of motion indicates degenerative changes, even in the absence of roentgen changes.

B. Weight-bearing x-rays are important in both the AP and lateral projections. An intermetatarsal angle greater than 13° between the first and second rays indicates metatarsus primus varus, a structural development that must be taken into account when planning surgery. The AP will also indicate the condition of the MTP joint, whether there is lateral subluxation of the sesamoids, and the relative length of the first ray compared to the other rays.

C. Conservative treatment consists of shoes with adequate width and length and, in cases of diminished weight-bearing by the first ray, inserts that extend out under the first ray helping it to carry more load. Most patients deserve a trial of conservative therapy, since the degree of deformity does not always correlate well with symptoms and disability. In my experience, patients who require surgery can be divided into two broad categories—the older, more sedentary patient and the active patient of all ages. In the former group a Keller Procedure provides adequate relief of symptoms with minimal operative morbidity. Active patients can be divided into those with hallux rigidus changes (DJD of the first MTP joint) secondary to excessive loading of the first ray, but without severe hallux valgus deformity, and patients with a hallux valgus deformity.

D. Hallux rigidus frequently results from a long first ray, which takes an inordinate amount of weight-bearing loads and eventually leads to degenerative changes in the MTP joint.[4,6] Certain activities, such as teeing off in golf, stress the first MTP joint. Individuals involved in a life of high-impact loading can best be helped with an arthrodesis in about 30° of dorsiflexion. Individuals whose daily activities involve relatively low-impact loads may do well with a Keller Procedure or Silastic implants. The indications for Silastic implants are still somewhat controversial and viewed by me with caution, particularly in view of the generally excellent results from MTP arthrodesis.

E. Bunions associated with hallux valgus generally have some degree of metatarsus primus varus. Which comes first and predisposes to the other is a source of controversy. If the bunion is associated with degenerative changes of the MTP joint, a Keller Procedure is the procedure of choice. Silastic implants are also an alternative.[9] Most of the controversy is directed at the hallux valgus deformity with a normal MTP joint. Available procedures range from soft tissue releases and reefings, such as the McBride procedure[5] to combinations of soft tissue adjustments and osteotomies.[1,7,10] I believe that a number of procedures are probably compatible with good results, so long as allowances are made for a hypermobile short first ray or an abnormally long first ray. Weight-bearing adjustments can be accomplished by: (1) shortening the first ray, (2) plantar flexing the first ray, or (3) a combination of both. For a hypermobile short first ray, I prefer a proximal osteotomy or a lapidus-type tarso-metatarsal fusion, with soft tissue correction of the valgus deformity.[3] The normal or long first ray that is not hypermobile can be handled with a variety of distal osteotomies, such as the Mitchell or Chevron type.[1,2]

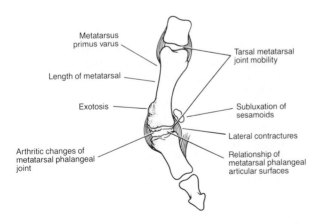

Factors to consider in the examination and treatment of bunions.

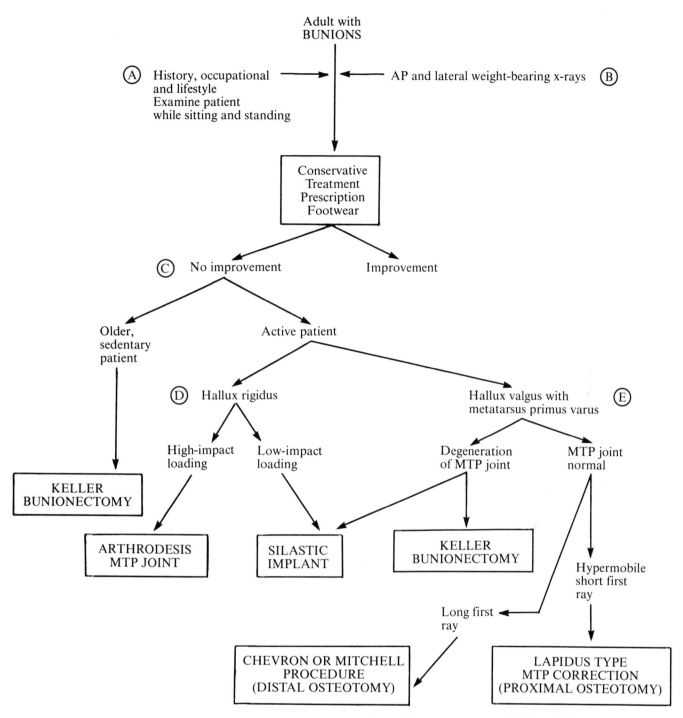

## REFERENCES

1. Carr C, Boyd B. Correctional osteotomy for metatarsus primus varus and hallux valgus. J Bone Joint Surg. l968;50-A:1353.
2. Johnson KA, Cofield RH, Morrey BF. Chevron osteotomy for hallux valgus. Clin Orthop Rel Res. 1979; 142:44–47.
3. Lapidus P. Operative correction of the metatarsus varus primus and hallux valgus. Surg Gynecol Obstet. l934;58:183.
4. Lipscomb PR. Arthrodesis of the first metatarsal phalangeal joint for severe bunions in hallux rigidus. Clin Orthop Rel Res. 1979; 142:48–54.
5. McBride E. The McBride bunion hallux valgus operation. J Bone Joint Surg. l967;49-A:1675.
6. McKeever DC. Arthrodesis of the first metatarsal phalangeal joint for hallux valgus, hallux rigidus and metatarsus primus varus. J Bone Joint Surg. l952;34-A:129.
7. Miller JW. Distal first metatarsal displacement osteotomy—its place in the scheme of bunion surgery. J Bone Joint Surg. l974;56-A:923:931.
8. Scranton RE, Rutkowski R. Anatomic variations in the first ray. Part I. Anatomic aspects related to bunion surgery. Clin Orthop Rel Res. l980;151:244.
9. Swanson AB, Lumsden RM, Swanson GD. Silicone implant arthroplasty of the great toe. A review of single stem and flexible hinge implants. Yr.,Vol.,Pp
10. Wagner WF. Technique and rationale of bunion surgery. Contemp Orthop. 1981:Vol 1040–1053.

# FEVER AND LOWER LIMB PAIN

## COMMENTS

A.  Young children who refuse to walk may have a spinal disorder (discitis).

B.  The classic posture for hip sepsis is flexion and abduction (to increase intracapsular volume; therefore, decrease pain). Patients with knee sepsis may adopt a similar posture. The infected knee is most comfortable in flexion. The child then externally rotates the limb to avoid pressure on the heel, which would force the knee into extension and cause pain. The resulting limb position (flexion, external rotation) is similar to that seen in hip sepsis.

C.  Examining a child with suspected joint sepsis or osteomyelitis while he is asleep provides a unique opportunity to *localize pain*. The child will wince and withdraw when the painful area is moved or palpated.

D.  A neonate may be afebrile, despite limb sepsis. Neonates who do not move their limbs normally or who "posture" a limb must be suspected of having joint sepsis or osteomyelitis, despite the absence of fever, elevated sedimentation rate, or an abnormal WBC and differential.

E.  In many cases of probable occult fracture, a clear diagnosis is never established. You are obligated to follow these patients carefully to be certain that they do not have an infection. Their spontaneous recovery from whatever caused the limp remains a mystery.

F.  Aspiration of first the periosteum and then the medullary cavity is best performed with image intensifier control. The thin metaphyseal cortex in a child can be readily penetrated, allowing aspiration of the medullary canal. If pus is not aspirated, any blood withdrawn should be gram stained and sent for culture. This bloody aspirate often produces a positive culture. A 16- or 18-gauge spinal needle with a stylet is ideal; however, a plain 14-gauge hypodermic needle is a practical substitute.

## REFERENCES

1.  Gillespie R. Septic arthritis of childhood. Clin Orthop. 1973; 96:152.
2.  Mollan RA, et al. Acute osteomyelitis in children. J Bone Joint Surg. 1977; 59(1):2.
3.  Morrey BF, et al. Hematogenous osteomyelitis in children. Orthop Clin N Am. 1975; 6(4):935.
4.  Rang M. *Children's Fractures*. Phildelphia: JB Lippincott, 1974.

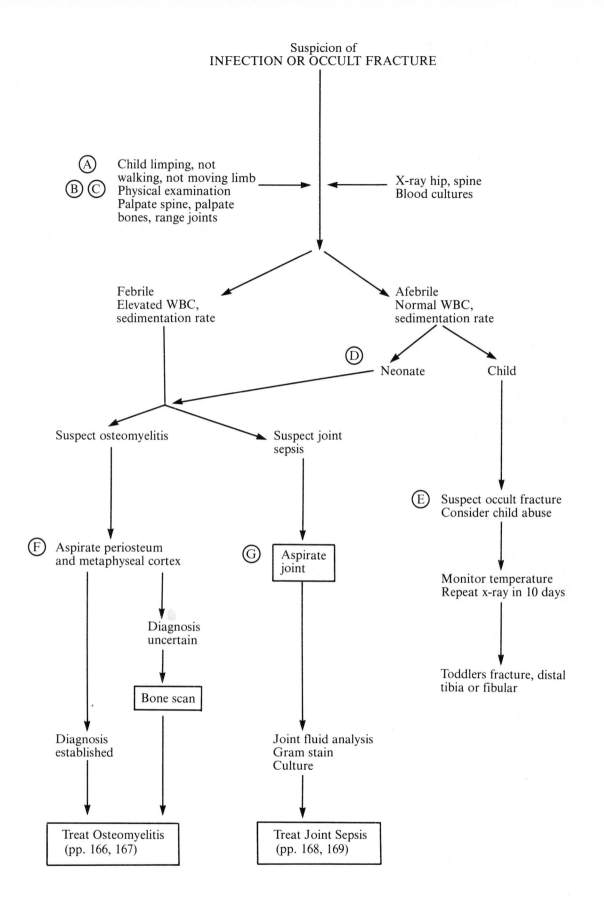

Suspicion of
**INFECTION OR OCCULT FRACTURE**

(A) Child limping, not
walking, not moving limb
(B) (C) Physical examination
Palpate spine, palpate
bones, range joints

X-ray hip, spine
Blood cultures

Febrile
Elevated WBC,
sedimentation rate

Afebrile
Normal WBC,
sedimentation rate

(D) Neonate        Child

Suspect osteomyelitis        Suspect joint
sepsis

(E) Suspect occult fracture
Consider child abuse

(F) Aspirate periosteum
and metaphyseal cortex

(G) Aspirate
joint

Monitor temperature
Repeat x-ray in 10 days

Diagnosis
uncertain

Bone scan

Toddlers fracture, distal
tibia or fibular

Diagnosis
established

Joint fluid analysis
Gram stain
Culture

Treat Osteomyelitis
(pp. 166, 167)

Treat Joint Sepsis
(pp. 168, 169)

# OSTEOMYELITIS

## COMMENTS

A. Because of improved awareness among orthopedists and pediatricians, as well as the aid of better diagnostic tools, osteomyelitis is often diagnosed very early. Despite the traditional axiom of "pus must be drained," certain children with osteomyelitis, diagnosed very early, do well with antibiotic treatment alone.

B. Antibiotics often must be selected prior to having definitive cultures. Synthetic penicillins or a cephalosporin will cover coagulase positive *S. aureus*.

C. If the patient does not respond to antibiotics alone, surgical drainage is indicated.

D. Surgical drainage relieves pressure and prevents further bone necrosis. I drill or window the cortex; however, some argue that since pus is already outside the metaphysis, the cortex has been biologically "windowed." The wound can be packed open or closed over a simple rubber drain which is pulled in 48 hours. Suction irrigation systems are complicated, rarely work, and have not been shown to provide better results than are achieved with a simple rubber drain.

E. The duration of the course of intravenous antibiotics for the treatment of acute osteomyelitis with or without surgical drainage remains controversial. Often the intravenous line is hard to keep in position and cut-downs are needed, making three to six weeks treatment very trying, both for the patient and the physician. Tetzlaff suggest early transfer to oral antibiotics if serum bacteriocidal levels can be monitored. The laboratory should have the infecting organism growing to perform serum bacteriocidal titers.

## REFERENCES

1. Cole WG, et al. Treatment of acute osteomyelitis in childhood. J Bone Joint Surg. 1982; 64B:2l8.
2. Morrey BF. Hematogenous osteomyelitis in children. Orthop Clin N Am. 1975; 6(4):935.
3. Prober CG. Oral antibiotic therapy for skeletal infections of children. Ped Inf Dis. 1982; 1:8.
4. Tetzlaff T, et al. Antibiotic concentration in pus and bone of children with osteomyelitis. J Ped. 1978; 92:135.

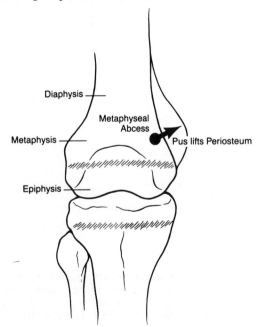

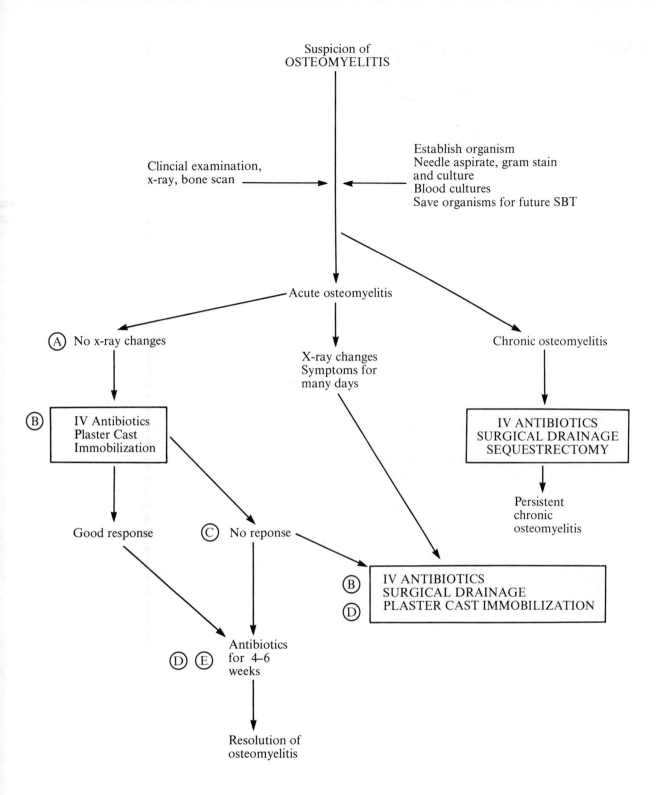

Suspicion of
OSTEOMYELITIS

Clincial examination,
x-ray, bone scan ⟶

Establish organism
Needle aspirate, gram stain
and culture
Blood cultures
Save organisms for future SBT

Acute osteomyelitis

Ⓐ No x-ray changes

X-ray changes
Symptoms for
many days

Chronic osteomyelitis

Ⓑ IV Antibiotics
Plaster Cast
Immobilization

IV ANTIBIOTICS
SURGICAL DRAINAGE
SEQUESTRECTOMY

Good response

Ⓒ No reponse

Persistent
chronic
osteomyelitis

Ⓑ
Ⓓ
IV ANTIBIOTICS
SURGICAL DRAINAGE
PLASTER CAST IMMOBILIZATION

Ⓓ Ⓔ Antibiotics
for 4–6
weeks

Resolution of
osteomyelitis

# SEPTIC ARTHRITIS

## COMMENTS

A. Neonates may have no fever, no systemic symptoms, and few findings. Most children who end up with a permanent handicap due to femoral head destruction are the result of either hip sepsis missed in a neonatology unit or hip sepsis associated with another illness during the first months of life.

B. Fluid from an infected joint is cloudy or purulent, has poor viscosity, and greater than 50,000 WBC with 90% PMNs. Fluid glucose is decreased and protein is increased. The fluid should be gram stained and cultured.

C. All septic hips must be drained surgically. The ossific nucleus is a delicate structure whose blood supply is obliterated by increased intracapsular pressure produced by an infection. Even organisms with limited virulence will damage the articular cartilage. Repeated aspirations are ineffective in completely decompressing the joint.

D. If the aspirated fluid is purulent and gram stain suggests *S. aureus*, surgical drainage is indicated for any joint. The powerful chondrolytic enzymes produced by *S. aureus* rapidly destroy articular cartilage.

E. Septic hips are best drained anteriorly, sometimes including percutaneous adductor tenotomy and intramuscular psoas tendon lengthening followed by immobilization in abduction to avoid residual hip subluxation. This is especially important in hips which are already subluxated at diagnosis. The frequent complication of hip subluxation following surgical drainage for hip sepsis has not been adequately emphasized. The posterior approach is an acceptable alternative for children diagnosed very early with no subluxation. Close the wounds over a plain rubber drain which is pulled in one to two days. Suction irrigation systems, which often include antibiotic solutions, function poorly and have not been proven effective. High does intravenous antibiotics provide an adequate level to the joint.

F. Antibiotic choice depends on definitive cultures (synovial fluid aspirate, blood). The initial choice is made with only gram stain evidence as the clinician cannot await cultures to initiate treatment. Children under age three years must be covered both for *S. aureus* and *H. influenza* (synthetic penicillin plus ampicillin or newer cephalosporins which cover both). Also, certain *H. influenza* strains are now resistent to ampicillin, requiring treatment with chloramphenicol. Children over age three years are covered for *S. aureus* alone (synthetic penicillin) until definitive cultures are available. Neonates may have streptococcus or a gram-negative organism. Consultation with a pediatrician will help you in both antibiotic selection and maintenance of an IV line.

G. Duration of intravenous antibiotics and total duration of antibiotic therapy (intravenous plus oral) remain controversial. Antibiotic therapy should be continued until the patient is clinically cured and the risks of relapse and future sequelae are minimized. Four to 6 weeks of antibiotic therapy is indicated for bone and joint infections. Traditionally, this entire course was given intravenously in hospital; however, in current practice intravenous therapy is given only until the acute signs and symptoms of infection are controlled. Early transitioin to oral antibiotics requires the use of serum bacteriocidal titers which in turn requires identification of the infecting organism. A child should be kept on intravenous antibiotics until the fever has resolved and the sedimentation rate has dropped significantly, followed by a cautious transition to oral antibiotics for a total therapeutic course of 4 to 6 weeks.

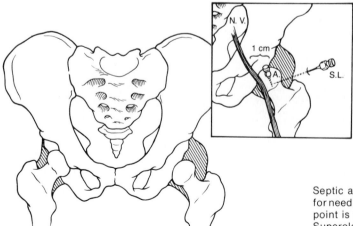

Septic arthritis, left hip. Inset demonstrates approaches for needle aspiration: A. Anterior approach. Note entrance point is 1 cm. lateral to neurovascular bundle (NV). S.L. Superolateral approach.

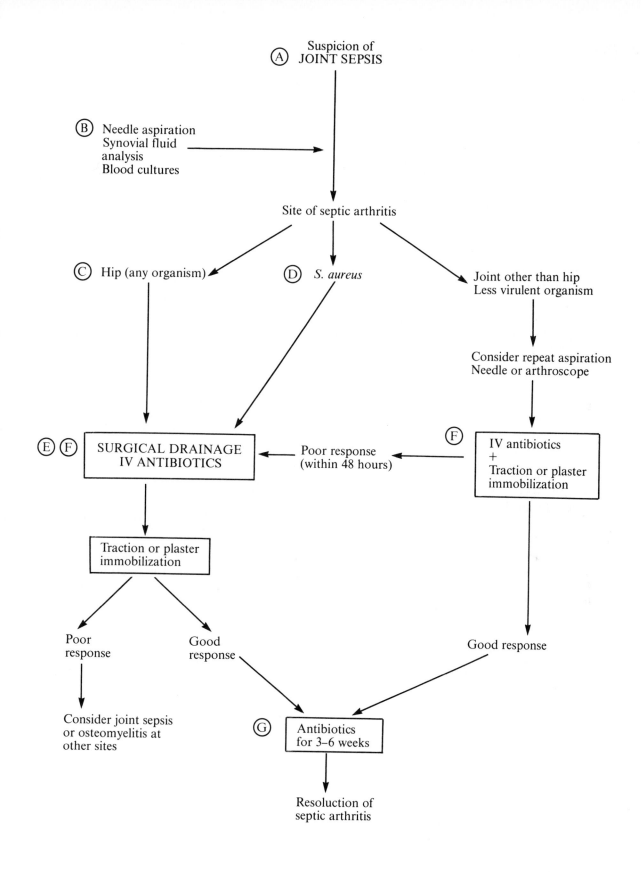

**REFERENCES**

1.  Gillespie R. Septic arthritis of childhood. Clin Orthop. 1973;96:152.

2.  Nelson JD, et al. Oral antibiotic therapy for skeletal infections of children. J. Ped. 1978;92:131.
3.  Prober, CG. Oral antibiotic therapy for bone and joint infections. Ped Inf Dis. 1982;1:8.

# SPINAL INFECTION (DISCITIS, OSTEOMYELITIS)

## COMMENTS

A. Young children presenting with discitis and refusal to walk are often mistakenly studied for a neurologic disorder.[1] Others presenting with abdominal pain are suspected of having appendicitis.

B. Disc-space narrowing may not occur until 2 to 3 weeks after the onset of symptoms.[2] The radioactive bone scan is extremely helpful in establishing the diagnosis during this period.

C. Discitis, intervertebral disc-space infection, and vertebral osteomyelitis form a spectrum of disorders with a probable common bacterial etiology.[3] The clinical and x-ray picture that develops is determined by the virulence and extent of the infection. With discitis, only the disc and adjacent end plates are involved. Vertebral osteomyelitis involves an entire vertebral body, perhaps with a more virulent organism. Because certain authors maintain that discitis is not bacterial in origin, they treat by immobilization rather than antibiotics. Young children with fever and an elevated sedimentation rate should be treated with antibiotics, which constitutes the specific treatment for bacterial infection.

D. In reported series, most patients with positive cultures have grown *S. aureus*. Initial empiric antibiotic therapy should therefore include a penicillinase-resistant penicillin or a cephalosporin. Duration of intravenous versus oral administration and total duration of antibiotic therapy are the same as for joint sepsis or osteomyelitis (intravenous until acute symptoms subside, oral for a *total* of 4–6 weeks).

E. Immobilization is advised only if the child remains symptomatic. Usually after 5 days of antibiotic therapy the child is much improved and quite comfortable. Older children (6–16 years) have protracted symptoms and often require a cast or brace.

F. Infants with vertebral osteomyelitis are often quite ill and may have several vertebral bodies involved. The radiographic appearance several years later is very similar to congenital kyphosis.

G. Localized kyphosis (gibbus) is common with severe vertebral osteomyelitis.

H. Antibiotic selection for vertebral osteomyelitis is similar to that in discitis. Chemotherapy with three agents (triple therapy) is advised for tuberculosis.

## REFERENCES

1. Eismont FJ. Vertebral osteomyelitis in infants. J Bone Joint Surg. 1982; 64B:32.
2. Spiegel PG, et al. Intervertebral disc-space inflammation in children. J Bone Joint Surg. 1972; 54A:284.
3. Wenger DR, et al. The spectrum of intervertebral disc-space infection in children. J Bone Joint Surg. 1978; 60A:100.

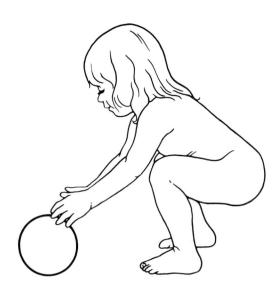

Child with discitis attempting to pick up ball. Spine remains stiff (loss of spinal rhythm).

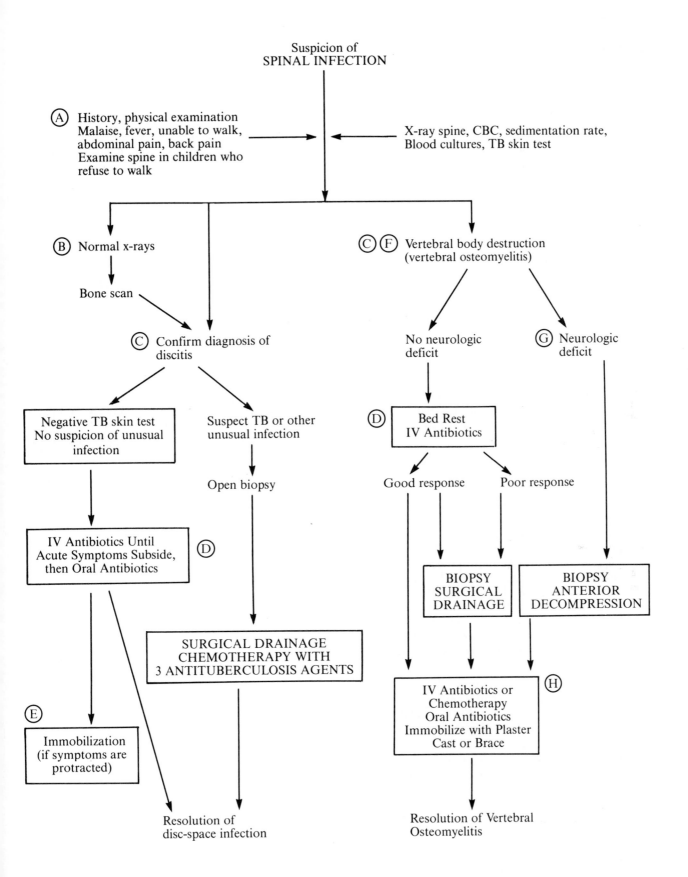

# TORTICOLLIS

## COMMENTS

A. Children with torticollis have a high incidence of hip dysplasia; thus, the hips must be examined.

B. Plain radiographs are satisfactory as an initial step. If basilar invagination or fixed rotatory subluxation is suspected, additional studies, including polytomography and cineradiography, are required.

C. Cervical adenitis, disc space infections, vertebral osteomyelitis, and even osteomyelitis of the rib are inflammatory causes of acute torticollis. Traumatic causes of torticollis include fixed rotatory subluxation, odontoid fracture, or other cervical fracture. Neurogenic causes of torticollis include syringomyelia, spinal cord tumors, cerebellar tumors, and vertebral body tumors which may impinge on neural elements (eosinophilic granuloma).

D. In addition to the Klippel-Feil syndrome, atlanto-occipital abnormalities, basilar impression, and odontoid anomalies may cause torticollis.

E. Extrinsic eye muscle imbalance (especially superior oblique palsy) is a common and often overlooked cause of head tilt in children.

F. The diagnosis of congenital muscular torticollis should be applied only after all other possible etiologies have been ruled out. The disorder is possibly caused by injury to the sternocleidomastoid muscle in the birth process, since many cases are associated with difficult deliveries (breech, forceps). The repair process causes fibrosis and contracture resulting in head tilt and rotation. The child often has a lump in the sternocleidomastoid muscle, appearing at age 2 to 4 weeks and disappearing by age 6 months. This feature is often overlooked unless the child is carefully examined during this age period.

G. In 90% of cases, congenital muscular torticollis resolves in the first year of life;[1] therefore, passive stretching is the only treatment advised at this age.

H. If correction has not occured by age 1 year, surgical release is indicated to prevent permanent facial asymmetry and head tilt. The facial asymmetry is partially related to the prone infant always sleeping with the head turned to the same side.

I. Distal release of both the sternal and clavicular attachments seems adequate for moderate cases. Some prefer a Z-lengthening to maintain neck contour; however, this procedure may prevent complete correction. A tansverse skin incision, well *above* the clavicle, following Langer's lines, is essential. Incisions directly over the bony prominence of the clavicle produce ugly scars.

J. Surgical treatment of torticollis is often applied too late with too little surgery, resulting in residual deformity. Severe cases benefit from both distal and proximal releases. The proximal release (mastoid incision) requires attention to the location of the spinal accessory nerve. The issue of postoperative immobilization remains unsettled, with many surgeons using no immobilization. More severe cases should probably be immobilized with a Minerva jacket in an overcorrected position.

## REFERENCES

1. Coventry MB, et al. Congenital muscular torticollis in infancy, some observations regarding treatment. J Bone Joint Surg. 1959; 41A: ; 815.
2. Ferkel RD et al. Muscular torticollis. A modified surgical approach. J Bone Joint Surg. 1983; 65A:894.
3. Hummer DC, Jr et al. The coexistence of torticollis and congenital dysplasia of the hip. J Bone Joint Surg. 1972; 54A:1255.
4. Ling CM. The influence of age on the results of open sternomastoid tenotomy in muscular torticollis. Clin Orthop. 1976; 116:142.

CHILD WITH HEAD TILT

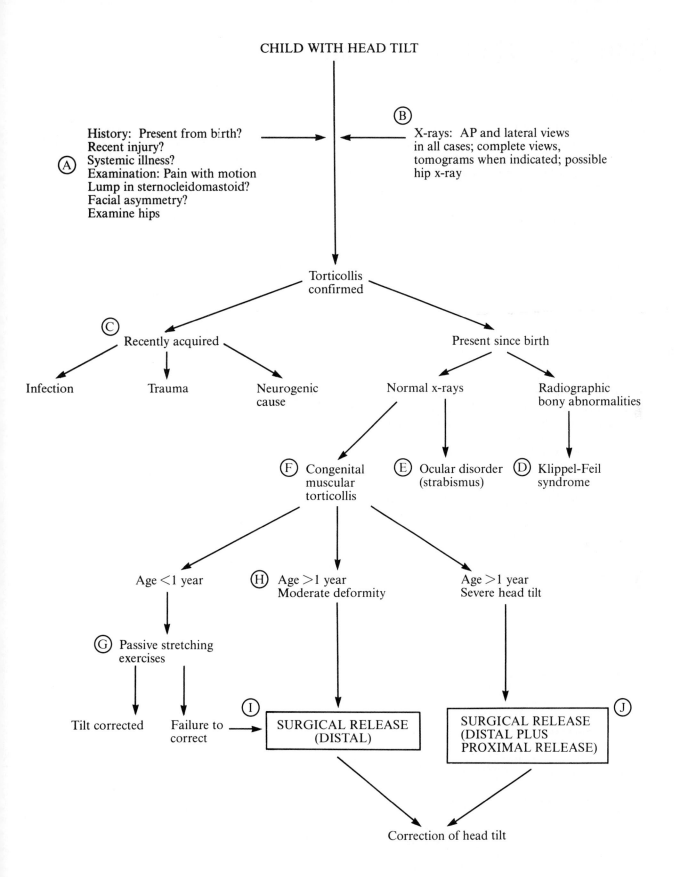

History: Present from birth?
Recent injury?
(A) Systemic illness?
Examination: Pain with motion
Lump in sternocleidomastoid?
Facial asymmetry?
Examine hips

(B) X-rays: AP and lateral views
in all cases; complete views,
tomograms when indicated; possible
hip x-ray

Torticollis
confirmed

(C) Recently acquired

Present since birth

Infection

Trauma

Neurogenic
cause

Normal x-rays

Radiographic
bony abnormalities

(F) Congenital
muscular
torticollis

(E) Ocular disorder
(strabismus)

(D) Klippel-Feil
syndrome

Age <1 year

(H) Age >1 year
Moderate deformity

Age >1 year
Severe head tilt

(G) Passive stretching
exercises

Tilt corrected

Failure to
correct

(I) SURGICAL RELEASE
(DISTAL)

(J) SURGICAL RELEASE
(DISTAL PLUS
PROXIMAL RELEASE)

Correction of head tilt

# CHILD WITH BACK PAIN

## COMMENTS

A.  Oblique radiographs are needed to evaluate suspected spondylolysis and spondylolisthesis. A bone scan is extremely helpful in evaluating a child with obscure back pain and normal plain radiographs. A technetium scan is quite adequate as a screening device.

B.  Abdominal disorders, particularly renal disease, may present with back pain. Percuss the renal area when evaluating back pain.

C.  If infection is suspected and other causes have been ruled out, perform a bone scan. Patients with discitis will have normal radiographs for 2 to 3 weeks whereas the scan will be abnormal much earlier.

D.  Spinal cord lesions usually present with neurologic symptoms or have neurologic deficit on physical examination.

E.  Modern myelography includes metrizamide dye and often concomitant CT scanning. The child must be supine to detect a tethered spinal cord. Send the child to a sophisticated neuroradiologic unit, when possible, to avoid unnecessary repetition of studies.

F.  Herniated discs occur reasonably often in adolescents and teenagers. The patient often has a severe trunk list (sciatic scoliosis) with back, hip, and radiating limb pain, especially with straight leg raising. Neurologic deficit, such as sensory or motor loss, or loss of reflexes, is rare, apparently because the nerve roots in children are more resistant to pressure. Treatment includes bed rest which, if unsuccessful, is followed by myelography and surgical excision of the herniated disc.

G.  Benign tumors producing back pain in children include osteoid osteoma, osteoblastoma, and aneurysmal bone cyst. Eosinophilic granuloma may produce the vertebral collapse seen in vertebra plana or Calve's disease.

H.  Malignant bony tumors that may involve the vertebral column include Ewing's sarcoma, osteosarcoma, and metastatic lesions, especially neuroblastoma.

## REFERENCES

1.  Tachdjian MO, et al. Orthopaedic aspects of intraspinal tumors in children. J Bone Joint Surg. 1965; 47A:223.
2.  Wenger DR, et al. The spectrum of intervertebral disc-space infection in children. J Bone Joint Surg. 1978; 60A:100.
3.  Lovell W, and Winter R. Pediatric Orthopaedics. Philadelphia: JB Lippincott, 1978.

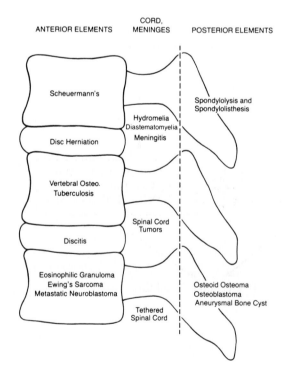

LOCATIONS OF DISORDERS PRODUCING
BACK PAIN IN CHILDREN

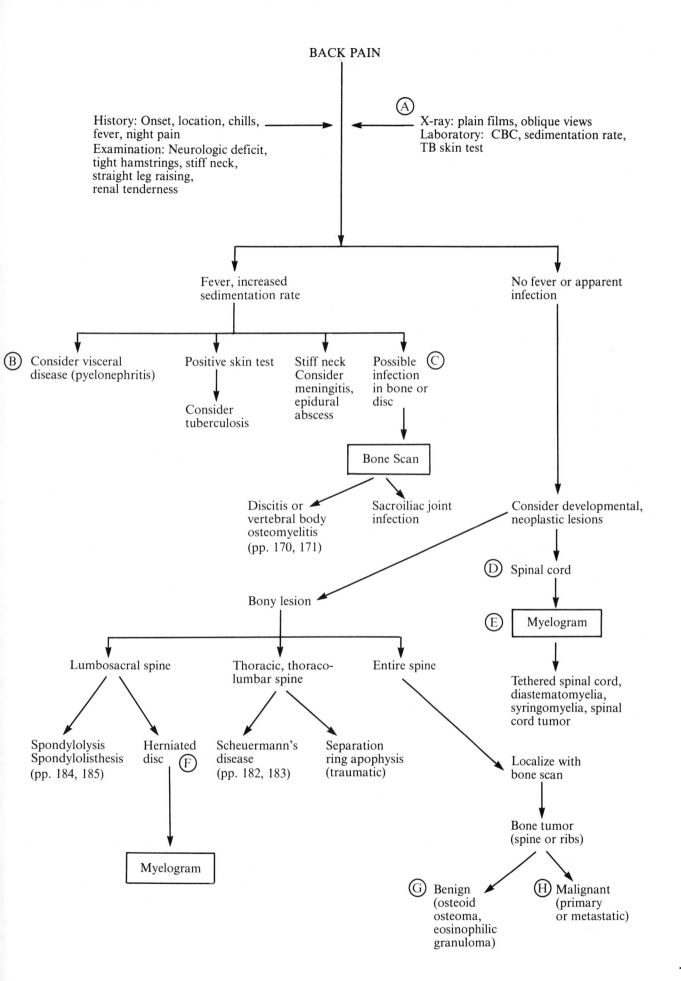

BACK PAIN

History: Onset, location, chills,
fever, night pain
Examination: Neurologic deficit,
tight hamstrings, stiff neck,
straight leg raising,
renal tenderness

Ⓐ X-ray: plain films, oblique views
Laboratory: CBC, sedimentation rate,
TB skin test

Fever, increased
sedimentation rate

No fever or apparent
infection

Ⓑ Consider visceral
disease (pyelonephritis)

Positive skin test

Stiff neck
Consider
meningitis,
epidural
abscess

Possible
infection
in bone or
disc Ⓒ

Consider
tuberculosis

Bone Scan

Discitis or
vertebral body
osteomyelitis
(pp. 170, 171)

Sacroiliac joint
infection

Consider developmental,
neoplastic lesions

Ⓓ Spinal cord

Bony lesion

Ⓔ Myelogram

Lumbosacral spine

Thoracic, thoraco-
lumbar spine

Entire spine

Tethered spinal cord,
diastematomyelia,
syringomyelia, spinal
cord tumor

Spondylolysis
Spondylolisthesis
(pp. 184, 185)

Herniated
disc Ⓕ

Scheuermann's
disease
(pp. 182, 183)

Separation
ring apophysis
(traumatic)

Localize with
bone scan

Bone tumor
(spine or ribs)

Myelogram

Ⓖ Benign
(osteoid
osteoma,
eosinophilic
granuloma)

Ⓗ Malignant
(primary
or metastatic)

# IDIOPATHIC SCOLIOSIS

## COMMENTS

A. Disorders with a high association of scoliosis include Marfan's syndrome, neurofibromatosis, and neuromuscular diseases. An extremely common cause for failing to pass school scoliosis screening is a minor limb length discrepancy producing a functional scoliosis. Pain is rare in idiopathic scoliosis and, when present, requires careful investigation.

B. Current concern about breast irradiation had led to the use of PA (posteroanterior) spine films rather than AP films for scoliosis evaluation, in order to decrease breast irradiation. A single PA view is adequate for school screening referrals who may or may not have scoliosis. True scoliosis requires a lateral view to evaluate for possible thoracic lordosis associated with scoliosis (hard to brace) or spondylolisthesis. Radiographs in the side bending position are rarely needed, except in preparation for surgical correction in problem cases.

C. Infantile idiopathic scoliosis is rare in the United States. Mehta's rib-vertebral angle difference is very useful in prognosticating curve progression.

D. Patients with juvenile idiopathic scoliosis, treated by bracing, are faced with 6 to 8 years of bracing. Tolo et al have found that part-time brace wear is effective once the curve is well controlled.

E. Not all skeletally immature adolescents with 15° to 30° curves progress, even though they are "supposed to." A recent trend in scoliosis management includes observing curves for a longer time to be certain that they are truly progressive. If you have radiographic evidence of progression from 10° to 20°, brace at 20°. If there are no prior films and the child has less than 25° curve, bracing can be withheld until the curve progresses. If the curve is over 25°, the child is braced on the first visit.

F. Underarm orthoses (Boston or variation) have cosmetic advantages and are now used for most curves. The apex of the thoracic curve should be at T9 or below for an underarm orthosis to be effective. Electrical stimulation of muscle (via surface or implanted electrodes) is being used on an investigational basis for maintenance and/or correction of idiopathic scoliosis. Its efficacy has not been determined.

G. Harrington instrumentation and spinal fusion, using distraction plus compression rods (plus transverse fixation between the rods), remains the standard of care for severe curves or curves not controlled by bracing. In most centers, thoracic curves of greater than 40° or double major curves of greater than 60° (in the skeletally immature child) are treated surgically. These guidelines are less rigidly applied in patients who are skeletally mature. The Luque method (sublaminar wires segmental spinal instrumentation) is reserved for difficult cases (adult scoliosis, neurofibromatosis, neuromuscular disease), in which the benefit of secure fixation with more certain union outweighs the greater risk for neurologic deficit inherent to sublaminar wiring.

## REFERENCES

1. Moe JH, Winter RB, Bradford DS, Lonstein JE. *Scoliosis and Other Spinal Deformities*. Philadelphia: WB Saunders, 1978.
2. Mehta MH. The rib-vertebral angle in the early diagnosis between resolving and progressive infantile scoliosis. J Bone Joint Surg. 1972; 54B:230.
3. Tolo V, et al. The characteristics of juvenile idiopathic scoliosis and the results of its treatment. J Bone Joint Surg. 1978; 60B:181.
4. Winter RB, et al. Excessive thoracic lordosis and loss of pulmonary function in patients with idiopathic scoliosis. J Bone Joint Surg. 1975; 57A:972.

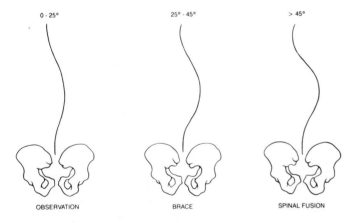

0 - 25°  25° - 45°  > 45°

OBSERVATION  BRACE  SPINAL FUSION

TREATMENT — IDIOPATHIC SCOLIOSIS

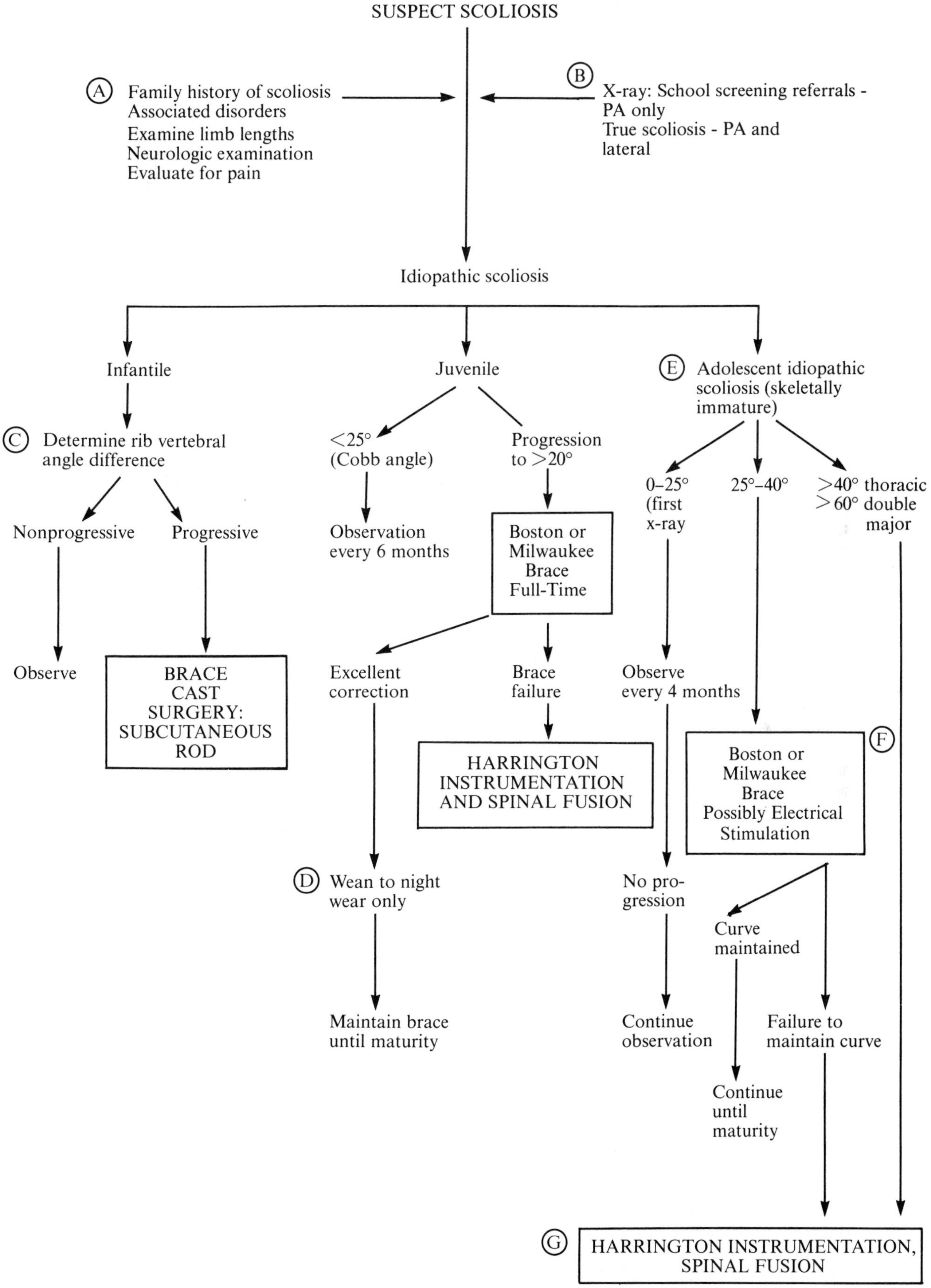

SUSPECT SCOLIOSIS

(A) Family history of scoliosis
Associated disorders
Examine limb lengths
Neurologic examination
Evaluate for pain

(B) X-ray: School screening referrals -
PA only
True scoliosis - PA and
lateral

Idiopathic scoliosis

Infantile

Juvenile

(E) Adolescent idiopathic
scoliosis (skeletally
immature)

(C) Determine rib vertebral
angle difference

<25°
(Cobb angle)

Progression
to >20°

0–25°
(first
x-ray

25°–40°

>40° thoracic
>60° double
major

Nonprogressive

Progressive

Observation
every 6 months

Boston or
Milwaukee
Brace
Full-Time

Observe

BRACE
CAST
SURGERY:
SUBCUTANEOUS
ROD

Excellent
correction

Brace
failure

Observe
every 4 months

Boston or
Milwaukee
Brace
Possibly Electrical
Stimulation

(F)

HARRINGTON
INSTRUMENTATION
AND SPINAL FUSION

(D) Wean to night
wear only

No pro-
gression

Curve
maintained

Maintain brace
until maturity

Continue
observation

Failure to
maintain curve

Continue
until
maturity

(G) HARRINGTON INSTRUMENTATION,
SPINAL FUSION

# NEUROMUSCULAR SCOLIOSIS

## COMMENTS

A. Inherited neuromuscular (NM) diseases include: Friedreich's ataxia, Duchenne muscular dystrophy, spinal muscular atrophy, and other types of muscle disease.

B. Failure of neural elements to develop on a congenital basis, as in spina bifida, is a common cause of paralytic scoliosis. Spina bifida patients also commonly have defects in segmentation of the bony elements of the spine and thus have a congenital component to their scoliosis.

C. Both cerebral palsy and traumatic paraplegia produce an upper motor neuron lesion and spasticity with a high incidence of associated scoliosis. Nonambulatory children with severe spastic quadriplegia secondary to cerebral palsy and children with complete thoracic level paraplegia secondary to trauma almost predictably develop scoliosis.

D. A custom-molded wheelchair insert may slow the progression of mild scoliosis. Spinal hyperextension, by a chair insert, is thought to lock the posterior elements and delay scoliosis progression.[5]

E. In contrast to idiopathic scoliosis, NM scoliosis may progress after skeletal maturity; therefore, yearly observation is prudent in significant neuromuscular scoliosis which has not been surgically stabilized.

F. Many orthoses are available. Most often a child with NM disease will require a custom-molded, rather than an "off the shelf" model (Boston), since these patients tend to have unusual shapes. A single anterior opening or bivalve plastic orthosis is satisfactory.[3] Milwaukee braces are not often used because children with NM disease may tend to hang on the neck piece. In certan cases, the spinal orthosis may be suspended from the wheelchair (Newington).[1]

G. Nonoperative treatment is futile in patients with paralytic scoliosis who, despite orthotic treatment, continue to have curve progression. If the child is young, a subcutaneous Moe rod can be considered, which allows instrumentation without fusion. This must be followed by full-time bracing and yearly reoperation to lengthen the rod.

H. Luque segmental spinal instrumentation (SSI),[4] using L-shaped rods wired to each vertebral segment, has become an almost standard method for instrumentation in neuromuscular scoliosis.[2] Prior to this advance, most NM scoliosis required anterior and posterior fusion. Now, guidelines are being established concerning NM curves that can be treated by posterior fusion alone, with SSI. Current suggested guidelines are included in the algorithm. When the curve is severe or rigid, or when posterior elements are absent, anterior disc excision and grafting is advised prior to posterior SSI. Dwyer instrumentation, along with the disc excision, is reserved for the more severe curves.

## REFERENCES

1. Drennan JC, Renshaw TS, Curtis BH. The thoracic suspension orthosis. Clin Orthop. 1979; 139:33.
2. Herring JA, Wenger DR. Segmental spinal instrumentation: a preliminary report of forty consecutive cases. Spine 1982; 7:285.
3. Johnson CJ, Hakala MW, Rosenberger R. Paralytic spinal deformity: orthotic treatment in spinal discontinuity syndromes. J Ped Orthop. 1982; 2:233.
4. Luque ER. The anatomic basis and development of segmental spinal instrumentation. Spine 1982; 7:256.
5. Wilkens KE, Gibson DA. The pattern of spinal deformity in Duchenne muscular dystrophy. J Bone Joint Surg. 1976; 58A:24.

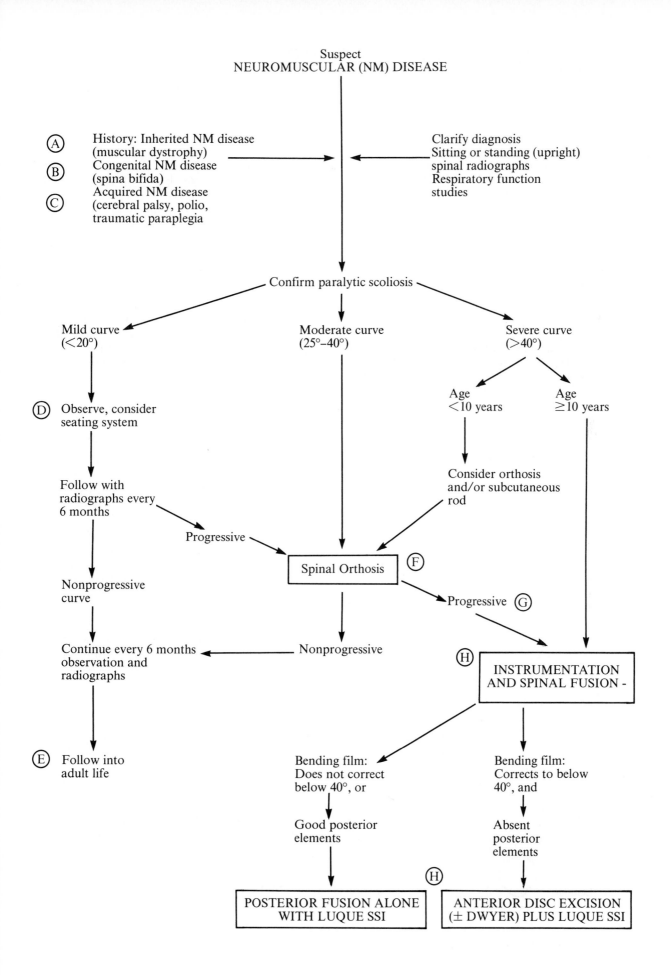

Suspect
NEUROMUSCULAR (NM) DISEASE

(A)  History: Inherited NM disease
     (muscular dystrophy)
(B)  Congenital NM disease
     (spina bifida)
(C)  Acquired NM disease
     (cerebral palsy, polio,
     traumatic paraplegia

Clarify diagnosis
Sitting or standing (upright)
spinal radiographs
Respiratory function
studies

Confirm paralytic scoliosis

Mild curve
(<20°)

Moderate curve
(25°–40°)

Severe curve
(>40°)

Age
<10 years

Age
≥10 years

(D)  Observe, consider
     seating system

Consider orthosis
and/or subcutaneous
rod

Follow with
radiographs every
6 months

Progressive

Spinal Orthosis    (F)

Nonprogressive
curve

Progressive  (G)

Continue every 6 months
observation and
radiographs

Nonprogressive

(H)  INSTRUMENTATION
     AND SPINAL FUSION -

(E)  Follow into
     adult life

Bending film:
Does not correct
below 40°, or

Bending film:
Corrects to below
40°, and

Good posterior
elements

Absent
posterior
elements

(H)

POSTERIOR FUSION ALONE
WITH LUQUE SSI

ANTERIOR DISC EXCISION
(± DWYER) PLUS LUQUE SSI

# CONGENITAL SCOLIOSIS

## COMMENTS

A. Congenital scoliosis is commonly associated with soft tissue anomalies of the spine, such as diastematomyelia or a tethered spinal cord, disorders that present as deformity or dysfunction in the lower extremity (e.g., equinovarus foot).

B. The association between congenital spinal anomalies and anomalies of the genitourinary (GU) system has been well described, with abnormalities in the IVP or cystogram noted in 20% of cases.[2] As a minimum, a careful history regarding the GU system should be taken and urinalysis, BUN, and creatinine performed. Ideally, an IVP and cystogram should be performed to screen for these abnormalities.

C. Intraspinal soft tissue anomalies associated with congenital scoliosis are often manifested by overlying skin abnormalities. These range from a hair patch, a dimple, or hemangioma to a subcutaneous lipoma. Their presence should alert you to the possibility of a diastematomyelia or another anomaly, and if associated with progressive neurologic defect, it constitutes an indication for a myelogram.

D. Unilateral unsegmented bars almost always result in curve progression and, when clearly documented in a growing child, form an indication for in-situ fusion.

E. When performing an in-situ fusion in a young child, only the affected region is fused to allow spinal growth in the remaining segments. Some children remain unbalanced and require subsequent spinal bracing. In certain cases, the compensatory curves above and below the fused segment slowly progress, requiring a longer spinal fusion in adolescence.

F. Although the congenital scoliosis itself will not be improved by a brace, bracing is often effective in controlling compensatory curves.[4]

G. Although careful observation and documentation are required, not all congenital curves are progressive, with only about 50% requiring specific treatment (bracing or surgery). The remaining patients maintain a balanced trunk and spine despite their vertebral anomalies.

H. Most spinal fusions for congenital scoliosis are performed in-situ without instrumentation. In certain cases, when long compensatory curves above and below the deformed segment also need to be included in the fusion, consideration can be given to using a Harrington rod, which provides some correction and greater internal stability.[1] In such cases, a myelogram should be performed prior to instrumentation, and the distraction forces at surgery should be minimal.

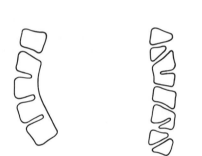

HEMIVERTEBRA     UNSEGMENTED BAR     COMBINED DEFECT

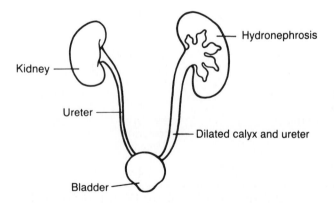

Kidney

Ureter

Bladder

Hydronephrosis

Dilated calyx and ureter

Top, Types of congenital scoliosis. Bottom, Associated GU anomalies.

## REFERENCES

1. Hall JE, Herndon WA, Levine CR. Surgical treatment of congenital scoliosis with or without Harrington instrumentation. J Bone Joint Surg. 1981;63(A):608.
2. MacEwen GD, Winter RB, Hardy JH. Evaluation of kidney anomalies in congenital scoliosis. J. Bone Joint Surg. 1972; 54(A):1451.
3. Winter RB, Moe JH, Eilers VE. Congenital scoliosis, a study of 234 patients treated and untreated. J Bone Joint Surg. 1968; 50(A):1.
4. Winter RB, MacEwen GD, Moe JH, Peon H. Milwaukee brace in congenital scoliosis. Spine 1976; 1:85.

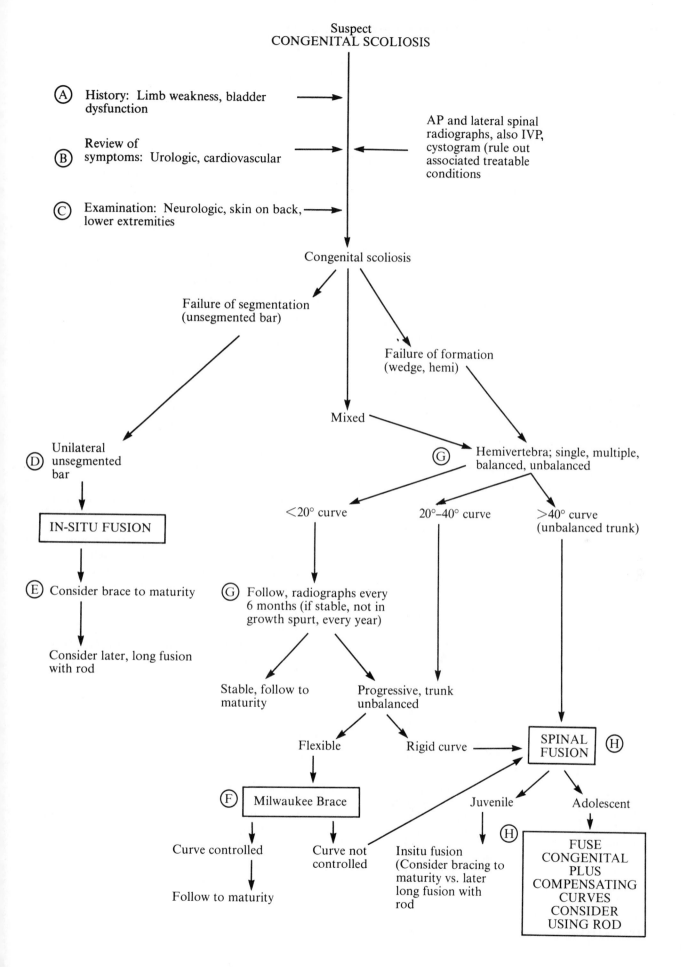

Suspect
CONGENITAL SCOLIOSIS

(A) History: Limb weakness, bladder dysfunction

(B) Review of symptoms: Urologic, cardiovascular

AP and lateral spinal radiographs, also IVP, cystogram (rule out associated treatable conditions

(C) Examination: Neurologic, skin on back, lower extremities

Congenital scoliosis

Failure of segmentation (unsegmented bar)

Failure of formation (wedge, hemi)

Mixed

(D) Unilateral unsegmented bar

(G) Hemivertebra; single, multiple, balanced, unbalanced

IN-SITU FUSION

<20° curve

20°–40° curve

>40° curve (unbalanced trunk)

(E) Consider brace to maturity

(G) Follow, radiographs every 6 months (if stable, not in growth spurt, every year)

Consider later, long fusion with rod

Stable, follow to maturity

Progressive, trunk unbalanced

Flexible

Rigid curve

SPINAL FUSION (H)

(F) Milwaukee Brace

Juvenile

Adolescent

Curve controlled

Curve not controlled

Insitu fusion (Consider bracing to maturity vs. later long fusion with rod

(H)

Follow to maturity

FUSE CONGENITAL PLUS COMPENSATING CURVES CONSIDER USING ROD

# SCHEUERMANN'S DISEASE (ADOLESCENT ROUNDBACK)

## COMMENTS

A. Scheuermann's disease has been reported to be transmitted in an autosomal dominant mode[3]; therefore, look at the parents. Distinguishing "normal" from "abnormal" is very difficult in adolescent roundback. Significant pain during adolescence is uncommon, except for lumbar Scheuermann's, which is characteristically painful. Other disorders that might cause roundback and vertebral wedging include trauma, rickets, osteogenesis imperfecta, idiopathic juvenile osteoporosis, neurofibromatosis, as well as bone dysplasias (achondroplasia, Morquio's, spondylopiphyseal dysplasia).[4] Patients with roundback often have tight hamstrings, a factor believed by some to be the cause of the roundback (tight hamstrings produce pelvic extension, which in turn causes truck extension and a need to adopt flexion of the thorax (increased kyphosis) to maintain postural balance. Also, tight pectorals contribute to associated round shoulders.

B. Radiographs include an AP to evaluate for scoliosis, an associated deformity noted in 25% of cases which, fortunately, is rarely progressive. The lateral view rules out known causes of kyphosis (congenital, bone dysplasias) and allows the kyphosis to be measured (Cobb method) as well as wedging to be assessed. Hyperextension lateral views are used to determine flexibility (and correctability) of the kyphosis. Schmorl's nodes (end-plate erosions) are commonly seen in Scheuermann's disease.

C. Patients with a rigid deformity, greater than 40° kyphosis, and wedging of greater than 5° at three levels have Scheuermann's disease. Patients with a significant roundback deformity who remain flexible and have no wedged vertebra on radiograph are said to have postural roundback.[1]

D. Children with mild deformity can be treated by a physical therapy program which focuses on stretching (hamstrings, pectorals, anterior longitudinal ligament) as well as strengthening (spine extensor muscles).

E. A modified Milwaukee brace (see figure) provides a three-point corrective force which is extremely effective in treating both Scheuermann's disease and adolescent roundback.[1] The brace must be used prior to vertebral end-plate closure (skeletal maturity) and is worn 23 hours per day for one year, followed by nighttime wear only for another year.

F. Surgical correction is rarely indicated for adolescent roundback because the long-term natural history of the disease is not predictably severe enough to warrant surgical correction in any but the most severe cases. Patients who fail brace treatment, refuse brace wear, or are skeletally mature when first seen should be considered for surgical correction only if three indications are met: (1) severity (greater than 70°), (2) severe pain, (3) severe cosmetic need. Successful surgery is demanding and includes anterior disc excision plus bone grafting, followed by posterior Harrington compression instrumentation 2 weeks later.[2]

## REFERENCES

1. Bradford DS, et al. Scheuermann's kyphosis and roundback; results of Milwaukee brace treatment. J Bone Joint Surg. 1974;56-A:740.
2. Bradford DS, et al. Scheuermann's kyphosis; results of surgical treatment by posterior spine arthrodesis in twenty-two patients. J Bone Joint Surg. 1975;57-A:439.
3. Halal F, et al. Dominant inheritance of Scheuermann's juvenile kyphosis. Am J Dis Child. 1978;132:1105.
4. Kling TF, et al. Adolescent round back deformity. Ortho Surv. 1982; 5:340

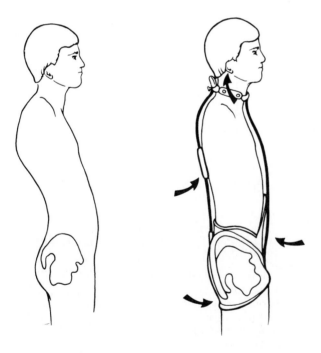

Modified Milwaukee brace used to correct roundback.

ADOLESCENT WITH ROUNDBACK

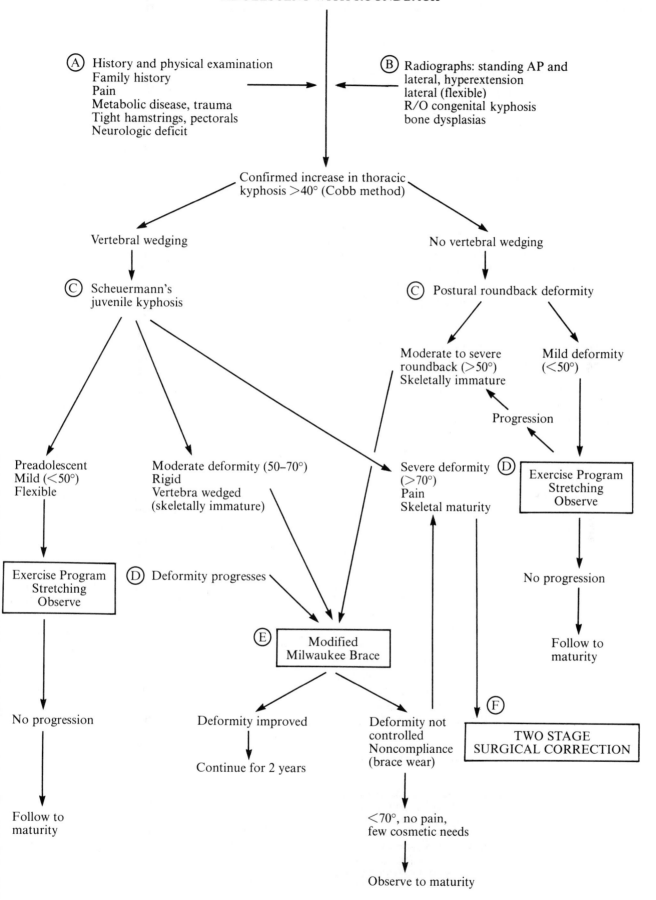

Ⓐ History and physical examination
Family history
Pain
Metabolic disease, trauma
Tight hamstrings, pectorals
Neurologic deficit

Ⓑ Radiographs: standing AP and
lateral, hyperextension
lateral (flexible)
R/O congenital kyphosis
bone dysplasias

Confirmed increase in thoracic
kyphosis >40° (Cobb method)

Vertebral wedging

No vertebral wedging

Ⓒ Scheuermann's
juvenile kyphosis

Ⓒ Postural roundback deformity

Moderate to severe
roundback (>50°)
Skeletally immature

Mild deformity
(<50°)

Progression

Preadolescent
Mild (<50°)
Flexible

Moderate deformity (50–70°)
Rigid
Vertebra wedged
(skeletally immature)

Severe deformity
(>70°)
Pain
Skeletal maturity

Ⓓ Exercise Program
Stretching
Observe

Exercise Program
Stretching
Observe

Ⓓ Deformity progresses

No progression

Ⓔ Modified
Milwaukee Brace

No progression

Follow to
maturity

Deformity improved

Deformity not
controlled
Noncompliance
(brace wear)

Ⓕ
TWO STAGE
SURGICAL CORRECTION

Follow to
maturity

Continue for 2 years

<70°, no pain,
few cosmetic needs

Observe to maturity

# SPONDYLOLYSIS AND SPONDYLOLISTHESIS

## COMMENTS

A. According to Wiltse, the incidence of spondylolysis is about 4.5% in preadolescent children, but rises to 12% in gymnasts. Thus, vigorous athletic activity in children may produce a fracture of a pars interarticularis, which is already weak on a genetic basis.[5] Scoliosis is commonly associated with spondylolisthesis; however, each disorder is addressed individually for treatment purposes.[3] Patients with significant spondylolisthesis have a classic appearance of a short torso and flat buttocks, often standing with their knees held in modest flexion. Neurologic status, including bladder function, must be assessed, although neurologic deficit is uncommon.

B. The pars defect appears as a band or break in the "scotty dog's neck" (pars interarticularis) of L5 on the oblique view. A standing spot lateral view of L5-S1, performed initially and at follow-up, allows an accurate assessment of possible slip progression. Bone scans will show increased activity on one or both sides in symptomatic spondylolysis,[4] but are not routinely required. Myelograms are rarely needed, except perhaps in preparing for surgery in a child with a neurologic deficit.

C. Wiltse describes five types of spondylolisthesis (dysplastic, isthmic, degenerative, traumatic, pathologic).[5] Most cases in children are of the dysplastic or isthmic type.

D. Patients with acute symptoms and a pars defect may actually heal the defect, much as any fracture would heal, after 10 to 12 weeks of immobilization in a plaster body jacket or a Boston type spinal orthosis. More chronic cases are instructed in back care, abdominal muscle strengthening, with a brace or corset used for persistent symptoms. In general, once symptoms resolve, the child can resume normal activities, although advice regarding return to rigorous spine-bending athletic events (gymnastics, down lineman in football) is controversial. Conservative physicians restrict the children; however, most allow self-limiting pain or slip progression which is treated by fusion to determine activity levels.

E. Slip severity is graded according to the amount that the body of L5 has slipped on S1 (see figure). In addition, a more severe *slip angle* (see figure) increases the probability of further slip and is considered a risk factor.[1]

F. Children with slips who have persistent tight hamstrings have pain despite eight months of conservative therapy, or have slip progression should be surgically stabilized by insitu lateral mass fusion, *without* removal of the L5 posterior elements. Moderate slips are fused from L5 to the sacrum. Severe slips, due to the geometry of the deformity encountered intraoperatively, must be fused from L4 to the sacrum.[6] Many surgeons use no postoperative immobilization or at most a corset. I advise 12 weeks in a lumbar body jacket with the cast extended to just above the knee on one side.

G. Patients with very severe deformities (grades 4 and 5) have a severe cosmetic deformity, but look surprisingly better after successful in-situ fusion, which alleviates hamstring spasm, knee flexion, and other causes of the cosmetic deformity. Because the incidence of pseudoarthrosis after fusion attempt is higher in this group, surgical reduction plus anterior and posterior fusion may be considered in extremely severe cases.[2]

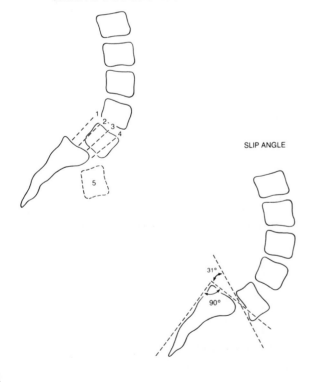

SEVERITY OF SPONDYLOLISTHESIS

SLIP ANGLE

## REFERENCES

1. Boxall D, et al. Management of severe spondylolisthesis in children and adolescents. J Bone Joint Surg. 1979;61-A:479.
2. Bradford DS, et al. Treatment of severe spondylolisthesis; a combined approach for reduction and stabilization. Spine 1979;4:423.
3. Fisk JR, et al. Scoliosis, spondylosis, and spondylisthesis; their relationship as reviewed in 539 patients. Spine 1978; 3:234.
4. Gelfand MJ, et al. Radionuclide bone imaging in spondylolysis of the lumbar spine in children. Radiology 1981;140:191.

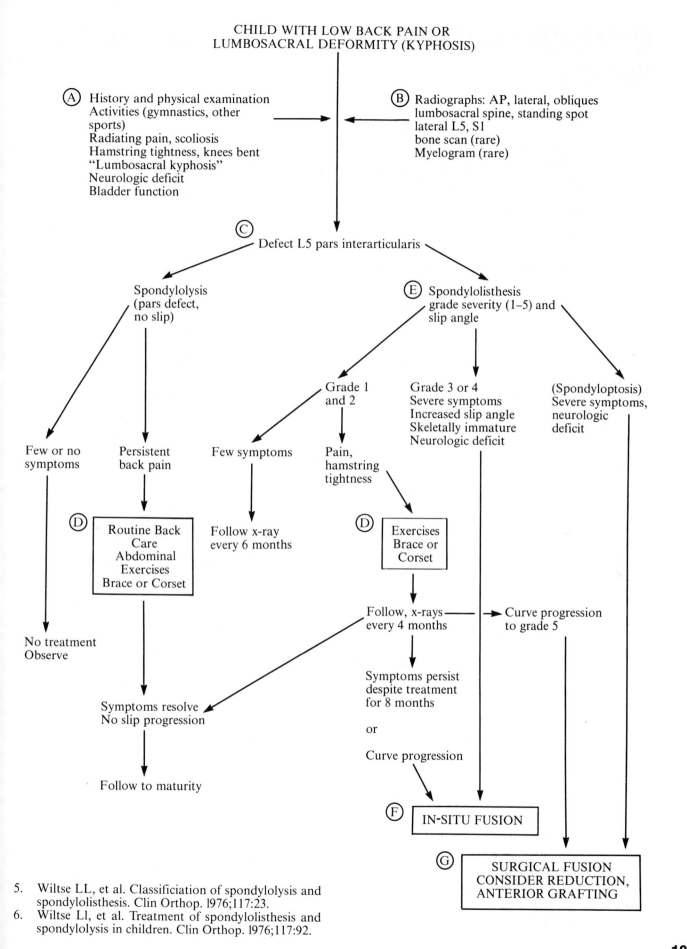

CHILD WITH LOW BACK PAIN OR
LUMBOSACRAL DEFORMITY (KYPHOSIS)

(A) History and physical examination
Activities (gymnastics, other
sports)
Radiating pain, scoliosis
Hamstring tightness, knees bent
"Lumbosacral kyphosis"
Neurologic deficit
Bladder function

(B) Radiographs: AP, lateral, obliques
lumbosacral spine, standing spot
lateral L5, S1
bone scan (rare)
Myelogram (rare)

(C) Defect L5 pars interarticularis

Spondylolysis
(pars defect,
no slip)

(E) Spondylolisthesis
grade severity (1–5) and
slip angle

Grade 1
and 2

Grade 3 or 4
Severe symptoms
Increased slip angle
Skeletally immature
Neurologic deficit

(Spondyloptosis)
Severe symptoms,
neurologic
deficit

Few or no
symptoms

Persistent
back pain

Few symptoms

Pain,
hamstring
tightness

(D) Routine Back
Care
Abdominal
Exercises
Brace or Corset

Follow x-ray
every 6 months

(D) Exercises
Brace or
Corset

No treatment
Observe

Follow, x-rays
every 4 months

Curve progression
to grade 5

Symptoms resolve
No slip progression

Symptoms persist
despite treatment
for 8 months

or

Curve progression

Follow to maturity

(F) IN-SITU FUSION

(G) SURGICAL FUSION
CONSIDER REDUCTION,
ANTERIOR GRAFTING

5. Wiltse LL, et al. Classificiation of spondylolysis and
spondylolisthesis. Clin Orthop. 1976;117:23.
6. Wiltse Ll, et al. Treatment of spondylolisthesis and
spondylolysis in children. Clin Orthop. 1976;117:92.

# CONGENITAL HIP DISLOCATION IN THE INFANT

### COMMENTS

A. CDH (congenital dislocation of the hip) is more common in breech delivered, female, first-born infants (uterus "tighter") and in families with a history of CDH. The Ortolani test, during which the femoral head is reduced and then redislocated over the acetabular rim (Fig. 1A), should be performed on all infants to establish the diagnosis. The baby must be relaxed and warm (preferably asleep) for a valid examination. A general examination should precede the hip examination and include neurologic assessment (paralytic ?, arthrogryposis ?), neck examination (torticollis associated with CDH), spine examination (spina bifida or variants), and foot examination (CDH associated with metatarsus varus). Infants with hip sepsis often have few systemic findings (fever, etc). Be certain that what you are calling a dislocated hip is truly congenital and not a septic condition. A congenital dislocation is never painful or stiff, whereas a septic hip in infancy usually is.

B. Because much of the hip is cartilaginous in infancy, radiographs are of limited value. The Von Rosen view (hips extended and abducted 45°, internally rotated) makes the malalignment of the involved femur more evident and is preferred by some.[5] The clinical examination is more important than the radiograph.

C. "Not reducible" means that the Ortolani test is no longer elicitable; thus, the hip is now fixed in the dislocated position. This is more common in an older infant or in a child with teratologic dislocation. Radiographically, the metaphysis (femoral head) is laterally positioned and directed *above* the triradiate cartilage, even in the hyperflexed Pavlik position. Despite this irreducibility, a several-week trial of the Pavlik harness is indicated because in many cases the hip does reduce, despite the initial fixed dislocation.

D. The Pavlik harness (Fig. 1B) has become a standard for treating CDH in children up to age 4 to 6 months. The reason for its wide acceptance is that with the harness the hip can be hyperflexed, and thus even difficult dislocated hips can be directed toward the triradiate cartilage. Hyperflexion is safe; however, the excessive tightening of the abduction straps (posterior) may lead to avascular necrosis. Even though the radiograph initially shows the femoral head to be lateralized, the position is accepted as long as the head is directed toward the triradiate cartilage. Subsequent visits should demonstrate "penetration" of the femoral head into the acetabulum or, occasionally, failure to reduce. The Pavlik harness is complicated, and most failures are due to failure of physicians and parents to understand and use the device properly. In difficult social situations, hospital admission for initial instruction should be considered. The physician should see the child weekly for 2 weeks and then monthly until the outcome has been established.

E. Most infants achieve a reduction and begin to develop a more normal acetabulum in 3 months. Older children require longer treatment. Initial monthly check radiographs are taken in the hyperflexed Pavlik position. After 3 months of treatment, a hip extension film should be performed to confirm that the reduction is stable.

F. Newborns often have normal hips after 3 months of treatment. Older infants may require much longer treatment. Eventually, the child is weaned to nap- and nighttime wear. Abduction splinting, at least part-time, should be continued until the hip is radiographically normal. In older infants, this is made easier by switching from the Pavlik harness to a Lorenz, Camp, Ilfeld, or other type of abduction device.

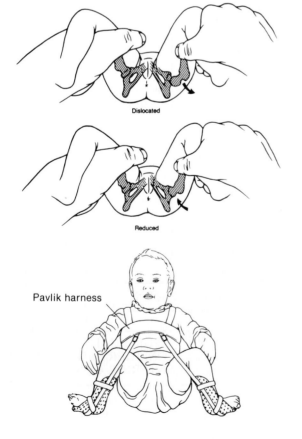

Ortolani maneuver to diagnose CDH in infancy

Dislocated

Reduced

Pavlik harness

# INFANT WITH SUSPECTED HIP DISORDER

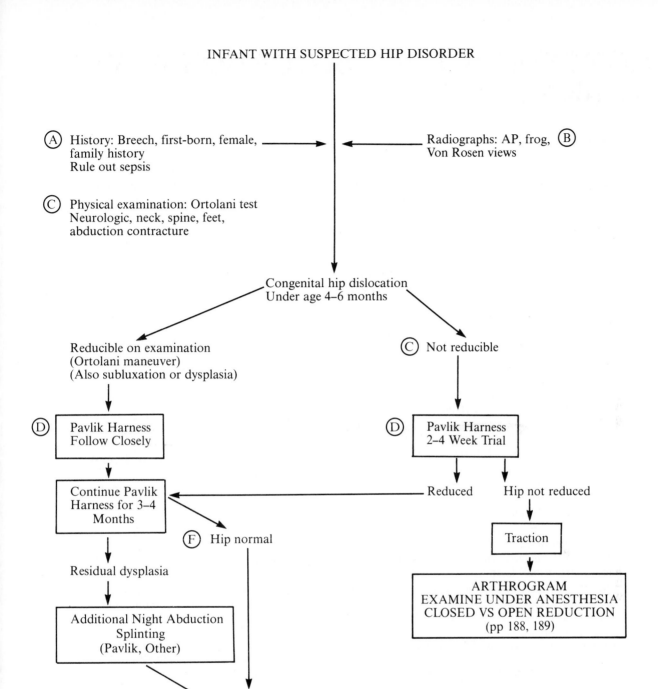

(A) History: Breech, first-born, female,
family history
Rule out sepsis

(B) Radiographs: AP, frog,
Von Rosen views

(C) Physical examination: Ortolani test
Neurologic, neck, spine, feet,
abduction contracture

Congenital hip dislocation
Under age 4–6 months

Reducible on examination
(Ortolani maneuver)
(Also subluxation or dysplasia)

(C) Not reducible

(D) Pavlik Harness
Follow Closely

(D) Pavlik Harness
2–4 Week Trial

Continue Pavlik
Harness for 3–4
Months

Reduced

Hip not reduced

(F) Hip normal

Traction

Residual dysplasia

ARTHROGRAM
EXAMINE UNDER ANESTHESIA
CLOSED VS OPEN REDUCTION
(pp 188, 189)

Additional Night Abduction
Splinting
(Pavlik, Other)

Normal hip

## REFERENCES

1. Coleman SS. *Congenital Dysplasia and Dislocation of the Hip*. St. Louis: CV Mosby, 1978.
2. Hensinger RN. Treatment in early infancy: birth to two months. In *Congenital Dislocation of the Hip*. Edited by MO Tachdjian. New York: Churchill Livingstone, 1982.
3. MacEwen GD, Ramsey DL. The hip. In *Pediatric Orthopaedics*. Edited by WW Lovel and R.B. Winter. Philadelphia: JB Lippincott, 1978.
4. Mubarak SJ. Pitfalls in the use of the Pavlik harness for congenital dysplasia, subluxation, and dislocation of the hip. J Bone Joint Surg. 1981; 63A:1239.
5. Von Rosen S. Early diagnosis and treatment of congenital dislocation of the hip joint. Acta Orthop Scand 1957; 26:136.

# CONGENITAL HIP DISLOCATION IN THE YOUNG CHILD

## COMMENTS

A. Within a few months after birth, a congenitally dislocated hip can no longer be reduced and redislocated (Ortolani maneuver). The hip is now in a fixed, dislocated position, and physical findings include limited hip abduction and a short thigh when both hips are flexed (Galeazzi sign).

B. After about the age of 6 months, the Pavlik is less effective in treating a fixed, dislocated hip. These patients require hospitalization for skin traction to stretch the capsule, ligaments, and muscles to prepare for a safe closed reduction under anesthesia. The type of traction used differs from center to center. Variations of Bryant's traction are effective; however, the physician and nursing staff must be well acquainted with the traction method used to avoid the complications of skin and compartmental slough. A few centers have used home traction successfully.[2] Many centers use traction for an arbitrary 2 weeks, whereas others require radiographic documentation of improved femoral head position or "stations" before reduction is attempted.[1]

C. The decision for closed versus open reduction is made in the operating room after examination under anesthesia, arthrogram, and adductor tenotomy. The sense of clinical stability with a wide "safe zone" is the most important determinant in proceeding with closed reduction. The "safe zone" refers to the degrees between maximal abduction and adduction to the point that the femoral head redislocates. A percutaneous adductor tenotomy usually improves the "safe zone".

D. The human position implies hyperflexion of the hips (120°) with only modest abduction (50°). This position is less likely to place excessive pressure on the femoral head and is advised to avoid avascular necrosis. This is in contrast to the traditional Lorenz or frog position (90° flexion, 90° abduction), which has been indicted as contributing to avascular necrosis.

E. The goals of open reduction are different in young children (less than 15 months) than older children. In the younger child with an arthrographically documented block to reduction, release of this obstruction (capsular constriction, psoas tendon) by the medial (Ludloff) approach is all that is needed. The capsule is not opened excessively, as this may lead to residual subluxation. The remainder of treatment is the same as with closed reduction, since capsulorrhaphy or internal stability is not provided. Thus, the human position cast is required for at least 3 months. Because the anatomy in the depths of the adductor region is not familiar to many surgeons, the medial approach should be used only by those trained in the method. Older children (more than 15 months) are better served by anterior open reduction, which allows capsulorrphaphy.

F. Children over the age of 2 years should have open reduction without an attempt at closed reduction. Traditionally, these children have been treated with preliminary skin or skeletal traction followed by open reduction, often including innominate osteotomy. Recent experience has demonstrated that older children (4 years old and older) can be safely treated by primary open reduction, including femoral shortening, thus avoiding the need for preoperative traction. As experience expands, some younger children (2 to 4 years of age) have been treated by means of femoral shortening without traction. Whether or not the femur is shortened, an effective capsulorrhaphy is the key to maintaining reduction.[5]

## REFERENCES

1. Gage J, Winter RB. Avasclar necrosis of the capital femoral epiphysis as a complication of closed reduction of congenital dislocation of the hip. J Bone Joint Surg. 1972; 54A:373.
2. Keenan J, MacEwen GD, et al. Home traction in the management of congenital dislocation of the hip. Clin Orthop. 1982; 165:83
3. Mau H, et al. Open reduction of congenital dislocation of the hip by Ludloff's method. J Bone Joint Surg. 1971; 53A:1281.
4. Renshaw T. Inadequate reduction of congental dislocation of the hip. J Bone Joint Surg. 1981; 63A:1114.
5. Salter RB, et al. The first fifteen years' personal experience with innominate osteotomy in the treatment of congenital dislocation and subluxation of the hip. Clin Orthop. 1974; 98:72.

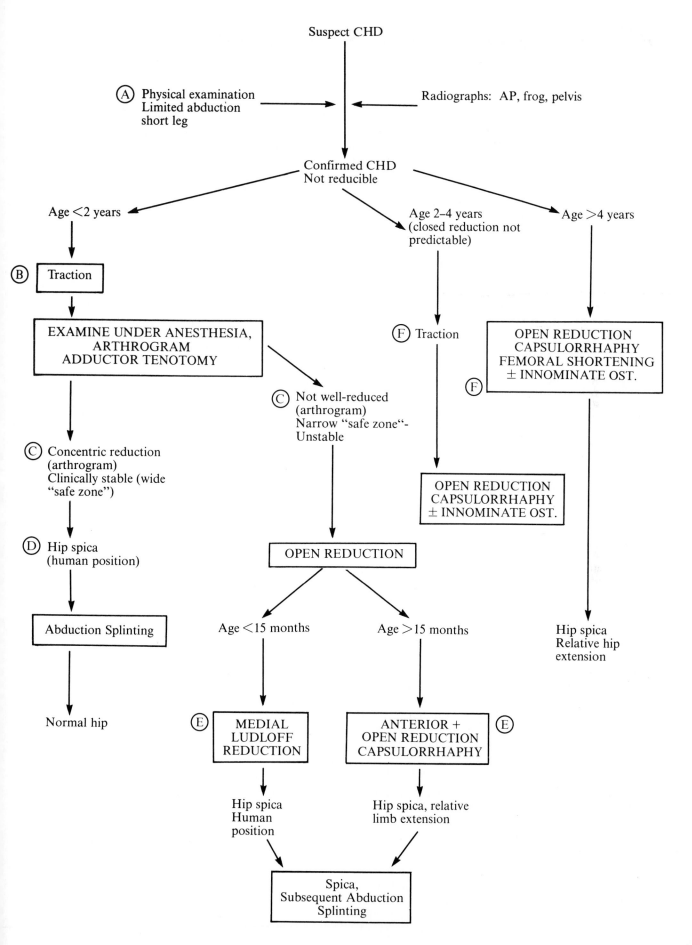

# ACUTE TRANSIENT SYNOVITIS

## COMMENTS

A. Acute transient synovitis of the hip, also known as toxic synovitis, transient arthritis, irritable hip syndrome, and observation hip is a poorly understood cause of childhood limp or refusal to walk. The condition often parallels or follows a viral upper respiratory infection and has been considered by some to represent a viral or perhaps "viral-immune response" disorder affecting the hip. The treating physician's main responsibility is to clearly establish whether he can just observe the patient or whether the child may have hip sepsis (clearly not an observation hip). Legg-Perthes disease and monoarticular rheumatoid arthritis must also be considered.

B. Transient synovitis is most common between the ages of 2 and 10 years and occurs more frequently in males. In severe cases, the child refuses to walk and has markedly limited hip motion. In less severe cases the child limps and guards his hip when examined.

C. The hip range of motion examination helps to distinguish transient synovitis from hip sepsis. An experienced examiner can usually differentiate the guarded, partially limited motion of transient synovitis from the severely restricted, extremely painful motion associated with hip sepsis. Because the foregoing applies only to "standard" cases, laboratory studies (temperature, white blood cell count, sedimentation rate) are vital.

D. Occasionally, in experienced hands, and more frequently in inexperienced hands, the final distinction between transient synovitis hip sepsis is determined by needle aspiration under image intensifier, including an injection of radiopaque dye into the joint to confirm the intra-articular position of the needle tip.

E. Laboratory data in transient synovitis include mild temperature elevation, mild increase in WBC, mild sedimentation rate elevation (usually normal). If the physical examination and blood analysis are not convincing, hip aspiration may need to be considered. Aspirated fluid in transient synovitis may be clear, cloudy, or even bloody (traumatic hip), but is always sterile.

F. Initial treatment is bed rest, usually at home. Home traction can be used in more persistent cases. Occasionally, hospitalization is required to perform the studies needed to rule out sepsis and thus allay parental and physician concern.

G. Failure to resolve with rest should lead to a more extensive work-up. the bone scan is useful to rule out rare disorders such as sacroiliac joint infection, osteomyelitis of the ilium, osteoid osteoma, and other conditons that may mimic transient synovitis of the hip.

H. A few patients with transient synovitis (2 to 5%), especially those with recurrent episodes, go on to develop Legg-Perthes disease during the subsequent year. This is probably the result of increase intracapsular pressure producing vascular tamponade. Therefore, patients with transient synovitis should have their hips examined once or twice in the year following the episode of transient synovitis. Radiographs are unnecessary if hip motion is full.

## REFERENCES

1. Nachemson A, Scheller S. A clinical and radiographic follow-up study of transient synovitis of the hip. Acta Orthop Scand. 1969;40:479.
2. Sharwood PF. The irritable hip syndrome in children. A long-term follow-up. Acta Orthop Scand. 1981;52(6):633.
3. Valderrama JAF. The observation hip syndrome and its late sequelae. J Bone Joint Surg. 1963;45B:462.

HIP SYNOVITIS

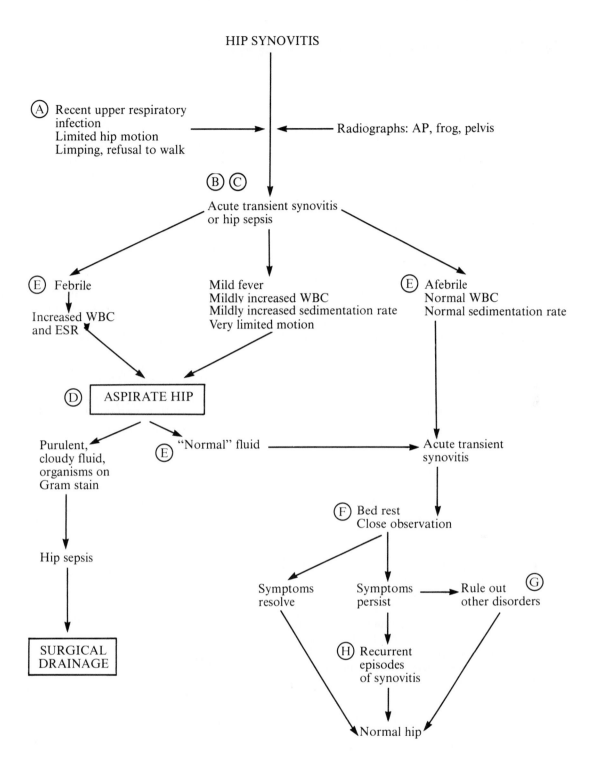

Ⓐ Recent upper respiratory infection
Limited hip motion
Limping, refusal to walk

Radiographs: AP, frog, pelvis

Ⓑ Ⓒ Acute transient synovitis or hip sepsis

Ⓔ Febrile

Increased WBC and ESR

Mild fever
Mildly increased WBC
Mildly increased sedimentation rate
Very limited motion

Ⓔ Afebrile
Normal WBC
Normal sedimentation rate

Ⓓ ASPIRATE HIP

Purulent, cloudy fluid, organisms on Gram stain

Ⓔ "Normal" fluid

Acute transient synovitis

Hip sepsis

Ⓕ Bed rest
Close observation

SURGICAL DRAINAGE

Symptoms resolve

Symptoms persist

Rule out other disorders Ⓖ

Ⓗ Recurrent episodes of synovitis

Normal hip

191

# LEGG-PERTHES DISEASE

## COMMENTS

A. Legg-Perthes disease is the result of avascular necrosis of the femoral head in a growing child. The reason for the avascular necrosis is unknown. Children with this disorder are often small for age, wiry, and hyperactive, with a bone age that is delayed by 1 to 2 years. They often present with pain referred to the knee and may arrive with knee radiographs, performed by an unwary physician. Decreased hip abduction and internal rotation are the classic physical findings.

B. In the earliest radiographic stage (Waldenström), only widening of the cartilage space is noted. Later, the ossific nucleus appears more dense (avascular stage). The "45° frog" radiograph (frog position, but flexed only 45° and abducted only 45°) is the best view to demonstrate the "crescent sign" or fracture between the normal cartilage-subchondral bone and the avascular epiphysis. The extent of this line is an early indicator of the extent of head involvement.

C. Age is an important indicator of outcome. Children under 5 years very often do well without specific treatment. Children over age 10 years react like adults, with avascular necrosis, and often fare badly no matter how well you treat them. Severe loss of hip motion is also an important guide to outcome, both at diagnosis and throughout treatment.

D. Catterall has classified Legg-Perthes disease according to the percentage of the femoral head that is avascular (1=25%, 2=50%, 3=75%, 4=100%) (see figure).[1] The circumstance has been compared to a myocardial infarction. A small infarction of the femoral head produces a Catterall 1, whereas a severe infarction results in a Catterall 4. With more complete head involvement, the patient is more likely to develop permanent femoral head shape change, thus increasing the risk for adult arthritis.

E. Catterall also describes "at risk" factors. When two or more are present, the patient is "at risk" for head shape change and, therefore, should be treated. The "at risk" factors are predictably more common in older children with Catterall 3 or 4 involvement. They include: (1) lateral subluxation, (2) lateral calcification, (3) large metaphyseal cyst, (4) Gage's sign (triangular lucency—lateral physis and epiphysis due to repair tissue), and (5) horizontal growth plate.

F. As implied earlier, the treatment goal is to maintain hip range of motion—and thus maintain a round femoral head—during the temporary period of avascularity and healing when the head is biologically plastic. This is achieved by an abduction device, which contains the "at risk" femoral head within the acetabulum. Choices for abduction bracing include the Craig Splint, Toronto brace, Atlanta brace, and others. The Atlanta brace is currently most popular because children find it more acceptable.

G. Examination under anesthesia plus arthrogram provides important information regarding head deformity, flattening, and subluxation. An adductor release improves hip abduction. An optional intramuscular psoas tendon release—anterior approach, just below inguinal ligament, just lateral to the femoral nerve—improves extension and internal rotation. Postoperative Petrie casts maintain the improved motion that has been gained. Petrie casts (two long leg casts with broomsticks between them to maintain abduction) are remarkably effective in Legg-Perthes disease.[3] Their weight alone provides a ballast—which the irritated hip is unable to resist—with resulting abduction and containment.

H. There is no certain *medical* indication for surgical containment because even difficult patients can be contained by a combination of releases, Petrie casts, and braces. There are other sociologic and psychologic reasons for surgical containment (refusal to wear brace, living in mobile home, already a teenager). The distinct advantage of surgical containment is its permanence, since the patient cannot remove it. A proximal femoral osteotomy (varus, derotation, extension) fixed with an AO blade plate is my preference, as it decompresses an irritated joint. Complications are common following surgical containment[5] and should be understood.

## REFERENCES

1. Catterall A. The natural history of Perthes disease. J Bone Joint Surg. 1971;53B:37.
2. Moseley C. The biomechanics of the pediatric hip. Orthop Clin Am. 1980;11:3.
3. Petrie JG, et al. The abduction weight-bearing treatment in Legg-Perthes disease. J Bone Joint Surg. 1971;53B:54.
4. Salter RB. The pathogenesis of deformity in Legg-Perthes disease. J Bone Joint Surg. 1966;48B:389.
5. Wenger DR. Selective surgical containment for Legg-Perthes disease: Recognition and management of complications. J Ped Orthop. 1981;1:153.

Suspected
LEGG-PERTHES DISEASE

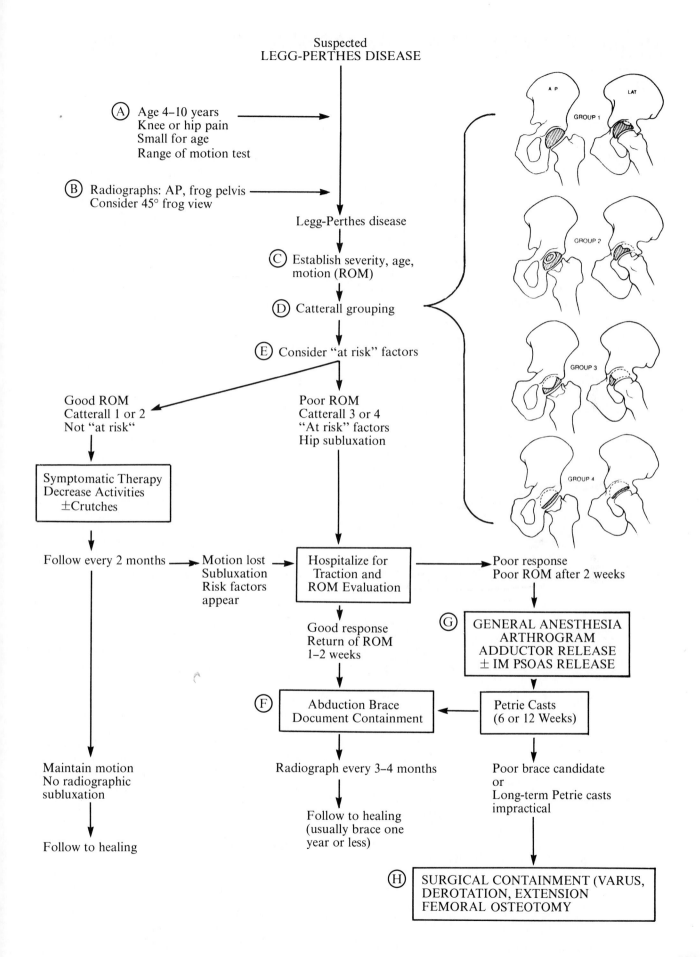

Ⓐ Age 4–10 years
Knee or hip pain
Small for age
Range of motion test

Ⓑ Radiographs: AP, frog pelvis
Consider 45° frog view

Legg-Perthes disease

Ⓒ Establish severity, age,
motion (ROM)

Ⓓ Catterall grouping

Ⓔ Consider "at risk" factors

Good ROM
Catterall 1 or 2
Not "at risk"

Poor ROM
Catterall 3 or 4
"At risk" factors
Hip subluxation

Symptomatic Therapy
Decrease Activities
±Crutches

Follow every 2 months → Motion lost
Subluxation
Risk factors
appear

Hospitalize for
Traction and
ROM Evaluation

Poor response
Poor ROM after 2 weeks

Good response
Return of ROM
1–2 weeks

Ⓖ GENERAL ANESTHESIA
ARTHROGRAM
ADDUCTOR RELEASE
± IM PSOAS RELEASE

Maintain motion
No radiographic
subluxation

Ⓕ Abduction Brace
Document Containment

Petrie Casts
(6 or 12 Weeks)

Radiograph every 3–4 months

Poor brace candidate
or
Long-term Petrie casts
impractical

Follow to healing

Follow to healing
(usually brace one
year or less)

Ⓗ SURGICAL CONTAINMENT (VARUS,
DEROTATION, EXTENSION
FEMORAL OSTEOTOMY

# SLIPPED CAPITAL FEMORAL EPIPHYSIS (SCFE)

## COMMENTS

A. Kline's line and the metaphyseal blur are important clues to early SCFE on the AP view (see figure); however, a lateral view is vital to confirm the diagnosis. A cross-table lateral is preferred in severe cases (patients have trouble getting into the frog position) and in patients with acute symptoms (the forced frog position could precipitate further slipping). Radiographs are important in distinguishing between an acute and a chronic slip. Chronic slips demonstrate metaphyseal "rounding-off" (remodeling).

B. Acute slips are rare (less than 10% of total) and must be recognized because they are the only type that can be reduced with reasonable safety. Any attempt to reduce a chronic slip will produce avascular necrosis. Acute slips follow specific trauma, and the patients have severe pain, similar to that in an adult with a hip fracture.

C. Acute slips can be reduced by two methods. The most gentle is to place a stout, threaded distal femoral traction pin with 7 to 10 pounds longitudinal traction and 2 to 3 pounds attached to the lateral extension of the pin to provide an internal rotation moment. This usually reduces an acute slip (or the acute component of a sub-acute slip) overnight, and the slip can then be pinned. A second method, acceptable for true acute slips only, is manipulative reduction under general anesthesia, followed by pin fixation.

D. Large threaded Steinman pins or AO epiphyseal screws are the best choices for pinning. Hagie pins, Knowles pins, and others are not removable—they break when removal is attempted because of the large threaded head and narrow shaft. Clear radiographic control is vital to keep the pins well away from the articular surface. Many cases of chondrolysis are the result of pins left permanently protruding into the hip joint. Read Walter's account and be certain you understand the "hidden pin in the three-quarter position" concept.[4]

E. Acute slip on a pre-existing chronic slip is a difficult diagnosis to establish with certainty. It is usually made by careful correlation of the history and radiographic findings. In these rare cases, the acute component of the slip can be reduced by the method described in C with the chronic component pinned insitu. The hip may be "over-reduced", with resulting avascular necrosis; thus, undercorrection or partial correction is advised.

F. Most slips are chronic and must not be reduced, as reduction produces avascular necrosis. The head has been in the "slipped position" for a long time and cannot be safely reduced. Even severe slips can be pinned or bone grafted insitu with subsequent remodeling, resulting in excellent hip motion and function.[1]

G. Because of the many reported complications with pin fixation (pin protrusion with chondrolysis, inability to remove pins), bone grafting is again becoming popular.[2] No pins are needed; thus, pin removal is avoided. The method is effective, but the surgical procedure is more extensive.

H. Southwick's corrective triplane proximal femoral osteotomy can be considered in very severe slips.[3] Most conservative centers prefer to pin or graft even the severe cases, and corrective osteotomy is performed electively one year later only in patients with residual deformity (fixed external rotation). This philosophy nearly obviates corrective osteotomy.

## REFERENCES

1. Boyer D, et al. Slipped capital femoral epiphysis. Long-term follow-up study of 121 patients. J Bone Joint Surg. 1981;63A:85.
2. Melby A, et al. Treatment of chronic slipped capital femoral epiphysis by bone graft epiphyseodesis. J Bone Joint Surg. 1980;62:119.

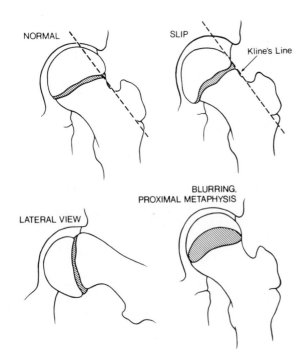

Radiographic changes in slipped capital femoral epiphysis.

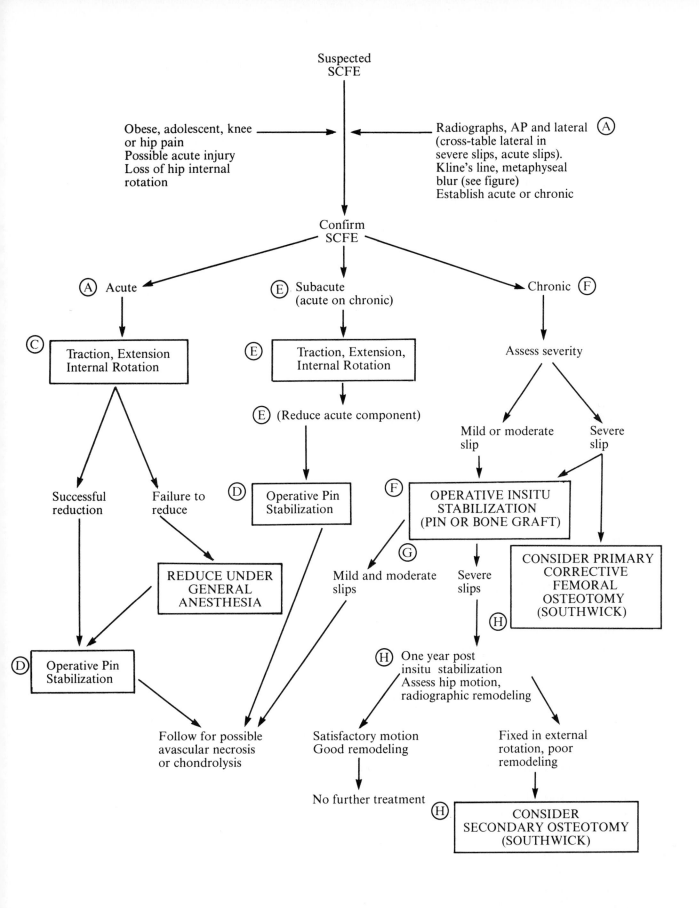

Suspected
SCFE

Obese, adolescent, knee
or hip pain
Possible acute injury
Loss of hip internal
rotation

Radiographs, AP and lateral (A)
(cross-table lateral in
severe slips, acute slips).
Kline's line, metaphyseal
blur (see figure)
Establish acute or chronic

Confirm
SCFE

(A) Acute     (E) Subacute     Chronic (F)
              (acute on chronic)

(C) Traction, Extension     (E) Traction, Extension,     Assess severity
Internal Rotation           Internal Rotation

(E) (Reduce acute component)

Successful    Failure to     Mild or moderate     Severe
reduction     reduce         slip                 slip

(D) Operative Pin     (F) OPERATIVE INSITU
Stabilization         STABILIZATION
                      (PIN OR BONE GRAFT)

REDUCE UNDER
GENERAL          (G)
ANESTHESIA

Mild and moderate     Severe          CONSIDER PRIMARY
slips                 slips           CORRECTIVE
                                      FEMORAL
                                  (H) OSTEOTOMY
                                      (SOUTHWICK)

(D) Operative Pin
Stabilization

(H) One year post
insitu stabilization
Assess hip motion,
radiographic remodeling

Follow for possible      Satisfactory motion     Fixed in external
avascular necrosis       Good remodeling         rotation, poor
or chondrolysis                                  remodeling

                         No further treatment

                                             (H) CONSIDER
                                                 SECONDARY OSTEOTOMY
                                                 (SOUTHWICK)

3. Southwick WO. Osteotomy through the lesser trochanter for slipped capital femoral epiphysis. J Bone
Joint Surg. 1967;49A:807.
4. Walters R, Simon SS. Joint destruction: a sequela of
unrecognized pin penetration in patients with slipped
capital femoral epiphysis. In *The Hip. Proceedings of
the Eighth Open Scientific Meeting of The Hip Society*.
St. Louis: CV Mosby, 1980.

# KNEE PAIN IN THE ADOLESCENT

## COMMENTS

A. Patients with hip disease present with knee pain due to referred pain. Always perform a hip range of motion examination in patients with supposed knee pain. *Never* arthroscopically examine a knee without a prior careful physical examination of the entire patient, with particular attention paid to the hip examination.

B. First, look at all tissues (bone, soft tissue) to rule out tumors, hemangiomas, and other lesions. Then think about specific knee pathology. Four views are required to completely evaluate the knee. The physical examination should be performed first, however, and if the disease is obvious (ie., Osgood-Schlatter), AP and lateral views may suffice. The tunnel or notch view is essential to diagnose osteochondritis dissecans. The sunrise or tunnel view may aid in assessing patellar alignment. Specific variants of this view (Merchant, Laurin) should be studied. Then select one as a standard for your radiographer.

C. Careful physical examination should localize the disorder (patellar, joint line, intra-articular). The usual tests for intra-articular disorders (McMurray, Apley tests), as well as tests for knee ligament stability, are performed. Chronicity is determined by measuring thigh and calf diameters on the normal and symptomatic sides. Patients with serious disease (especially tumors) have atrophy.

D. A congenital discoid meniscus produces a characteristic lateral joint line clunk or click with flexion and extension. The abnormal meniscus may be torn. Partial surgical excision of the torn portion or the portion medial to the lateral condyle relieves symptoms in patients who have pain. No treatment is required if the child has no symptoms.

E. Popliteal cysts (Baker's cysts) are common in children. In contrast to adults, the disorder in children usually is *not* associated with intra-articular disease. Thus, further assessment (i.e., arthroscopy) is not warranted, unless there are complaints or findings to suggest an internal derangement. The soft tissue detail on the lateral radiograph should be scrutinized for calcifications that can be seen in hemangiomas or synovial sarcomas. Popliteal cysts are not treated initially, but followed regularly. They often disappear with time. If the cyst persists or enlarges, surgical excision is performed.

F. Both patellar tendinitis and patellar traction epiphysitis (Sinding-Larson-Johansson disease) may be due to overuse. So-called "overuse" syndromes are common in adolescent athletes, who may be pushed beyond their individual musculo-skeletal system's capacity. Activity restriction is often effective in relieving symptoms.

## REFERENCES

1. Burkson RJ, et al. Popliteal cyst; a clinicopathologic survey. J Bone Joint Surg. 1956;38A:1265.
2. Highgenboten CL. Children's knee problems. Orthop Rev. 1981;10:37.
3. Insall J. Patellar pain — current concepts review. J Bone Joint Surg. 1982;64A:147.
4. Munzinger U, et al. Internal derangement of the knee joint due to pathologic synovial folds: the mediopatellar plica syndrome. Clin Orthop. 1981; 155:59.
5. Murdock G. Congenital discord medial semilunar cartilage. J Bone Joint Surg. 1956; 38-B:564.

KNEE PAIN

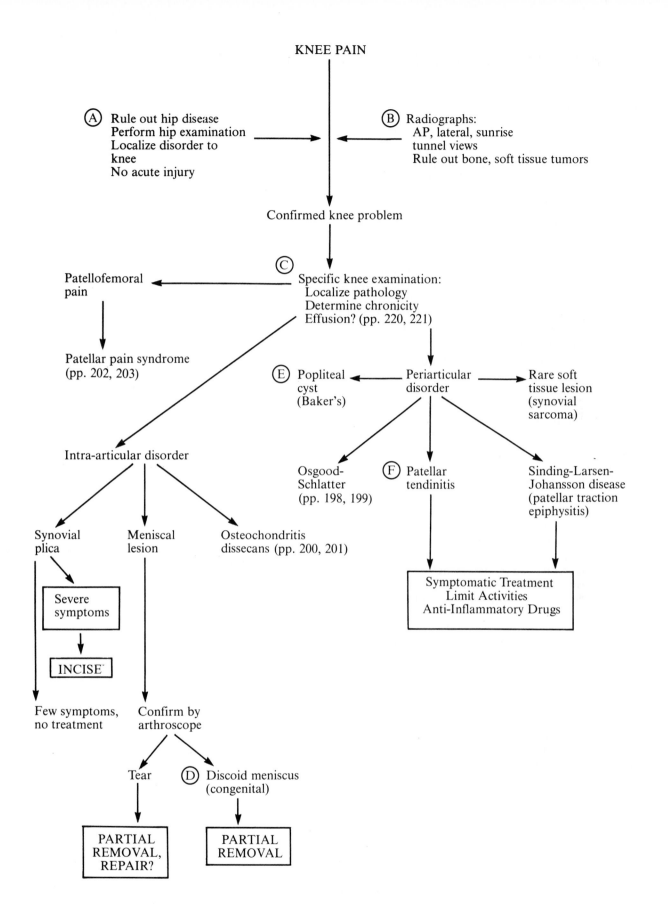

Ⓐ Rule out hip disease
Perform hip examination
Localize disorder to knee
No acute injury

Ⓑ Radiographs:
AP, lateral, sunrise tunnel views
Rule out bone, soft tissue tumors

Confirmed knee problem

Patellofemoral pain

Ⓒ Specific knee examination:
Localize pathology
Determine chronicity
Effusion? (pp. 220, 221)

Patellar pain syndrome
(pp. 202, 203)

Ⓔ Popliteal cyst (Baker's)

Periarticular disorder

Rare soft tissue lesion (synovial sarcoma)

Intra-articular disorder

Osgood-Schlatter
(pp. 198, 199)

Ⓕ Patellar tendinitis

Sinding-Larsen-Johansson disease (patellar traction epiphysitis)

Synovial plica

Meniscal lesion

Osteochondritis dissecans (pp. 200, 201)

Severe symptoms

INCISE

Symptomatic Treatment
Limit Activities
Anti-Inflammatory Drugs

Few symptoms, no treatment

Confirm by arthroscope

Tear

Ⓓ Discoid meniscus (congenital)

PARTIAL REMOVAL, REPAIR?

PARTIAL REMOVAL

# OSGOOD-SCHLATTER DISEASE

## COMMENTS

A. Patients with suspected Osgood-Schlatter disease should have knee radiographs performed, not so much for the suspected problem—Osgood-Schlatter disease can be diagnosed by physical examination —but to rule out other bony or soft tissue lesions (especially malignant bone tumors such as osteosarcoma[3]. The classic radiographic finding in Osgood-Schlatter disease is a fragmented, irregular tibial tubercle.

B. Osgood-Schlatter disease is an inflammatory response in the area where the patellar tendon inserts into the tibial tubercle. Partial, temporary separation of a portion of the tubercle growth center may initiate the response. There is no evidence for avascular necrosis.

C. Most patients with this disorder have few symptoms and require no treatment. Once they and their parents understand the disorder, they are perfectly happy to live with the moderate discomfort that may persist sporadically until skeletal maturity. Sometimes wrapping the area with one, or even two, 6-inch Ace bandages gives symptomatic relief and prevents complete knee flexion, a position that exacerbates symptoms. The child is not restricted from sports.

D. Most persistent, severe cases may require temporary restriction from sports and temporary immobilization with a knee immobilizer or, rarely, a cast. When symptoms resolve, the patient is allowed to resume activities, including athletics, as tolerated. Bowers has reported patellar tendon avulsion as a complication of Osgood-Schlatter disease; however, this complication is exceedingly rare, and the incidence may not be any greater than that of tibial tubercle avulsion in adolescent athletes without Osgood-Schlatter disease (noted in high jumpers—"jumper's knee").

E. In most patients, symptoms resolve at skeletal maturity when the tubercle fuses to the main body of the tibia. In certain patients, a separate ossicle fails to unite and produces persistent protracted symptoms. Surgical excision of this ununited ossicle provides predictable pain relief.

## REFERENCES

1. Bowers KD. Patellar tendon avulsion, as a complication of Osgood-Schlatter's disease. Am J Sports Med. 1981;9:356.
2. Levine J. A new conservative treatment of Osgood-Schlatter disease. Clin Orthop. 1981;158:126.
3. Mital M, et al. The so-called unresolved Osgood-Schlatter lesion. J Bone Joint Surg. 1980;62A:732.

PAIN IN TIBIAL TUBERCLE AREA

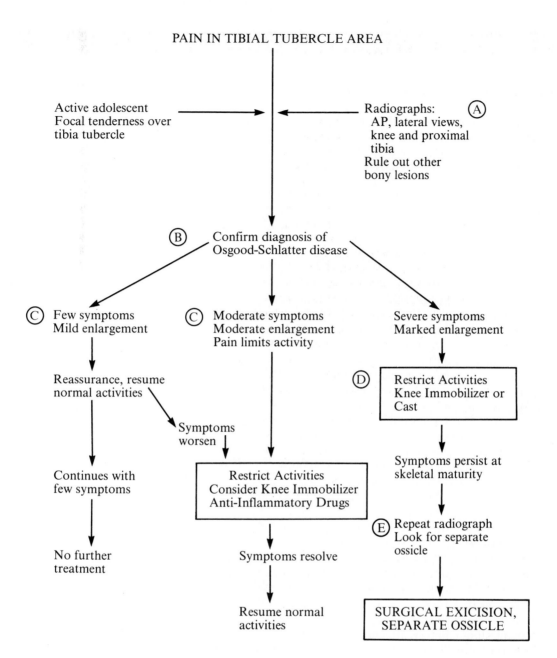

Active adolescent
Focal tenderness over
tibia tubercle

Radiographs: (A)
AP, lateral views,
knee and proximal
tibia
Rule out other
bony lesions

(B) Confirm diagnosis of
Osgood-Schlatter disease

(C) Few symptoms
Mild enlargement

(C) Moderate symptoms
Moderate enlargement
Pain limits activity

Severe symptoms
Marked enlargement

Reassurance, resume
normal activities

(D) Restrict Activities
Knee Immobilizer or
Cast

Symptoms
worsen

Continues with
few symptoms

Restrict Activities
Consider Knee Immobilizer
Anti-Inflammatory Drugs

Symptoms persist at
skeletal maturity

No further
treatment

Symptoms resolve

(E) Repeat radiograph
Look for separate
ossicle

Resume normal
activities

SURGICAL EXICISION,
SEPARATE OSSICLE

# OSTEOCHONDRITIS DISSECANS: KNEE

## COMMENTS

A.  The tunnel view is often the only view that clearly demonstrates the lesion, most commonly located in the posterior portion of the medial femoral condyle. Care should be taken not to overinterpret irregularities in normal ossification of the femoral condyles.[3] Tomograms or arthrograms were occasionally used in the past; however, arthroscopy has supplanted these methods.

B.  The etiology of osteochondritis dissecans is unclear. Trauma due to impingement by an elongated anterior tibial spine has been suggested. Occasionally, lesions are seen in locations other than the medial condyle, especially massive lateral condyle lesions present in both knees.

C.  Most younger children have a benign course with little treatment other than activity restriction. Linden has reported excellent long-term function in younger children with osteochondritis dissecans. The arthroscopic era has perhaps provided more attention to this disorder than it merits, especially in young children. A few weeks of activity restriction and perhaps a knee immobilizer are appropriate initial treatment.

D.  Beyond adolescence, the lesions are often larger and less likely to heal spontaneously. Patients of this age with a significant radiographic lesion and symptoms should have arthroscopic examination to establish the severity of the lesion. If the lesion is nearly or completely detached, loose bodies should be sought and removed.

E.  Large lesions that are intact can be drilled either open or preferably via an arthroscope. Partially detached lesions can be reattached. The method of Lipscomb,[4] using smooth Kirschner wires, which are left long (subcutaneous) proximally and removed in 6 to 8 weeks, is preferred to bone pegs or screws, which can become loose in the joint.

F.  Very large, nearly loose, or completely loose segments usually fit poorly in the crater and have little chance of reuniting with drilling. They should be removed and the base or crater drilled to encourage the development of fibrocartilage. These patients have surprisingly good early function but, if the lesion is large, may develop osteoarthritis later.

## REFERENCES

1.  Bunch WH. Decision analysis of treatment choices in the osteochondroses. Clin Orthop. 1981;158:91.
2.  Caffey J. Ossification of the distal femoral epiphysis. J Bone Joint Surg. 1958;40A:647.
3.  Linden BJ. Osteochondritis dissecans of the femoral condyles; a long-term follow-up study. J Bone Joint Surg. 1977;59A:769.
4.  Lipscomb PR Jr., et al. Osteochondritis dissecans of the knee with loose fragments. Treatment by replacement and fixation with readily removed pins. J Bone Joint Surg. 1978;60A:235.
5.  Pappas AM. Osteochondritis dissecans. Clin Orthop. 1981;158:59.

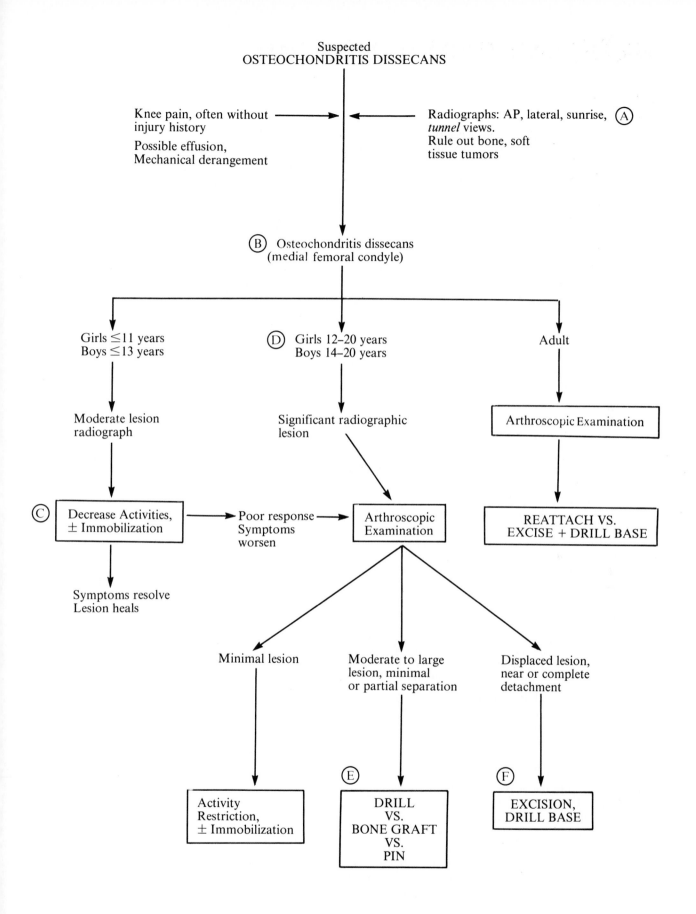

# PATELLAR PAIN SYNDROME

## COMMENTS

A. Chondromalacia, although commonly used as a clinical diagnosis, is truly a pathologic diagnosis describing softening, fibrillation, and degeneration of the articular cartilage. Few children with patellar pain truly have chondromalacia. Thus, a more accurate and preferred description of the clinical problem is "patellar pain syndrome."

B. The classic examination to elicit the patellar pain syndrome is compression of the patella into the intercondylar notch with the knee extended. The patient is then asked to contract the quadriceps. If the maneuver elicits pain, the process is localized to the patellar region. Careful palpation of the patellofemoral joint is also useful. Malalignment or a tendency toward lateral subluxation is suspected if the patient becomes anxious when you try to subluxate the patella laterally (Fairbank's sign).

C. Standard sunrise views are of little use. Choose one of the more specific methods[4,5] to assess patellar alignment.

D. Try not to settle for the nonspecific diagnosis of patellar pain syndrome. Determine the specific cause, if possible. However, this is not meant to encourage arthroscopy on every patient. Once you are certain that the patient does not have a serious or disabling conditon, start treatment with quadriceps strengthening and activity modification, even if the specific diagnosis is unclear. Many patients will resolve their symptoms without your knowing the exact cause. Only persistent, recalcitrant problems demand expensive further work-ups.

E. "Overuse" patellar malalignment, and excessive lateral patellar pressure syndromes are commonly related to so-called chondromalacia and will be further discussed on page 204.

F. A bipartite patella is usually a painless, normal variation of ossification. Rarely, the separate superolateral ossicle remains partially separated from the patella, resulting in chronic pain. Focal tenderness is characteristic, and occasionally the separate ossicle requires removal.[1]

G. Severe angular or rotatory malalignment of the entire limb (genu valgum, severe femoral torsion) may produce patellar pain.

H. Definitive treatment for "patellar pain syndrome" should include specific measures to correct the biomechanical anomaly affecting the patellofemoral joint and causing fibrillation. Shaving off fibrillated cartilage without addressing the primary cause is unreasonable, unlikely to give lasting relief, and comparable to treating a high fever with aspirin alone, only to find that the true cause of the fever was appendicitis.

## REFERENCES

1. Green WT Jr. Painful bipartite patellae. A report of three cases. Clin Orthop. 1975;110:197.
2. Highgenboten CL. Children's knee problems. Orthop Rev. 1981;10:37.
3. Insall J. Patellar pain—current concepts review. J Bone Joint Surg. 1982;64A:147.
4. Laurin CA, et al. The tangential x-ray investigation of the patellofemoral joint. Clin Orthop. 1979;144:16.
5. Merchant AC, et al. Roentgenographic analysis of patellofemoral congruence. J. Bone Joint Surg. 1974;56A:1391.

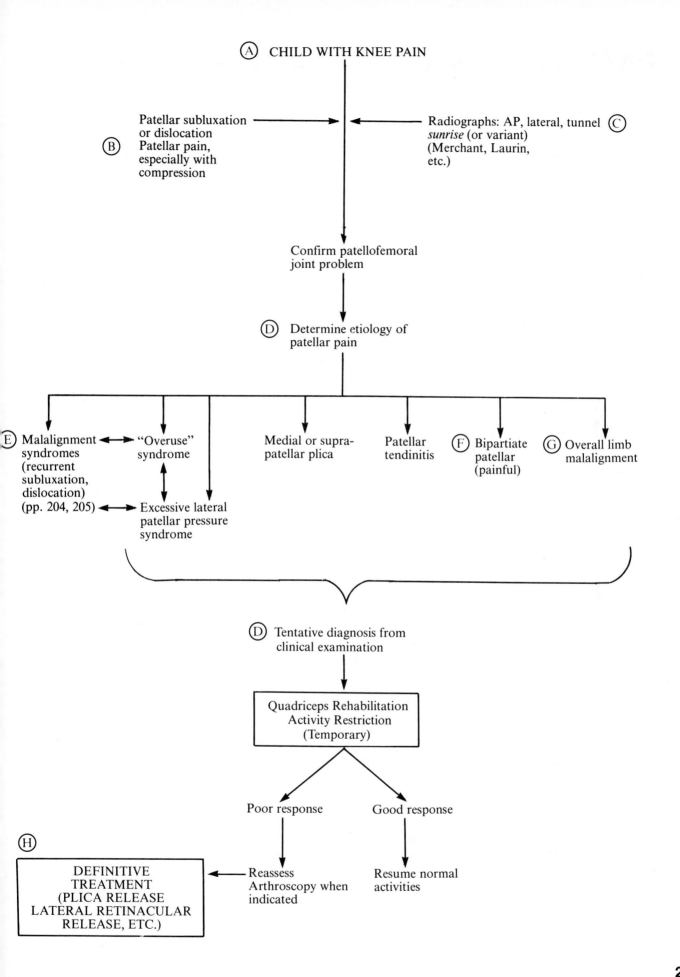

Ⓐ CHILD WITH KNEE PAIN

Ⓑ Patellar subluxation ⟶ ← Radiographs: AP, lateral, tunnel Ⓒ
or dislocation *sunrise* (or variant)
Patellar pain, (Merchant, Laurin,
especially with etc.)
compression

Confirm patellofemoral
joint problem

Ⓓ Determine etiology of
patellar pain

Ⓔ Malalignment ◄─► "Overuse"    Medial or supra-    Patellar    Ⓕ Bipartiate    Ⓖ Overall limb
syndromes    syndrome    patellar plica    tendinitis    patellar    malalignment
(recurrent                                                                  (painful)
subluxation,
dislocation)
(pp. 204, 205) ◄─► Excessive lateral
patellar pressure
syndrome

Ⓓ Tentative diagnosis from
clinical examination

Quadriceps Rehabilitation
Activity Restriction
(Temporary)

Poor response           Good response

Ⓗ

DEFINITIVE    ← Reassess           Resume normal
TREATMENT        Arthroscopy when      activities
(PLICA RELEASE    indicated
LATERAL RETINACULAR
RELEASE, ETC.)

# PATELLAR DISLOCATION IN THE CHILD

## COMMENTS

A. Patients with acute patellar dislocations usually present with a clear history of dislocation; however, the patella may have spontaneously reduced by the time you examine the child. Accurate diagnosis of recurrent dislocation or subluxation is more difficult. These patients often give a history of "giving way" and "pseudo-locking," thus mimicking a meniscal injury.

B. Choose a specific sunrise view (Merchant, Laurin), and use it consistently. In acute dislocation, look for bony avulsion from the medial patella and/or loose bodies.

C. Look for factors that may predispose a child to patellary dislocation or subluxation. They include: deficient medial patellar facet, patella alta, vastus medialis weakness, excessive lateral retinacular tightness, genu valgum, excessive femoral anteversion (in-torsion), and others.

D. Surgeons who open the knee medially in an acute dislocation should be aware that the retinaculum may have avulsed from the adductor tubercle region rather than tearing within the substance of the retinaculum adjacent to the patella. Unwary surgeons have missed the tear because they did not recognize this pattern. Any bony fragments must be removed (or reattached), the lateral retinaculum released, and the medial retinaculum tightened (realignment).

E. Recurrent patellar dislocation (with spontaneous reduction) and recurrent subluxation are hard to distinguish. Findings include medial tenderness, apprehension (Fairbanks's test), and quadriceps atrophy.

F. There are more than 100 different types of operations that can be used for quadriceps and patellar realignment. Choosing one is rather like choosing a religion. I prefer both a lateral release and a medial reefing plus vastus med ialis advancement. The Hauser procedure (moving patellar tendon medially including a tibial bone block) is contraindicated in a child with open growth plates because the procedure will cause growth arrest.

G. Arthroscopic lateral retinacular releases are currently performed rather indiscriminately for unexplained patellar pain in adolescents. Reserve this overused technique for the few patients who do not respond to lengthy, vigorous quadriceps rehabilitation and in whom you have good reason to suspect excessive lateral pressure.

## REFERENCES

1. Highgenboten CL. Children's knee problems. Orthop Rev. 1981;10:37.
2. Hughston JC. Subluxation of the patella. J Bone Joint Surg. 1968;50A:1003.
3. Laurin CA, et al. The tangential x-ray investigation of the patellofemoral joint. Clin Orthop. 1979;144:16.
4. Merchant AC, et al. Roentgenographic analysis of patellofemoral congruence. J Bone Joint Surg. 1974;56A:1391.

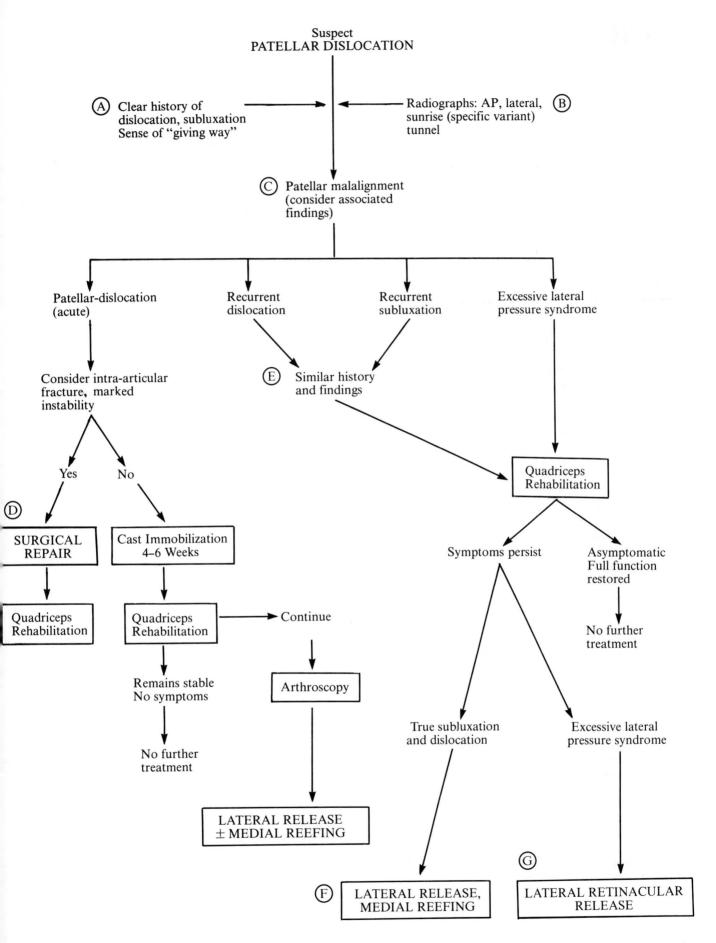

# TIBIAL BOWING

## COMMENTS

A. Infants and children with specific tibial bowing (not genu varum) present with three classic directions of bowing, each representing a disorder with an entirely different prognosis. Careful physical examination and study of the tibial radiographs should lead to the correct diagnosis.

B. Anterolateral bow is almost always associated with congenital pseudoarthrosis of the tibia, which in turn is commonly associated with neurofibromatosis. Thus, a careful assessment of family history (autosomal dominant) and examination of the child's skin for cafe-au-lait spots are indicated. The tibia is often bowed but intact initially (prepseudoarthrosis), but usually progresses to a fracture that will not heal. Bracing is indicated to prevent bow progression and development of fracture.

C. Patients with an established congenital pseudoarthrosis often eventually require amputation. Milder forms can be treated surgically with some chance of achieving union. I prefer resection of the pseudoarthrosis, intramedullary tibial and fibular rods, bone grafting, and sometimes electrical stimulation as well.

D. Posteromedial tibial bowing is an odd, unsightly tibial deformity, noted at birth. Radiographs demonstrate the direction of the bow and confirm that the bone is normal. The etiology is unknown and the prognosis is excellent for complete spontaneous correction, despite the severe appearance at birth. Both the parents and the physician sometimes find it hard to believe that spontaneous correction will occur. Very severe forms with associated foot deformity may benefit from a short period of corrective casting. The only long-term problem is a moderate limb length discrepancy, as reported by Hofmann et al.[2] Thus, the parents must be advised of this possibility and the child followed to determine the need for possible subsequent contralateral epiphyseodesis.

E. Anteromedial bow is seen in association with fibular shortening or fibular hemimelia. The short fibula allows the foot to develop in a valgus position and the tibia to be bowed antermedially. In more severe forms, lateral rays of the foot are absent. Treatment for fibular hemimelia varies according to severity, ranging from observation of possible limb length discrepancy with possible contralateral epiphyseodesis to Syme's amputation of the foot on the hemimelic side in severe cases.

## REFERENCES

1. Achterman C, et al. Congenital deficiency of the fibular. J Bone Joint Surg. 1979;61B:133.
2. Hofmann A, Wenger D. Posteromedial bowing of the tibia. Progression of discrepancy in leg lengths. J Bone Joint Surg. 1981;63A:384.
3. Morrissy RT, et al. Congenital pseudoarthrosis of the tibia. J Bone Joint Surg. 1981;63B:367.

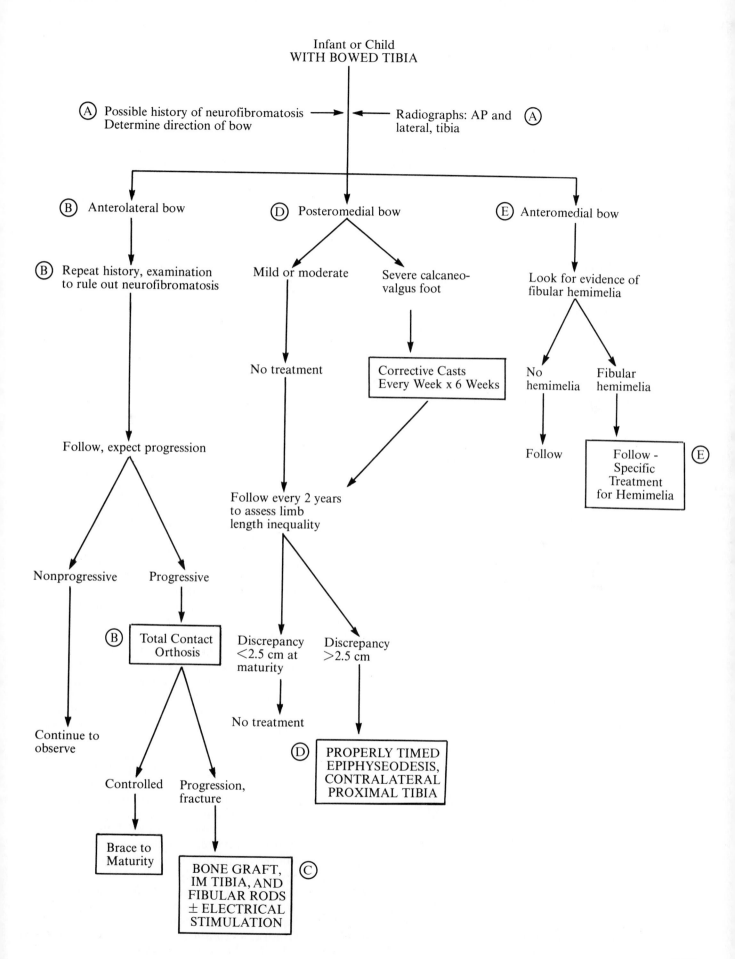

Infant or Child
WITH BOWED TIBIA

Ⓐ Possible history of neurofibromatosis → ← Radiographs: AP and Ⓐ
Determine direction of bow              lateral, tibia

Ⓑ Anterolateral bow          Ⓓ Posteromedial bow          Ⓔ Anteromedial bow

Ⓑ Repeat history, examination          Mild or moderate    Severe calcaneo-          Look for evidence of
to rule out neurofibromatosis                               valgus foot              fibular hemimelia

Follow, expect progression          No treatment          Corrective Casts          No          Fibular
                                                          Every Week x 6 Weeks      hemimelia    hemimelia

Nonprogressive    Progressive                                                        Follow       Follow -
                                                                                                  Specific
                 Ⓑ Total Contact              Follow every 2 years                               Treatment    Ⓔ
                    Orthosis                   to assess limb                                     for Hemimelia
                                              length inequality

Continue to                        Discrepancy    Discrepancy
observe                            <2.5 cm at     >2.5 cm
                                   maturity

            Controlled    Progression,          No treatment
                          fracture

            Brace to                        Ⓓ PROPERLY TIMED
            Maturity                           EPIPHYSEODESIS,
                                               CONTRALATERAL
                          BONE GRAFT,    Ⓒ     PROXIMAL TIBIA
                          IM TIBIA, AND
                          FIBULAR RODS
                          ± ELECTRICAL
                          STIMULATION

# TOEING IN AND OUT

## COMMENTS

A.  The natural evolution of rotational alignment must be understood. Most children are born with internal (medial) tibial torsion that is masked by an external rotation contracture of the hip secondary to intrauterine position. Rarely, if ever, do children have true bony femoral retroversion. Instead, the external limb rotation seen at initial standing is due to contracture of the external rotator muscles of the hip. These contractures stretch out as the child begins to walk, and then the internal tibial torsion becomes apparent.

B.  Staheli's rapid method for rotational assessment is superb for documentation (see figure).[3,4] Watch the child walk and document whether the feet are pointing *out* (positive foot progression angle—PFA) or *in* (negative PFA). The child lies *prone* with the knee bent 90°, and you assess the foot (adducted, neutral, abducted). The thigh-foot angle documents tibial torsion (positive values = external or lateral torsion; negative values = internal or medial torsion). Finally, femoral rotation is documented (the prone position is best for this test because the hip is extended, as it is in weightbearing).

C.  External rotation contracture of the hip is very common and not well recognized. Many children first stand (age 9 to 12 months) with their feet pointed out 90°. The passive hip examination shows no internal rotation of the hip (often contracted in external rotation). This condition spontaneously corrects with 9 to 12 months of independent walking and requires no treatment —not even a Denis-Browne bar. In severe protracted cases, prone frog-leg sleeping may delay spontaneous correction. Maintenance of prone frog-leg sleeping and failure to correct severe toeing-out is somewhat more common in children with developmental delay.

D.  The Denis-Browne brace is used only rarely for severe torsional problems in children of very concerned parents—perhaps one of 20 patients with torsional problems. The night brace, by changing foot position during sleep, is very effective in aiding nature's spontaneous correction of tibial torsion. Parents are told that the torsion will almost certainly correct without treatment by school age, but that a brace will hasten this process, providing correction within one year if worn faithfully each night. Few parents have the discipline to keep their child in the brace, and the protesting kicks of vigorous children have been known to demolish crib slats. To avoid overuse, I insist that children walk independently for 6 months—to allow spontaneous correction— before prescribing a Denis-Browne splint.

E.  Excessive medial femoral torsion or anteversion improves spontaneously until age 12 years and rarely requires treatment. These children adopt a W position for sitting, a position most comfortable for them. They walk with characteristic excessive pelvic rotation because they lack one of the parameters of normal gait, that is, adequate hip external rotation in swing phase. Spontaneous correction should continue until age 12 years, and night braces are ineffective. The W-sitting position is discouraged; however, the relationship between avoiding this position and improved spontaneous correction is empiric.

F.  Many European and selected North American authors have suggested that maintenance of increased anteversion predisposes to premature hip arthritis. Consequently, these centers advise femoral derotation in severe cases to avoid arthritis. More conservative centers perform

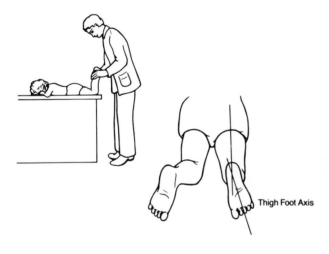

| TORSIONAL PROFILE | | |
|---|---|---|
| | R | L |
| INTERNAL ROTATION | | |
| EXTERNAL ROTATION | | |
| THIGH-FOOT AXIS | | |
| FOOT | | |

Thigh Foot Axis

Top: Torsional profile, as described by Staheli, can be documented on this form. Internal rotation and external rotation refer to rotation of the femur (anteversion). Bottom: Thigh-foot axis describes tibial torsion while foot description is either "abducted," "straight," or "adducted."

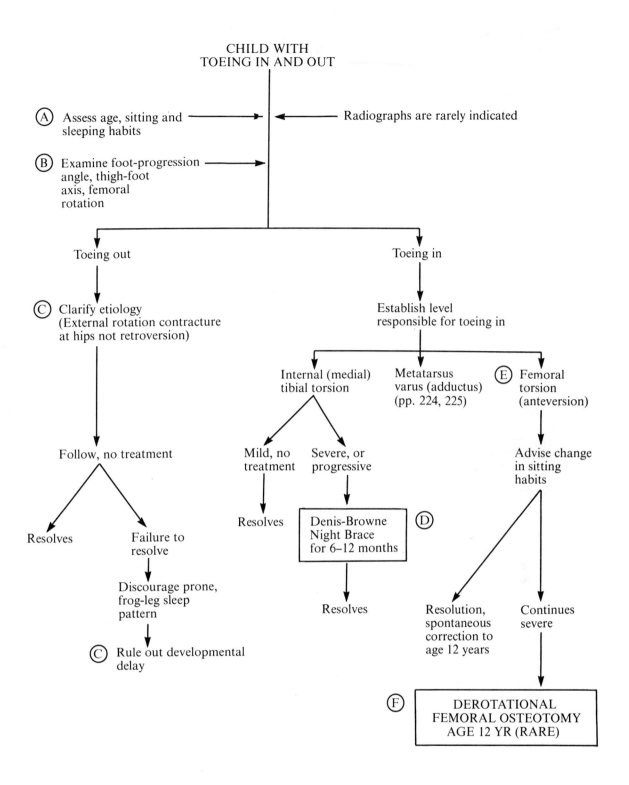

CHILD WITH
TOEING IN AND OUT

(A) Assess age, sitting and sleeping habits → ← Radiographs are rarely indicated

(B) Examine foot-progression angle, thigh-foot axis, femoral rotation →

**Toeing out**

(C) Clarify etiology (External rotation contracture at hips not retroversion)

Follow, no treatment

Resolves

Failure to resolve

Discourage prone, frog-leg sleep pattern

(C) Rule out developmental delay

**Toeing in**

Establish level responsible for toeing in

Internal (medial) tibial torsion

Mild, no treatment

Resolves

Severe, or progressive

Denis-Browne Night Brace for 6–12 months (D)

Resolves

Metatarsus varus (adductus) (pp. 224, 225)

(E) Femoral torsion (anteversion)

Advise change in sitting habits

Resolution, spontaneous correction to age 12 years

Continues severe

(F) DEROTATIONAL FEMORAL OSTEOTOMY AGE 12 YR (RARE)

femoral derotation only in rare teenage girls who have a very ugly gait due to extreme anteversion. Perhaps one in 500 patients with excessive anteversion requires this procedure. The results are excellent and the patients are happy.

**REFERENCES**

1.  Khermosh O, et al. Tibial torsion in children. Clin Orthop. 1971;79:26.

2.  Staheli LT, et al. Tibial torsion: a method of assessment and a survey of normal children. Clin Orthop. 1972;86:183.

3.  Staheli LT, et al. Femoral anteversion and physical performance in adolescent and adult life. Clin Orthop. 1977;129:213.

4.  Staheli LT. Medial femoral torsion. Orthop Clin N Am. 1980;11:39.

# BOWLEGS AND KNOCK-KNEES

## COMMENTS

A. Most normal children temporarily have bowed legs (physiologic bowing), which spontaneously correct by age 18 months to 3 years. Your attention should be focused on very severe cases or those that fail to correct. A family history of short stature may tip you off to an inherited disorder (vitamin D resistant rickets, sex-linked dominant) which may be causing the bowing. At about 3 years of age, most children develop normal physiologic valgus (see figure).

B. Children with physiologic bowing have a gentle bow throughout the tibia and femur. Children with tibia vara (Blount's disease) have a sharp, angular deformity at the knee (see figure).

C. Radiographs should be ordered only in very severe bowing, in asymmetric bowing (possible Blount's), and when the history suggests a metabolic disorder.

D. Normally, children develop physiologic valgus at the age of 3 years, which corrects by about age 6 years. If the valgus is severe or not self-correcting, consider metabolic disorders, renal failure, or other possibilities. Unfortunately, not all normal children correct their juvenile physiologic valgus, particularly obese, flatfooted children. Medial distal femoral physeal stapling, crucially timed, is remarkably effective in correcting severe cases.[4]

E. Severe physiologic bowing may occasionally proceed to Blount's disease, especially in black children. Remember that all children who develop Blount's disease at one time had normal knee radiographs (physiologic varus). Long-leg orthoses, worn during the daytime to correct abnormal varus forces of weightbearing, are effective in preventing the occasional progression of severe physiologic varus to Blount's disease. Night braces (mermaid splint) are not effective, since the daily weight-bearing varus stress continues.

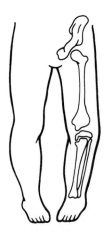

Blount's disease. Physiologic varus fails to correct and sharp angular deformity, focal at knee, results. Condition is sometimes bilateral.

F. The most common metabolic disease that causes significant genu varum or valgum is vitamin D-resistant rickets. There is usually a family history, and laboratory studies (low serum phosphorus, elevated serum alkaline phosphatase) clinch the diagnosis. Metaphyseal dysostosis has a similar radiographic presentation, but normal serum chemistries. Abnormal serum phosphorus, creatinine, and blood urea nitrogen point to rickets due to renal failure.

G. Tibia vara (Blount's disease) is a growth disturbance of the proximal medial tibial physis that develops in children age 18 months to 3 years. The Langenskiold classifications are chronologic; in other words, all patients begin with stage I and progress to stage V and VI (permanent, irreversible growth plate bridging medially) unless the cycle of progressive varus-growth-suppression-further varus is broken.[2] In early stages this can be done by orthoses (long-leg, worn during day with weightbearing; night-time braces are ineffective). A much less common adolescent variant of tibia vara appears in adolescence and is treated by corrective osteotomy.

H. Patients may rapidly progress to stages III and IV and then must be promptly treated with corrective osteotomy of the tibia and fibula *below* the growth plates to avoid progression to permanent growth plate closure. In rare cases, patients with medial bony bridging (stages V and VI) can be considered for excision of the bony bar with cranioplast or Silastic spacer replacement plus corrective osteotomy.

Normal progression from bowlegs in first year to knock-knees at 3 years to straight lower limbs at 6 years.

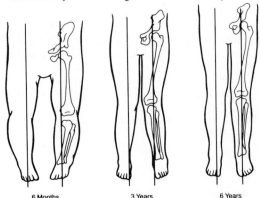

6 Months          3 Years          6 Years

## REFERENCES

1. Klassen RA, Peterson HA. The physeal bar resection: the Mayo Clinic experience. Orthop Trans. 1982;6:65.

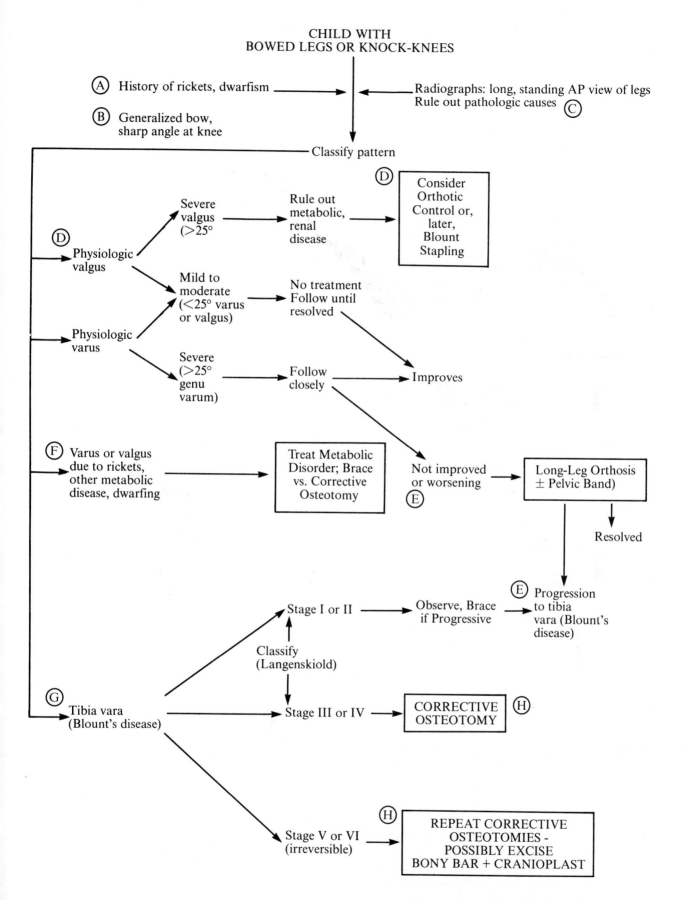

CHILD WITH
BOWED LEGS OR KNOCK-KNEES

(A) History of rickets, dwarfism ⟶ ⟵ Radiographs: long, standing AP view of legs
Rule out pathologic causes (C)

(B) Generalized bow,
sharp angle at knee

Classify pattern

(D)
┌─────────────┐
│ Consider    │
│ Orthotic    │
│ Control or, │
│ later,      │
│ Blount      │
│ Stapling    │
└─────────────┘

Severe
valgus
(>25°  ⟶  Rule out
         metabolic,
         renal
         disease

(D)
Physiologic
valgus

Mild to
moderate  ⟶  No treatment
(<25° varus   Follow until
or valgus)    resolved

Physiologic
varus

Severe
(>25°  ⟶  Follow
genu      closely  ⟶  Improves
varum)

(F) Varus or valgus
due to rickets,
other metabolic       ⟶  ┌──────────────────┐
disease, dwarfing        │ Treat Metabolic  │   Not improved  ⟶  ┌──────────────────┐
                         │ Disorder; Brace  │   or worsening      │ Long-Leg Orthosis│
                         │ vs. Corrective   │   (E)               │ ± Pelvic Band)   │
                         │ Osteotomy        │                     └──────────────────┘
                         └──────────────────┘                              │
                                                                           Resolved

                                                          (E) Progression
Stage I or II  ⟶  Observe, Brace  ⟶  to tibia
                  if Progressive      vara (Blount's
                                      disease)

Classify
(Langenskiold)

(G)                    Stage III or IV  ⟶  ┌──────────────────┐  (H)
Tibia vara                                 │ CORRECTIVE       │
(Blount's disease)                         │ OSTEOTOMY        │
                                           └──────────────────┘

(H)
┌──────────────────────────┐
Stage V or VI  ⟶  │ REPEAT CORRECTIVE        │
(irreversible)    │ OSTEOTOMIES -            │
                  │ POSSIBLY EXCISE          │
                  │ BONY BAR + CRANIOPLAST   │
                  └──────────────────────────┘

2.  Langenskiold A. Tibia vara: osteochondrosis
    deformans tibiae: Blount's desease. Clin Orthop,
    1981;158:77.
3.  Salenius P, et al. The development of the tibiofemoral

    angle in children. J Bone Joint Surg. 1975;57A:259.
4.  Zuege RC, Blount WP, et al. Epiphyseal stapling for
    angular deformity of the knee. J Bone Joint Surg.
    1979;61A:320.

# LIMB LENGTH INEQUALITY

## COMMENTS

A. The causes of limb length inequality in children are well known to orthopaedic surgeons. Congenital anomalies (femoral, tibial, fibular), neonatal osteomyelitis, and growth plate fracture with resulting growth arrest are the most common causes. Benign tumors (enchondromatosis), vascular disorders (Klippel-Trenaunay-Weber syndrome), neurofibromatosis, other neurologic disorders (cerebral palsy, polio, spinal dysraphism), and hemihypertrophy are also associated with, or responsible for, discrepancies.

B. Children with significant hemihypertrophy may have associated renal tumors and should be followed closely during the first 2 years of life. An intravenous pyelogram and/or renal scan should be considered to rule out tumor.

C. During the first few years of life, clinical measurements of discrepancy are satisfactory. After the age of 5 years, patients with significant, probably progressive discrepancies should have orthoroentgenograms, plus bone age films, taken yearly to allow accurate charting of discrepancy progression. Moseley's ingenious method of charting progression while simultaneously predicting final discrepancy has become an international standard.[3] The advantage of this method over the Green-Anderson method[1] is that with one simple plotting on each visit a graph depicting current discrepancy, percent inhibition, and predicted final discrepancy is developed.

D. Childhood is the ideal time to correct limb length discrepancy because the open physes can be used (arrested) to provide correction with minimal surgery and very short hospitalizations. Children with minor discrepancies (less than 3 cm) can be given a shoe lift, but few will wear it; and minor discrepancies have no proven deleterious effect on the spine or body.

E. Timing for epiphysiodesis is crucial and should be both cross-checked (Moseley and Green-Anderson methods) and rechecked just prior to surgery.[1,3] The Phemister method[4] is preferred to Blount's stapling method because the staples often irritate overlying tissues and require removal and thus a second operation.

F. Wagner's method and equipment have improved the results of tibial and femoral lengthening;[5] however, lengthening is still fraught with complications and should be performed in centers with experience in this method. Children should be 10 years of age prior to lengthening, as they need emotional maturity and stamina to adapt to the method. The joints at either end of the bone to be lengthened should be stable. Limbs with acquired discrepancies (infection, trauma) are easier to lengthen than those with congenital discrepancies.

G. Children with congenital anomalies (PFFD, severe fibular hemimelia) for whom severe final discrepancies are predicted are best treated by early amputation and prosthesis fitting.

H. Epiphysiodesis is no longer possible in skeletally mature patients. In patients with only moderate discrepancies, shortening osteotomy plus rigid internal fixation is greatly preferred to lengthening because healing is rapid, complications are few, and hospitalization is short.

## REFERENCES

1. Anderson M, Green WT, et al. Growth and predictions of growth in the lower extremities. J Bone Joint Surg. 1963;45A:1.
2. Mackie GG, et al. Hemihypertrophy and its association with intra-abdominal dysplasia and neoplasia. In *Symposium on Vascular Malformations and Vascular Lesions.* Edited by H Williams, St. Louis: CV Mosby, 1983, p 203.
3. Moseley CF. A straight line graph for leg-length discrepancies. J Bone Joint Surg. 1977;59A:174.
4. Phemister DB. Operative arrestment of longitudinal growth of bones in the treatment of deformities. J Bone Joint Surg. 1933;15:1.
5. Wagner H. Surgical lengthening or shortening of femur and tibia. Technique and indications. In *Progress in Orthopaedic Surgery.* Vol. 1. Berlin. Springer-Verlag, 1977; 71.

# LIMB LENGTH INEQUALITY

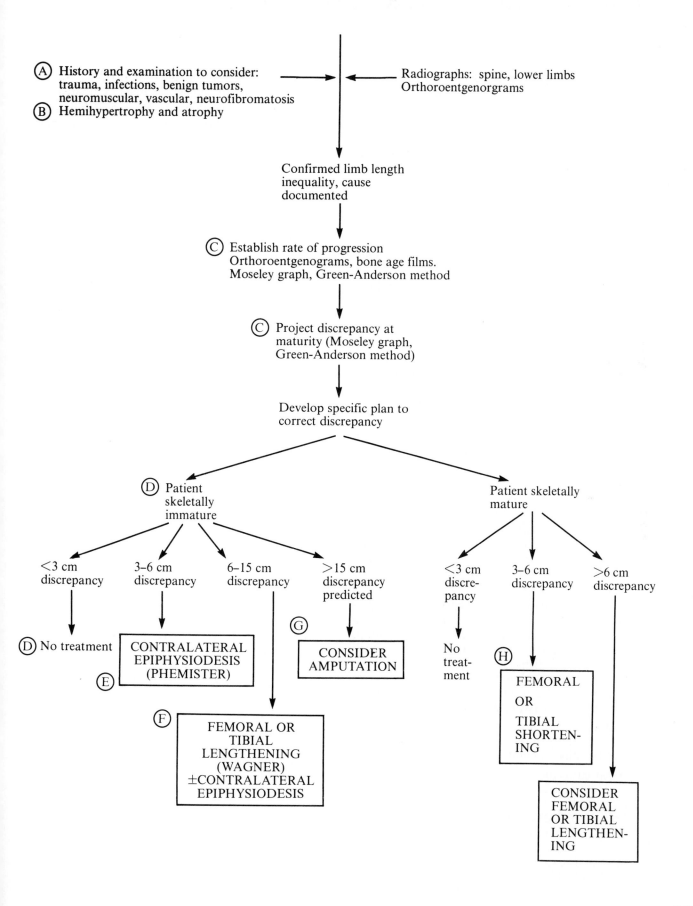

(A) History and examination to consider: trauma, infections, benign tumors, neuromuscular, vascular, neurofibromatosis
(B) Hemihypertrophy and atrophy

Radiographs: spine, lower limbs
Orthoroentgenorgrams

Confirmed limb length inequality, cause documented

(C) Establish rate of progression Orthoroentgenograms, bone age films. Moseley graph, Green-Anderson method

(C) Project discrepancy at maturity (Moseley graph, Green-Anderson method)

Develop specific plan to correct discrepancy

(D) Patient skeletally immature

<3 cm discrepancy
3–6 cm discrepancy
6–15 cm discrepancy
>15 cm discrepancy predicted

(D) No treatment

(E) CONTRALATERAL EPIPHYSIODESIS (PHEMISTER)

(F) FEMORAL OR TIBIAL LENGTHENING (WAGNER) ±CONTRALATERAL EPIPHYSIODESIS

(G) CONSIDER AMPUTATION

Patient skeletally mature

<3 cm discrepancy
3–6 cm discrepancy
>6 cm discrepancy

No treatment

(H) FEMORAL OR TIBIAL SHORTENING

CONSIDER FEMORAL OR TIBIAL LENGTHENING

# LIMPING CHILD (AGE 0–5 YEARS)

## COMMENTS

A. Cause of limp in a child can be categorized according to age. The common causes of limp in the 0- to 5-year age group are quite different from those in the 10- to 15-year age group. Children who are not yet able to walk may have these disorders, and signs other than limp must be sought, for example, children of this age may refuse to walk. Physical findings are occult and hard to localize; a careful history and physical examination are necessary. In many children who limp, you will never establish a specific diagnosis, and the limp will disappear spontaneously. Your job is to rule out osteomyelitis, joint sepsis, or other treatable conditions.

B. Infection or occult fracture is by far the most common cause of limp or refusal to walk. Thus, the history, examination, and initial laboratory work (CBC, sedimentation rate) are designed to differentiate between occult injury and infection. Physical examination while the child is asleep is often remarkably useful in localizing the disorder. Palpate the ankle, calf, and thigh; then, range the knee and hip. The sleeping child will wince when you palpate the involved area.

C. Child abuse should be considered when you see a limping child. Atypical bruising (genital area, back, buttocks,), presentation several days after injury, and conflicting histories from several parties are characteristic.

D. If initial radiographs are normal and you strongly suspect an occult fracture, repeat the radiograph in 7 days. By that time a fracture line or periosteal new bone may be present. Bone scans help with early diagnosis of osteomyelitis or occult fractures.

E. Mild cerebral palsy, particulary spastic hemiplegia, may not be detected until a child begins to walk and run. The parents then report a limp. Review the birth history and look for "tight" muscles (hamstrings, adductors, heel cord) on physical examination. Children with spinal cord tumors or congenital spinal anomalies (diastematomyelia) may present with a limp.

F. Toddlers with discitis (infected intervertebral disc) may limp or refuse to walk. Carefully examine the spine in children who refuse to walk.

G. As already mentioned, child abuse should be considered in children with fractures. A nondisplaced spiral fracture of the distal third of the tibia (so-called "toddler's fracture") may cause a child to limp. Initial radiographs may be normal and should be repeated in 7 days, at which time the fracture line may become apparent. Osteomyelitis and joint sepsis are ruled out if the child is afebrile and has a normal WBC and sedimentation rate. The distinction between probable occult fracture and sepsis must be made.

H. There are many mundane causes of childhood limp. New shoes, skin blisters, and foreign bodies in the foot (glass, thorn) are examples.

## REFERENCES

1. Kempe HC, et al. The battered child syndrome. J Am M A. 1962;181:17.
2. Salter RB. The limping child. Pediatric Portfolio 1973; Vol. 2.

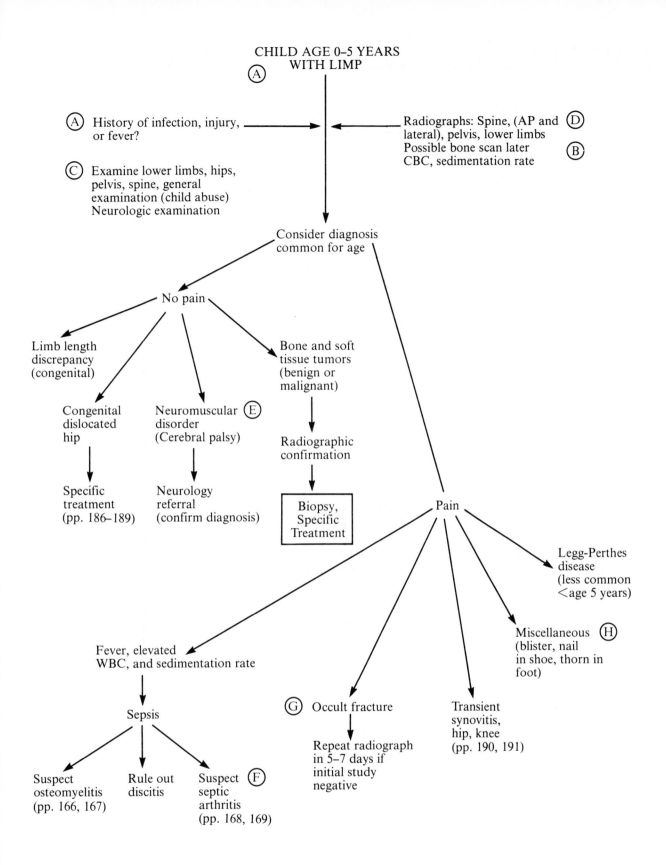

CHILD AGE 0–5 YEARS
WITH LIMP

Ⓐ

Ⓐ History of infection, injury,
or fever?

Ⓓ Radiographs: Spine, (AP and
lateral), pelvis, lower limbs
Ⓑ Possible bone scan later
CBC, sedimentation rate

Ⓒ Examine lower limbs, hips,
pelvis, spine, general
examination (child abuse)
Neurologic examination

Consider diagnosis
common for age

No pain

Limb length
discrepancy
(congenital)

Bone and soft
tissue tumors
(benign or
malignant)

Congenital
dislocated
hip

Neuromuscular Ⓔ
disorder
(Cerebral palsy)

Radiographic
confirmation

Specific
treatment
(pp. 186–189)

Neurology
referral
(confirm diagnosis)

Biopsy,
Specific
Treatment

Pain

Legg-Perthes
disease
(less common
<age 5 years)

Miscellaneous Ⓗ
(blister, nail
in shoe, thorn in
foot)

Fever, elevated
WBC, and sedimentation rate

Sepsis

Ⓖ Occult fracture

Transient
synovitis,
hip, knee
(pp. 190, 191)

Repeat radiograph
in 5–7 days if
initial study
negative

Suspect
osteomyelitis
(pp. 166, 167)

Rule out
discitis

Suspect Ⓕ
septic
arthritis
(pp. 168, 169)

# LIMPING CHILD (AGE 5-10 YEARS)

## COMMENTS

A. In a child 5 to 10 years of age, the likely causes of a previously undiagnosed limp are different from those in the 0- to 5-year-old group. Older children can communicate and localize their symptoms better. Osteomyelitis and joint sepsis are less common in this age group, but still are high on the list. Therefore, temperature, CBC, and sedimentation rate determinations remain mandatory. Congenital disorders (hip, spine, lower limb) are likely to have been diagnosed earlier, but must be sought since some become noticeable only with growth. Legg-Perthes disease and transient synovitis of the hip are very common in this age group. Also, knee(Osgood-Schlatter disease) and foot (Sever's disease) disorders are now more common.

B. Again, remember to examine the spine, pelvis, and hips in limping children, even though they have referred pain to the knee. Pelvic, spine, and hip disorders (especially spinal and pelvic infections or tumors) are characteristically diagnosed much later than is ideal because physicians look distally first.

C. Cerebral palsy probably will have been diagnosed earlier. Spinal cord tumors may present in this age group. Also, congenital spinal anomalies (diastematomyelia) may be seen at this time because of growth and progressive neurologic conditions, such as Charcot-Marie-Tooth disease and Friedreich's ataxia, also may appear at this age.

D. Occult fracture is now rare. Athletically active juveniles may suffer from stress fractures (metarsals, proximal tibia).

E. Knee disorders are much more common in 5- to 10-year-old children than in the younger group. Osgood-Schlatter disease is particularly common. Patellar malalignment problems (subluxation) begin to appear. Miscellaneous causes include discoid meniscus, synovial plica, and knee synovitis (rheumatoid and nonspecific).

F. Legg-Perthes disease most commonly appears in this age range. Occasionally, it follows serial bouts of transient hip synovitis. Limping and a complaint of hip or knee pain in an afebrile, wiry juvenile is Legg-Perthes disease until proven otherwise. Remember that knee pain may be referred from the hip.

## REFERENCES

1. Catterall A. The natural history of Perthes disease. J Bone Joint Surg. 1971;53B:37.
2. Salter RB. The limping child. Pediatric Portfolio 1973; Vol. 2.

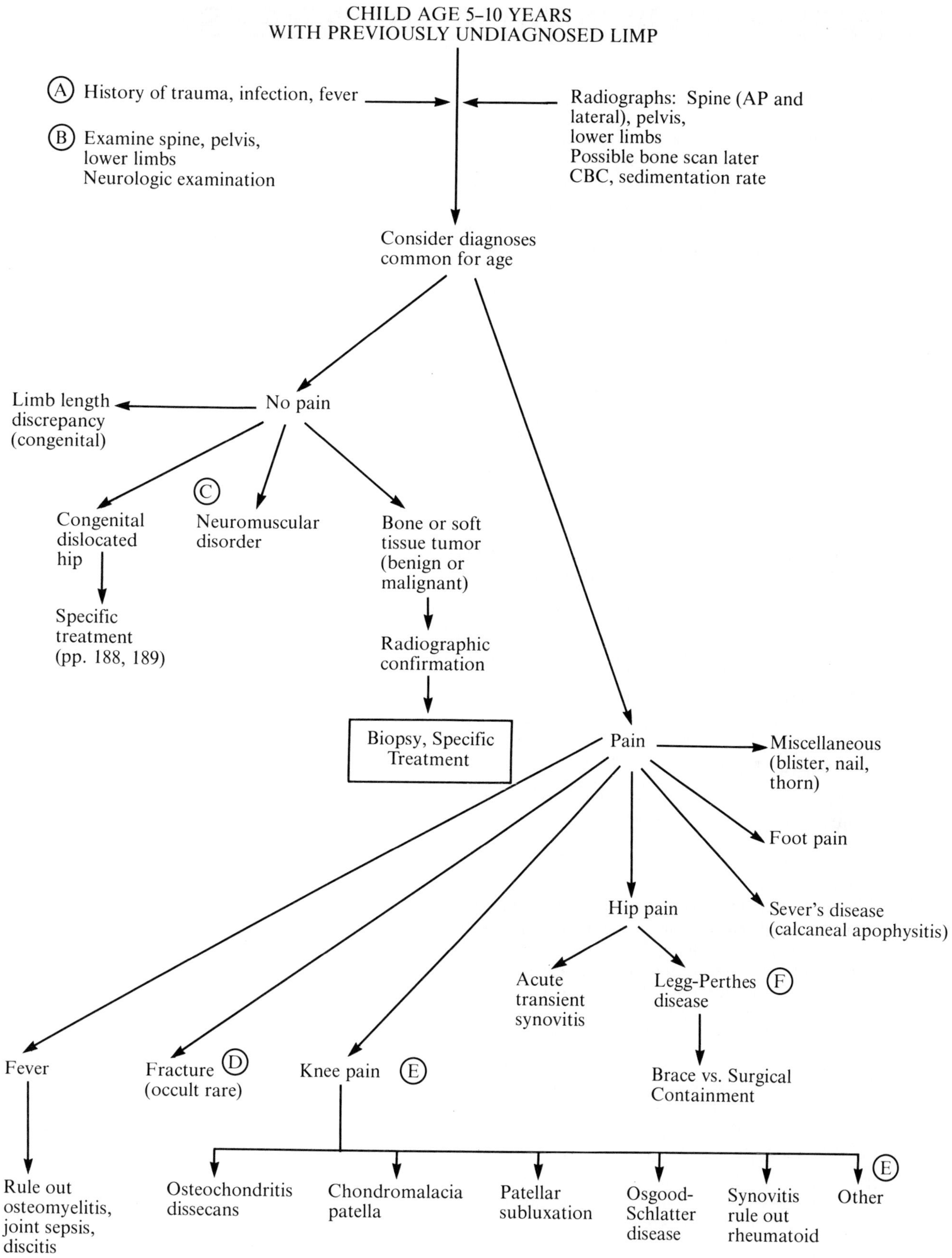

# CHILD AGE 5–10 YEARS
# WITH PREVIOUSLY UNDIAGNOSED LIMP

(A) History of trauma, infection, fever

(B) Examine spine, pelvis, lower limbs
Neurologic examination

Radiographs: Spine (AP and lateral), pelvis, lower limbs
Possible bone scan later
CBC, sedimentation rate

Consider diagnoses common for age

No pain

Limb length discrepancy (congenital)

Congenital dislocated hip

(C) Neuromuscular disorder

Bone or soft tissue tumor (benign or malignant)

Specific treatment (pp. 188, 189)

Radiographic confirmation

Biopsy, Specific Treatment

Pain

Miscellaneous (blister, nail, thorn)

Foot pain

Hip pain

Sever's disease (calcaneal apophysitis)

Acute transient synovitis

Legg-Perthes (F) disease

Fever

Fracture (D) (occult rare)

Knee pain (E)

Brace vs. Surgical Containment

Rule out osteomyelitis, joint sepsis, discitis

Osteochondritis dissecans

Chondromalacia patella

Patellar subluxation

Osgood-Schlatter disease

Synovitis rule out rheumatoid

Other (E)

# LIMPING CHILD (AGE 10–15 YEARS)

## COMMENTS

A. Adolescents and teenagers rarely present with a congenital disorder (CDH, limp length problem) as the cause of a previously undiagnosed limp. Furthermore, osteomyelitis and joint sepsis are distinctly less common in this age group, but they occasionally occur and therefore always must be considered. Instead of the aforementioned, these children usually have acquired disease that requires treatment. Spine, hip, and knee disorders are common, especially slipped capital femoral epiphysis.

B. Always consider spinal cord tumors with their associated evolving neurologic deficit as the cause of limp. Also, developmental lesions, such as diastematomyelia and tethered spinal cord, are commonly first diagnosed in adolescence.

C. Spinal causes of limp include discitis, disc herniation, spondylolysis, and spondylolisthesis.

D. Hip symptoms in the 10- to 15-year age group are very often secondary to slipped capital femoral epiphysis. These children often present with only knee pain. Classic findings include limited or no internal rotation of the hip, especially with hip flexion. A lateral radiograph is required to confirm the diagnosis. Treatment is always surgical stabilization. Legg-Perthes disease and transient synovitis are also seen in this age group, but are distinctly less common than in the 5- to 15-year-old group.

E. Adolescents are heavily involved in athletics; thus, in addition to the usual listed knee disorders common for this age group, they also suffer from overuse syndromes, which may be related to patellar malalignment or other causes. Their management is always complicated by the similarity between adolescent athletes and addicted adult joggers, in that neither group considers decreased activity as a reasonable treatment option.

## REFERENCES

1. Boyer D, et al. Slipped capital femoral epiphysis. Long-term follow-up study of 121 patients. J Bone Joint Surg. 1981; 63A:85.
2. Highgenboten CL. Children's knee problems. Orthop Rev. 1981; 10:37.
3. Insall J. Patellar pain—current concepts review. J Bone Joint Surg. 1982;64A:147.

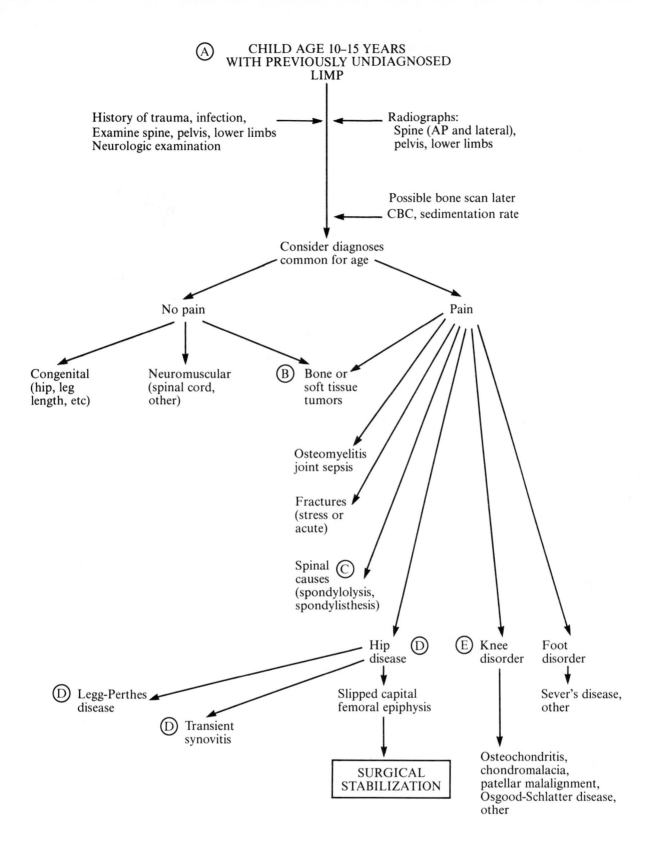

A CHILD AGE 10–15 YEARS
WITH PREVIOUSLY UNDIAGNOSED
LIMP

History of trauma, infection, → ← Radiographs:
Examine spine, pelvis, lower limbs     Spine (AP and lateral),
Neurologic examination     pelvis, lower limbs

Possible bone scan later
← CBC, sedimentation rate

Consider diagnoses
common for age

No pain          Pain

Congenital      Neuromuscular      B Bone or
(hip, leg       (spinal cord,        soft tissue
length, etc)    other)               tumors

Osteomyelitis
joint sepsis

Fractures
(stress or
acute)

Spinal C
causes
(spondylolysis,
spondylisthesis)

Hip D      E Knee      Foot
disease        disorder    disorder

D Legg-Perthes                              Sever's disease,
disease                                     other

D Transient      Slipped capital
synovitis        femoral epiphysis

SURGICAL          Osteochondritis,
STABILIZATION     chondromalacia,
                  patellar malalignment,
                  Osgood-Schlatter disease,
                  other

# JOINT EFFUSION

## COMMENTS

A. This chapter is meant to address the child who does not have a history, physical findings, or laboratory studies to suggest joint sepsis. The classic presentation is a juvenile with a fluid-filled knee, but no history of infection, trauma, or other disorder. The child often has little or no pain. The hip is not considered in this chapter because a hip effusion is not visible or palpable. Because the presentation and natural history of acute transient synovitis of the hip (observation hip syndrome) are better understood, that disorder will not be considered here.

B. The family history may be important in establishing a diagnosis of rheumatoid arthritis, hemophilia, gout, tuberculosis, and fungal infection.

C. In rheumatoid arthritis, the first radiographic changes are soft tissue swelling, capsular distention, and periarticular osteoporosis. Later, the articular cartilage space narrows. Adjacent bony and soft tissue lesions should be searched for as they may be the cause of the effusion. Classic examples are the sympathetic joint effusions produced by an osteoid osteoma or eosinophilic granuloma. Adjacent soft tissue hemangiomas may cause intra-articular bleeding.

D. An initial CBC and sedimentation rate are mandatory. If rheumatoid arthritis or another systemic disease is suspected, tests for C-reactive protein, rheumatoid factor, and antinuclear antibodies can be ordered. Unfortunately, there are no pathognomonic laboratory tests for rheumatoid arthritis, particularly in children, who usually have normal serum rheumatoid factors. Serum uric acid should be determined if gout is suspected, and appropriate hematologic studies (PTT) are indicated if hemophilia is suspected.

E. Joint fluid analysis is vital for assessment of an unexplained joint effusion. When intra-articular disease is suspected, the aspiration can be done in conjunction with arthroscopy, as can arthroscopic biopsy. In most cases, an initial needle aspiration is adequate and the expense of arthroscopy is avoided.

F. The pauciarticular form of rheumatoid arthritis, which involves a few large joints and produces minimal or no systemic symptoms, is the common final "explanation" for unexplained chronic joint effusion. There are two peak ages of onset—1 to 4 years and 9 to 14 years. Certain serum changes lead us, at our current state of knowledge, to refer to the disorder as an "auto-immune disease"; however, this is unlikely to be the primary cause. More likely, an invading organism (viral, protozoal, unusual bacteria) causes the secondary immune response; however, current knowledge and methods are inadequate to detect the etiologic agent. Patients with juvenile rheumatoid arthritis should have regular slit lamp examinations by an ophthalmologist because the eye is often involved, especially in the pauciarticular form. Failure to establish early diagnosis and treatment of this associated iridocyclitis can rapidly lead to blindness. The clinical course of pauciarticular arthritis is generally benign, usually resolving in 2 or 3 years.

G. A thorn or other foreign body can perforate the skin and enter a joint (especially the knee) in children, and the episode may not be remembered by the child or parent. Diagnosis is difficult. Arthroscopy may help. Sometimes the offending intruder is identified only at complete synovectomy.

H. Arthroscopic examination will help in cases in which an intra-articular problem—such as meniscal tear, loose body secondary to osteochondritis, synovial plica, and discoid meniscus—may be causing an effusion.

## REFERENCE

1. Tachjian MO. *Pediatric Orthopaedics.* Philadelphia: WB Saunders, 1972.

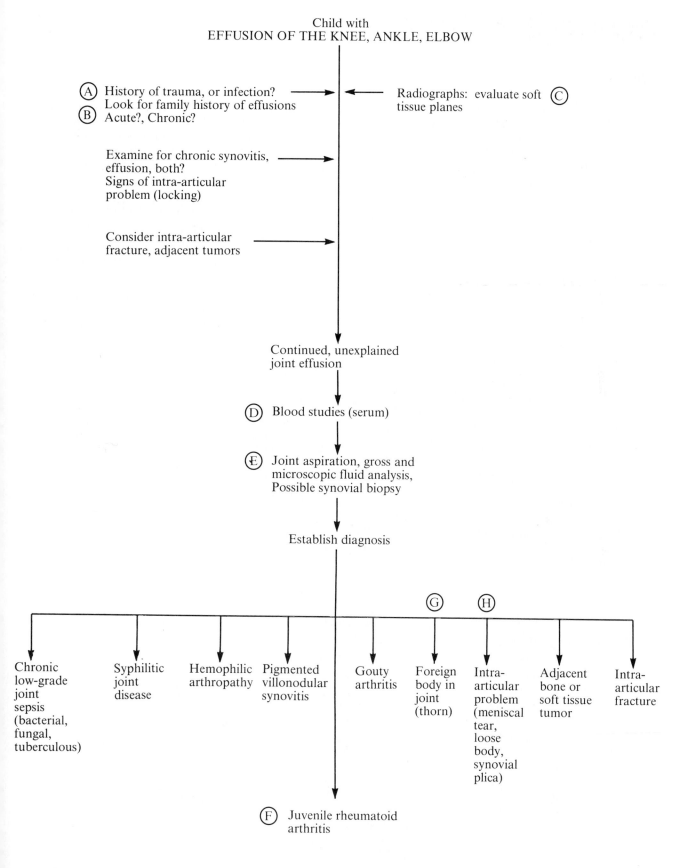

Child with
EFFUSION OF THE KNEE, ANKLE, ELBOW

(A) History of trauma, or infection?
(B) Look for family history of effusions
Acute?, Chronic?

Radiographs: evaluate soft (C)
tissue planes

Examine for chronic synovitis,
effusion, both?
Signs of intra-articular
problem (locking)

Consider intra-articular
fracture, adjacent tumors

Continued, unexplained
joint effusion

(D) Blood studies (serum)

(E) Joint aspiration, gross and
microscopic fluid analysis,
Possible synovial biopsy

Establish diagnosis

(G)   (H)

Chronic
low-grade
joint
sepsis
(bacterial,
fungal,
tuberculous)

Syphilitic
joint
disease

Hemophilic
arthropathy

Pigmented
villonodular
synovitis

Gouty
arthritis

Foreign
body in
joint
(thorn)

Intra-
articular
problem
(meniscal
tear,
loose
body,
synovial
plica)

Adjacent
bone or
soft tissue
tumor

Intra-
articular
fracture

(F) Juvenile rheumatoid
arthritis

# CLUBFOOT

## COMMENTS

A. Neurologic disorders such as spina bifida, tethered cord, and diastematomyelia can produce foot deformity. Since children with clubfoot have a higher incidence of congenital hip dislocation, you should examine the entire child, particularly the spine and hips, *before* examining the foot.

B. Radiographs confirm the severity of deformity, allow later comparisons, and help in judging the type of surgical correction needed.

C. The adhesive strapping method of Hensinger and Jones is effective and much tidier in treating the neonate.[1] A neonate commonly has a more flexible clubfoot, which is readily corrected by manipulation-strapping.

D. Correct manipulation and casting of a clubfoot is an acquired skill that is becoming a lost art.[2,3,4] The need for extensive surgery is reduced if casting is early and effective. Casts should be changed at least weekly and when possible every 3–4 days. Casts should be long leg (knee bent to 90°) to maintain a corrective force on the forefoot and to keep them from falling off.

E. A skillfully performed heel cord tenotomy can be performed on an outpatient basis with only local anesthesia.[3] This maneuver prevents production of a "rocker-bottom" foot by forcing dorsiflexion. Turco advises that the tenotomy be performed open, under general anesthesia, at the musculotendinous junction to avoid scarring,

which might make subsequent posteromedial release more difficult. Certain patients may benefit from a complete posterior release performed under general anesthesia.

F. A careful, technically correct, complete yet not overdone posteromedial release is one of the most difficult procedures in orthopaedics.[5] Correct surgery is only half the battle; maintaining the correction in the cast is vital.

G. Maintenance of the correction obtained at surgery requires pins across the talonavicular and subtalar joints.

H. The child is kept in a Denis-Browne splint full-time until pulling to stand, followed by night and nap-time use for 2 years.

## REFERENCES

1. Hensinger RW, Jones ET. *Neonatal Orthopaedics.* New York: Grune & Stratton, 1981.
2. Kite JH. Some suggestions on the treatment of clubfoot by casts. J Bone Joint Surg. 1963;45A:406.
3. Ponseti IV. Congenital Clubfoot, the results of treatment. J Bone Joint Surg. 1963;45A:261.
4. Ponseti IV. *Nonoperative treatment of congenital clubfoot.* Chicago: American Academy of Orthopaedic Surgeons Film Library, 1972.
5. Turco V. *Clubfoot.* New York: Churchill-Livingstone, 1981.

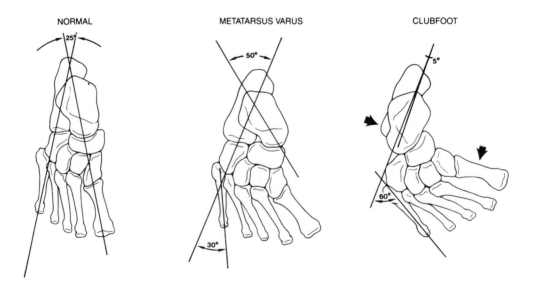

Note Kite's angle—increased in metatarsus varus
—decreased in club foot (after Ponseti).

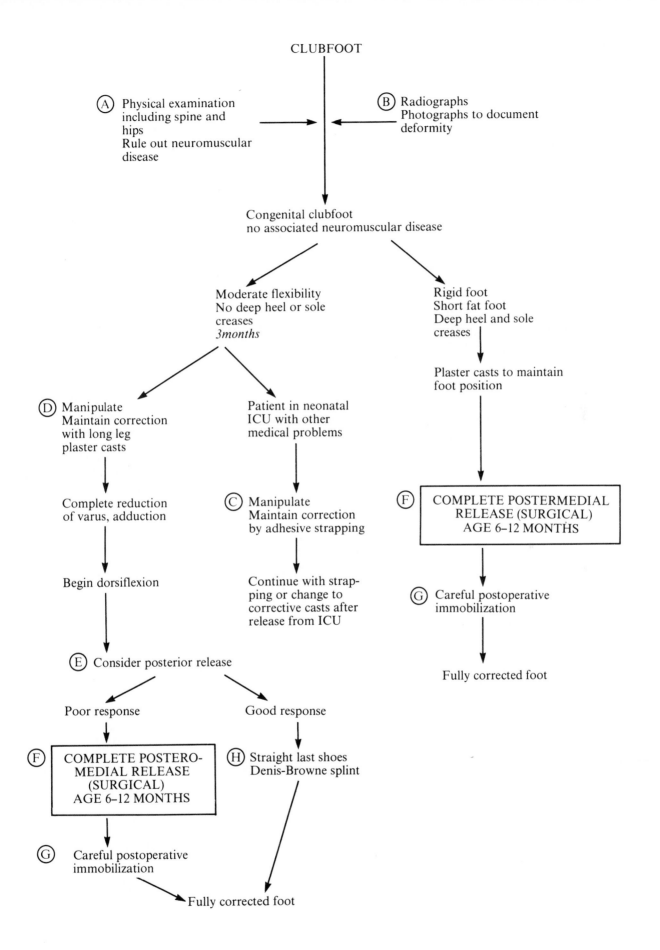

CLUBFOOT

(A) Physical examination including spine and hips
Rule out neuromuscular disease

(B) Radiographs
Photographs to document deformity

Congenital clubfoot
no associated neuromuscular disease

Moderate flexibility
No deep heel or sole creases
*3 months*

Rigid foot
Short fat foot
Deep heel and sole creases

Plaster casts to maintain foot position

(D) Manipulate
Maintain correction with long leg plaster casts

Patient in neonatal ICU with other medical problems

Complete reduction of varus, adduction

(C) Manipulate
Maintain correction by adhesive strapping

(F) COMPLETE POSTERMEDIAL RELEASE (SURGICAL) AGE 6–12 MONTHS

Begin dorsiflexion

Continue with strapping or change to corrective casts after release from ICU

(G) Careful postoperative immobilization

Fully corrected foot

(E) Consider posterior release

Poor response

Good response

(F) COMPLETE POSTERO-MEDIAL RELEASE (SURGICAL) AGE 6–12 MONTHS

(H) Straight last shoes Denis-Browne splint

(G) Careful postoperative immobilization

Fully corrected foot

# METATARSUS VARUS

## COMMENTS

A. The incidence of hip dysplasia is higher in patients with metatarsus varus than in the general population.[3] For this reason some clinics advise routine pelvic radiographs; however, a careful clinical examination should suffice.

B. The terms metatarsus varus and metatarsus adductus are used interchangeably. In patients requiring cast correction, special attention should be given to correction of the varus component of the forefoot. Residual heel valgus in severe untreated cases is more the result of failure to correct forefoot varus (supination) than from failure to correct forefoot adduction.

C. It is impossible to define "correctability." Only time will develop the clinical judgement necessary for the accurate categorization of patients. One helpful method is to stroke the foot medially, noting if the infant reflexly corrects the deformity.

D. Children with metatarsus varus requiring cast correction are best treated at age 2–4 months.[1] Only severe deformities should be considered for treatment at a younger age in order to avoid overtreating the many feet which initially appear to need correction but correct spontaneously. After age 6–8 months, the deformity is so rigid and the child so strong that cast correction is nearly impossible. At this age, alternatives include observation with hope that the foot will improve spontaneously. In rare cases, severe cases will require surgical correction at an older age. Corrective casts for metatarsus varus are quite different from clubfoot casts as distinguished in Ponseti's classic paper describing the mechanics of cast correction for metatarsus varus.[4] The heel must be held in varus with the fulcrum for forefoot correction at the cuboid laterally. Long leg casts (90°, knee bent) are preferable since (a) they will not slide off and (b) they provide rapid correction of both the foot deformity and the associated internal tibial torsion. Continue use of the cast correction until the deformity is overcorrected.[2]

E. Straight shoes will not correct a deformed foot but are sometimes used along with passive stretching by the parents as a sort of "milieu therapy" for mild cases. Feet requiring cast correction are maintained in the corrected position with straight last shoes until about age 2 years. A Denis-Browne splint is not advised because it tends to increase the already present excessive heel valgus.

F. Surgical correction for metatarsus varus is rarely indicated. When needed, Heyman-Herndon soft tissue releases are advised in children under age 4 years; multiple metatarsal osteotomies are recommended for older children. Avoid injury to the proximally located physis in the first metatarsal. Both procedures are technically demanding. In severe cases requiring surgical correction, associated heel valgus is common and must be addressed or the child will be further disabled because correction of the forefoot alone will remove the stable tripod of the foot.

## REFERENCES

1. Kite JH. Congenital metatarsus varus: report of 300 cases. J Bone Joint Surg. 1950;32A:500.
2. Kite JH. Congenital metatarsus varus. J Bone Joint Surg. 1967;49A:388.
3. Kurmar JS, MacEwen GD. The incidence of hip dysplasia with metatarsus adductus. Clin Orthop. 1982;164:234.
4. Ponseti IV. Congenital metatarsus adductus: the results of treatment. J Bone Joint Surg. 1966;48A:702.

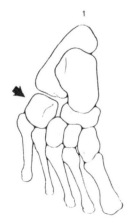 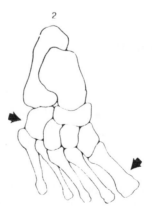 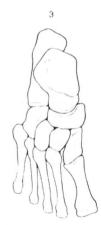

Correct application of forces for cast correction of metatarsus varus (after Ponseti).

METATARSUS VARUS

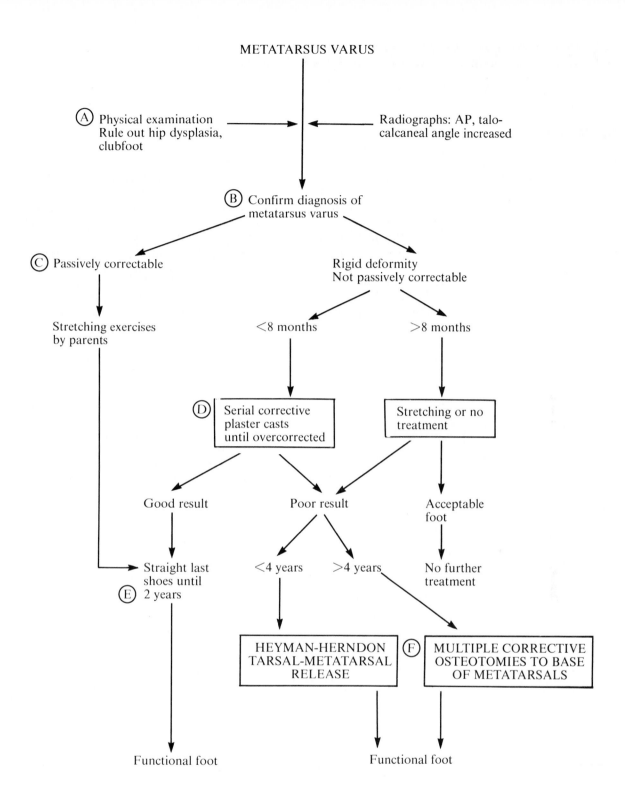

Ⓐ Physical examination
Rule out hip dysplasia,
clubfoot

Radiographs: AP, talo-
calcaneal angle increased

Ⓑ Confirm diagnosis of
metatarsus varus

Ⓒ Passively correctable

Rigid deformity
Not passively correctable

Stretching exercises
by parents

<8 months

>8 months

Ⓓ Serial corrective
plaster casts
until overcorrected

Stretching or no
treatment

Good result

Poor result

Acceptable
foot

Straight last
shoes until
Ⓔ 2 years

<4 years

>4 years

No further
treatment

HEYMAN-HERNDON
TARSAL-METATARSAL
RELEASE

Ⓕ MULTIPLE CORRECTIVE
OSTEOTOMIES TO BASE
OF METATARSALS

Functional foot

Functional foot

# VERTICAL TALUS (CONGENITAL CONVEX PES VALGUS)

## COMMENTS

A. About 50% of infants with a true vertical talus have an associated neuromuscular disorder such as spina bifida, arthrogryposis, or muscle disease. Physical examination should distinguish between a true vertical talus and a calcaneovalgus foot. In a true vertical talus the heel cord is contracted and the child has a rocker-bottom foot. Also, there is no "bone" felt when the heel is palpated because the tight heel cord has pulled the calcaneus out of the heel pad.

B. Vertical talus may be overdiagnosed radiologically. Any lateral view demonstrating a plantar directed talus should not necessarily be labeled a vertical talus. A diagnosis of vertical talus requires that the talus be in a fixed dislocated position on the dorsum of the talus. Forced plantar flexion lateral radiographs differentiate between talonavicular subluxation (oblique talus) and dislocation (vertical talus). The navicular is not yet ossified so the first metatarsal is used to assess alignment. If in forced plantar flexion the first metatarsal aligns with the talus, the navicular is reducible, the diagnosis of oblique talus is applied, and treatment is easier.

C. A true vertical talus has a fixed dislocation of the talonavicular joint; thus, the metatarsals do not align with the talus in the forced plantar flexion lateral radiograph. In addition, the subtalar joint is subluxated because the talus is directed medially with the remainder of the foot directed laterally.

D. Although an oblique talus is really a mild variation of vertical talus, the distinction is useful because most patients will respond to serial corrective casts plus a heel cord lengthening, whereas a true vertical talus requires extensive surgery to achieve correction.

E. Surgical correction of a severe vertical talus deformity is best performed at age 4–12 months. Because the disorder is rare and the surgical procedure is complex, only experienced surgeons should attempt it. The procedure can be performed in one[3] or two stages.[2] Variations are often needed in older children and include associated tendon transfers, bone-block procedures, medial column shortening, or navicular excision.[1]

F. Less severe cases that respond well to plaster cast correction can be considered for percutaneous pinning of the reduced talonavicular joint plus heel cord lengthening. The procedure is performed under image intensifier control. This much simpler procedure will give a satisfactory result only in feet with a moderate deformity.

## REFERENCES

1. Clark M, et al. Congenital vertical talus: Treatment by open reduction and navicular excision. J Bone Joint Surg. 1977;59A:816.
2. Coleman SS, et al. Pathomechanics and treatment of congenital vertical talus. Clin Orthop. 1970;70:62.
3. Tachdjian M. *Pediatric Orthopaedics*. Philadelphia: Saunders, 1972.

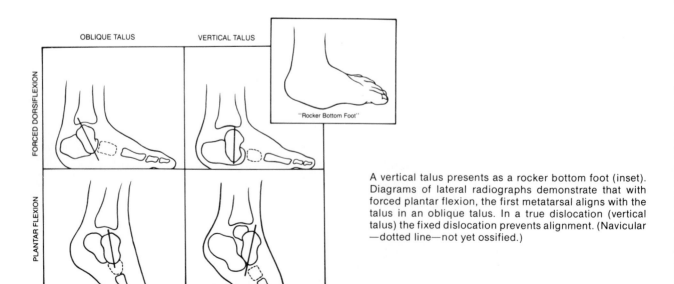

A vertical talus presents as a rocker bottom foot (inset). Diagrams of lateral radiographs demonstrate that with forced plantar flexion, the first metatarsal aligns with the talus in an oblique talus. In a true dislocation (vertical talus) the fixed dislocation prevents alignment. (Navicular—dotted line—not yet ossified.)

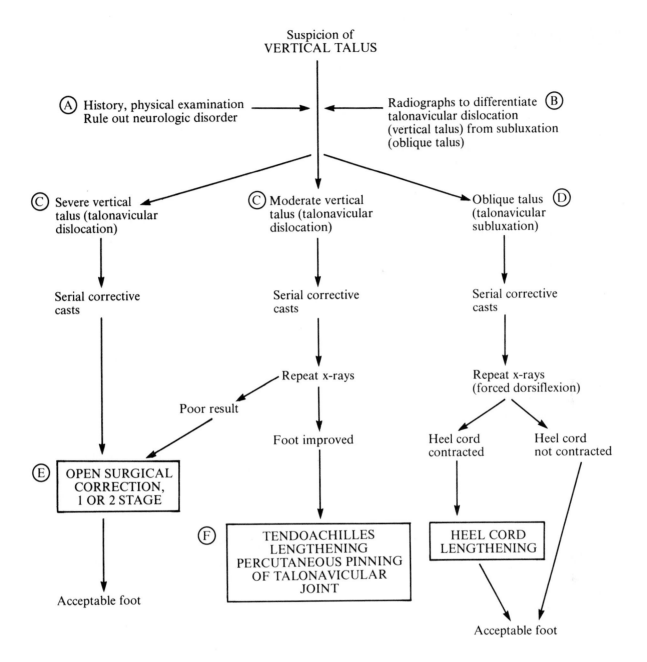

Suspicion of
VERTICAL TALUS

(A) History, physical examination
Rule out neurologic disorder

(B) Radiographs to differentiate
talonavicular dislocation
(vertical talus) from subluxation
(oblique talus)

(C) Severe vertical
talus (talonavicular
dislocation)

(C) Moderate vertical
talus (talonavicular
dislocation)

(D) Oblique talus
(talonavicular
subluxation)

Serial corrective
casts

Serial corrective
casts

Serial corrective
casts

Repeat x-rays

Poor result

Foot improved

Repeat x-rays
(forced dorsiflexion)

Heel cord
contracted

Heel cord
not contracted

(E) OPEN SURGICAL
CORRECTION,
1 OR 2 STAGE

(F) TENDOACHILLES
LENGTHENING
PERCUTANEOUS PINNING
OF TALONAVICULAR
JOINT

HEEL CORD
LENGTHENING

Acceptable foot

Acceptable foot

# CAVUS FOOT

## COMMENTS

A. Pes cavus is a fixed equinus and pronation deformity of the forefoot on the hindfoot, usually resulting from an underlying neuromuscular disorder: spinal dysraphism (spina bifida, lipoma, tethered cord, diastematomyelia), Charcot-Marie-Tooth disease, Friedreich's ataxia, cord tumor, and so on. Occasionally, cases are familial and/or idiopathic. When unilateral, a spinal disorder is almost always the cause.

B. The possible pathomechanical explanations for cavus deformity center on weakness of either extrinsic or intrinsic foot muscles initiating an imbalance in the delicate "windlass" mechanism, which provides normal balance between the forefoot and hindfoot. As the imbalance progresses, the plantar fascia contracts and clawing of the toes develops.

C. Current diagnosis and treatment of cavus foot requires a clear understanding of how loss of normal forefoot-hindfoot rotary mobility affects overall foot mechanics. All cavus feet demonstrate excessive plantar-flexion of the first ray with pronation of the forefoot in relation to the hindfoot. When the relative pronation is fixed (A), weight bearing forces the forefoot into supination (first metatarsal head strikes first) followed by obligatory heel varus (B). Coleman's lateral block test[1] (C), establishes whether the hindfoot is flexible or fixed and determines the type of surgical correction required.

D. Corrective shoes and/or inserts are not effective in correcting cavus feet.

E. Radical medial and plantar release—plantar fascia, short flexors, abductor hallucis—is best undertaken after age 4–5 years. Weekly cast changes are advised to gain full correction.

F. If hindfoot varus is fixed in the lateral block test and the first ray deformity is severe, lateral sliding or Dwyer calcaneal osteotomy plus dorsiflexion osteotomy of the first ray are added. These procedures are recommended for children age 10 or older with fixed deformity since the indications for, and results of, bony osteotomies in younger children are less clear.

G. Triple arthrodesis and Japas mid-foot osteotomy have nearly disappeared from the treatment scheme for cavus foot. In general, early aggressive soft tissue releases,[2] tendon transfers to maintain correction, and extra-articular osteotomies (Dwyer calcaneal, first metatarsal) render fusion of joints unnecessary.

H. Tendon transfers will maintain a deformity only after it has been corrected in some other manner. Thus, Coleman advises that they be performed, if necessary, 6 weeks after the initial procedure. I sometimes perform them at the initial procedure, after all correction has been achieved. Transfer of the posterior tibial tendon to the dorsum via the interosseous membrane is very effective. Other variations include transfer of the anterior tibial tendon laterally, peroneus longus to the brevis to reduce plantar flexion force of the first ray, extensor hallucis longus recession, and occasionally *en-masse* recession of the long toe extensors.

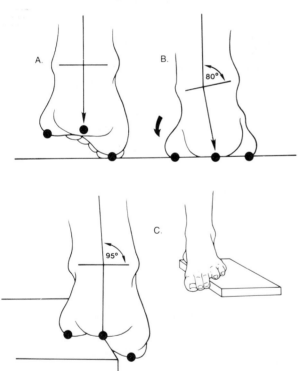

A Right cavus foot viewed from behind. First metatarsal is in fixed plantar flexion.
B With weight bearing, hindfoot is forced into obligatory varus.
C Coleman's block test. Hindfoot is correctable when first metatarsal hangs free from block.

## REFERENCES

1. Coleman SS, et al. A simple test for hindfoot flexibility in the cavovarus foot. Clin Orthop. 1977; 123:60
2. Paulos L, et al. Pes cavovarus: review of a surgical approach using selective soft tissue procedures. J Bone Joint Surg. 1980; 62A:942.

CAVUS FOOT

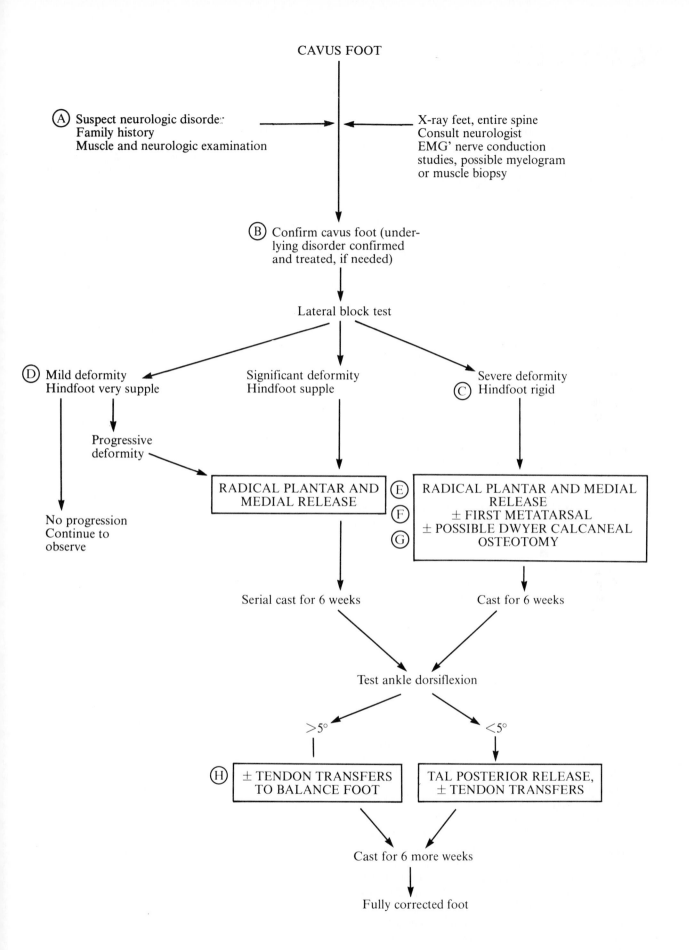

A) Suspect neurologic disorder
Family history
Muscle and neurologic examination

X-ray feet, entire spine
Consult neurologist
EMG' nerve conduction
studies, possible myelogram
or muscle biopsy

B) Confirm cavus foot (underlying disorder confirmed
and treated, if needed)

Lateral block test

D) Mild deformity
Hindfoot very supple

Significant deformity
Hindfoot supple

Severe deformity
C) Hindfoot rigid

Progressive
deformity

No progression
Continue to
observe

RADICAL PLANTAR AND
MEDIAL RELEASE

E)
F)
G)

RADICAL PLANTAR AND MEDIAL
RELEASE
± FIRST METATARSAL
± POSSIBLE DWYER CALCANEAL
OSTEOTOMY

Serial cast for 6 weeks

Cast for 6 weeks

Test ankle dorsiflexion

>5°

<5°

H) ± TENDON TRANSFERS
TO BALANCE FOOT

TAL POSTERIOR RELEASE,
± TENDON TRANSFERS

Cast for 6 more weeks

Fully corrected foot

# FLATFOOT

## COMMENTS

A. Most children with flexible flatfoot have loose ligaments, and thus their feet "sag" when they bear weight. As Salter states, if these children walked on their hands, they would have "flat" hands. Children with muscle disease may present with flatfoot. Use Gower's test to observe the child getting up from the floor. Also, children with cerebral palsy may present with a flatfoot secondary to heel cord tightness. The tiptoe test is another portion of the flatfoot screening process. When observed from behind, the flatfooted child has significant heel valgus. Then, when he stands on tiptoe, the hindfoot corrects into varus if the flatfoot is flexible and subtalar motion is not limited.

B. Tarsal coalition is a rare cause of flatfoot. When suspected because of limited subtalar motion, appropriate oblique and subtalar radiographic views are required.

C. Tight heel cords cause mid-foot breakdown or rockering which presents as a flatfoot. If tight, the heel cords should be stretched and may require surgical lengthening. Cerebral palsy should be considered in children with persistent tight heel cords.

D. Although widely prescribed by pediatricians and orthopaedic surgeons, the efficacy of so-called corrective footwear and/or inserts in changing the natural history of flexible flatfoot has not been established,[2] but is under investigation.[3] An active child is in the stance phase of weight bearing for only one hour of each day, considering sleeping, sitting, lounging, and swing phases. The only clear indications for treatment are severe shoe wear problems or severe foot or calf pain. Most shoes are prescribed to satisfy the parent's or physician's need to "do something". A medial heel wedge combined with a lateral sole wedge theoretically pronates the forefoot in relation to the hindfoot and thus provides correction. The University of California Biomechanics Laboratory (UCBL) insert is often used for severe deformities.[1] Corrective footwear is usually empirically discontinued by school age, a convenient and practical point at which the physician hopes the arch has improved and the child refuses to wear "orthopaedic shoes".

E. Surgical correction is rarely indicated for flexible flatfoot, but is occasionally needed when heel valgus and forefoot pronation are so severe that shoes cannot be worn. Extra-articular medial sliding calcaneal osteotomy plus medial soft tissue reefing with advancement of the posterior tibial tendon and spring ligament is partially effective in these severe cases.

## REFERENCES

1. Bleck EE, et al. Conservative management of pes valgus with plantar flexed talus, flexible. Clin Orthop. 1977;122:85.
2. Staheli L, et al. Corrective shoes for children: a survey of current practice. Pediatrics 1980;66:1.
3. Wenger D, et al. Prospective analysis comparing treatment methods for flexible flatfoot. Ongoing study, Texas Scottish Rite Hospital, Dallas, Texas, 1979.

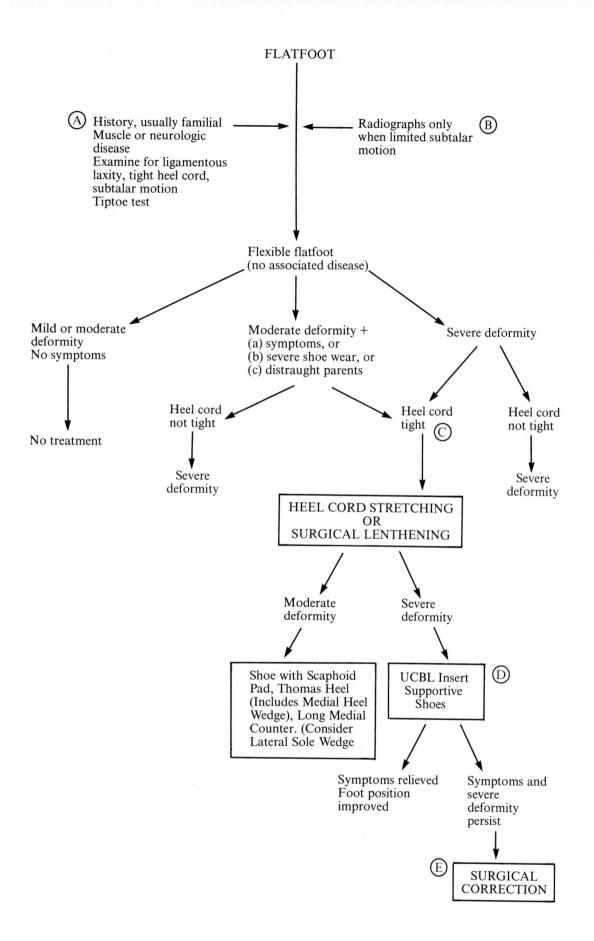

FLATFOOT

(A) History, usually familial
Muscle or neurologic
disease
Examine for ligamentous
laxity, tight heel cord,
subtalar motion
Tiptoe test

Radiographs only
when limited subtalar
motion (B)

Flexible flatfoot
(no associated disease)

Mild or moderate
deformity
No symptoms

Moderate deformity +
(a) symptoms, or
(b) severe shoe wear, or
(c) distraught parents

Severe deformity

No treatment

Heel cord
not tight

Heel cord
tight (C)

Heel cord
not tight

Severe
deformity

Severe
deformity

HEEL CORD STRETCHING
OR
SURGICAL LENTHENING

Moderate
deformity

Severe
deformity

Shoe with Scaphoid
Pad, Thomas Heel
(Includes Medial Heel
Wedge), Long Medial
Counter. (Consider
Lateral Sole Wedge

UCBL Insert
Supportive
Shoes (D)

Symptoms relieved
Foot position
improved

Symptoms and
severe
deformity
persist

(E) SURGICAL
CORRECTION

# TARSAL COALITION

## COMMENTS

A. Tarsal coalition is a misnomer since the conditon results from failure of segmentation of the tarsal bones. A term used almost synonymously with tarsal coalition is "peroneal spastic flatfoot".[2] Patients with calcaneonavicular coalitions in particular have a synovitis in the sinus tarsi area which causes increased reflex activity in the peroneal tendons, a probable protective mechanism. Quick forced varus or a reflex hammer tap on the peroneal tendons elicits spasticity.

B. Special x-rays are needed to demonstrate tarsal coalitions. AP and lateral x-rays will demonstrate neither of the classic types. The Canadian Army Foot Series includes AP, lateral, oblique, and axial (Harris) subtalar views. The axial view is required to demonstrate a talocalcaneal bar which forms medially in the area of the sustentaculum tali (A and B). The lateral oblique view will demonstrate a calcaneonavicular coalition (C). These two coalitions are by far the commonest. CT scanning is invaluable in difficult cases for diagnosis and preoperative planning.

C. Plain AP and lateral x-rays may demonstrate the secondary changes resulting from tarsal coalitions, namely narrowing of the posterior subtalar joint and osteophyte formation on the dorsum of the talus. It is important to rule out other causes of limited subtalar motion such as rheumatoid arthritis, osteomyelitis, osteoid osteoma, and other benign tumors such as aneurysmal bone cyst.

D. Symptoms usually do not occur until age 8–10 years when the cartilaginous or fibrous coalition begins to ossify.

E. Surgical excision of a calcaneonavicular bar often relieves symptoms. The short toe extensor muscle mass is sutured into the area from which the bar is removed to prevent regrowth.

F. Excision of a talocalcaneal bar is rarely successful in relieving symptoms. Thus, prolonged conservative treatment is advised; triple arthrodesis is performed if symptoms persist.

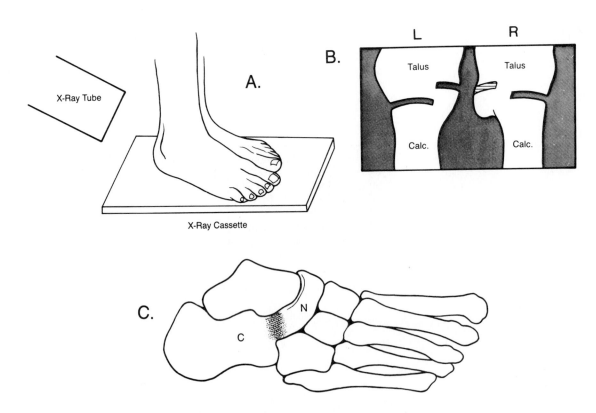

A   Diagram of the Harris axial view.
B   Radiograph of the Harris axial view demonstrating right tarsal coalition (talocalcaneal).
C   Lateral oblique radiograph demonstrating calcaneonavicular coalition.

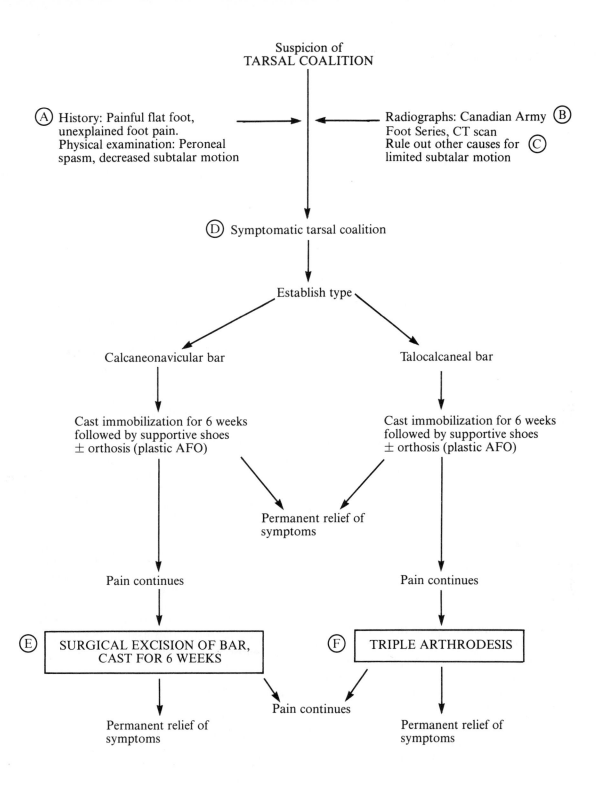

Suspicion of
TARSAL COALITION

(A) History: Painful flat foot,
unexplained foot pain.
Physical examination: Peroneal
spasm, decreased subtalar motion

Radiographs: Canadian Army (B)
Foot Series, CT scan
Rule out other causes for (C)
limited subtalar motion

(D) Symptomatic tarsal coalition

Establish type

Calcaneonavicular bar

Talocalcaneal bar

Cast immobilization for 6 weeks
followed by supportive shoes
± orthosis (plastic AFO)

Cast immobilization for 6 weeks
followed by supportive shoes
± orthosis (plastic AFO)

Permanent relief of
symptoms

Pain continues

Pain continues

(E) SURGICAL EXCISION OF BAR,
CAST FOR 6 WEEKS

(F) TRIPLE ARTHRODESIS

Permanent relief of
symptoms

Pain continues

Permanent relief of
symptoms

## REFERENCES

1. Cowell HR. Talocalcaneal coalition and new causes of peroneal spastic flatfoot. Clin Orthop. 1972; 85:16.

2. Harris RI, et al. Etiology of peroneal spastic flatfoot. J Bone Joint Surg. 1948; 30B:624.

# CEREBRAL PALSY

## COMMENTS

A. Neurologists refer to cerebral palsy as *static encephalopathy*. Take a careful history and, with follow-up examinations, confirm that the neurologic deficit is truly static. Unusual disorders, such as brain and cervical spine tumors, can mimic cerebral palsy.

B. Types of cerebral palsy include spastic, athetoid, hypotonic, mixed, and others. Children with the pure athetoid form rarely benefit from surgery. Severity refers to proportion of body involved—hemipelgic, diplegic, quadriplegic, total body (head also involved). Infants with cerebral palsy are often floppy and hypotonic. When the nerves become myelinated (6 months to 2 years), spasticity appears. Cerebral palsy patients have three stages in progression to fixed joint deformity; first, no dynamic or passive contracture; second, dynamic contracture, but no fixed contracture; third, fixed contracture. The physical therapy and orthopaedic team should intervene so that a child will not reach the third stage.

C. Cerebral palsy patients have many problems. This algorithm will focus only on the three major areas (spine, hips, lower extremity deformities and their effect on gait) in which orthopaedic surgeons can have their greatest effect.

D. Children with mild curves are initially managed with wheel chair inserts or seating systems. If this proves inadequate, a custom-molded under-arm plastic jacket can be tried. Certain patients with manic, uncontrollable behavior may not tolerate a brace and can only be kept under observation, allowed to progress, and then treated by surgical fusion, using Segmental Spinal Instrumentation. Currently, almost any cerebral palsy patient with severe progressive scoliosis is treated by surgical correction, even if the child is institutionalized and severely retarded. This is justified because a child with a straight spine can sit up and thus is happier and can be cared for more economically.

E. The hips in all cerebral palsy patients should be maintained in the acetabulum, since *some* patients develop severe pain following dislocation. Mental status is not considered a factor in determining the need for maintenance of reduction—severely affected institutionalized patients also have pain. The best method for maintaining reduction is early soft tissue release (adductors, psoas), followed by nighttime abduction splinting. Obtruator neurectomies are no longer routinely advocated because denervation is thought to produce muscle fibrosis, which may hasten redevelopment of contracture. More severe subluxation or dislocation requires varus femoral osteotomy or femoral plus pelvic osteotomy.

F. Children with significant cerebral palsy have early physical therapy to improve gait. In some cases, bracing is also used, although the modern trend is toward physical therapy with well-conceived, well-timed surgery rather than bracing. Inhibitory casts or intramuscular alcohol injections may also help in the planning of surgery. When indicated, surgery should be performed after the age of 3 to 4 years and before the age of 8 years. The surgeon, physical therapist, and parents should have a generally consistent philosophy regarding the role of surgery in improving gait. If you are not sincerely interested in cerebral palsy, refer the child to someone who is. The occasional, partially interested surgeon rarely achieves good results.

G. All hemiplegic children will walk. Thus, surgery is designed to make the child look better. Often, TAL (tendo Achilles lengthening) is adequate; however, adding posterior tibial intramuscular lengthening, medial hamstring lengthening, and adductor release improves dynamic in-torsion.

H. Children with diplegia and mild quadriplegia with crouch deformity may benefit from well-planned three-level surgery. Tendo-Achilles lenthening alone may worsen crouch at the knee in a child with flexion deformities at the hips, knees, and ankles. Such errors are the reason for the healthy degree of suspicion among physical therapists concerning the value of surgical intervention in cerebral palsy. Consider simultaneous three-level releases in patients with crouch deformity (psoas and adductors, hamstrings, heel cords), followed by 6 weeks in *walking* casts and continued physical therapy for several months.

## REFERENCES

1. Bleck EE. Locomotor prognosis in cerebral palsy. Dev Med Child Neurol. 1075;17:18.
2. Bleck EE. *Orthopaedic Management of Cerebral Palsy*. Philadelphia: WB Saunders, 1979.
3. Drennan J. *Orthopaedic Management of Neuromuscular Disorders*. Philadelphia: JB Lippincott, 1983.

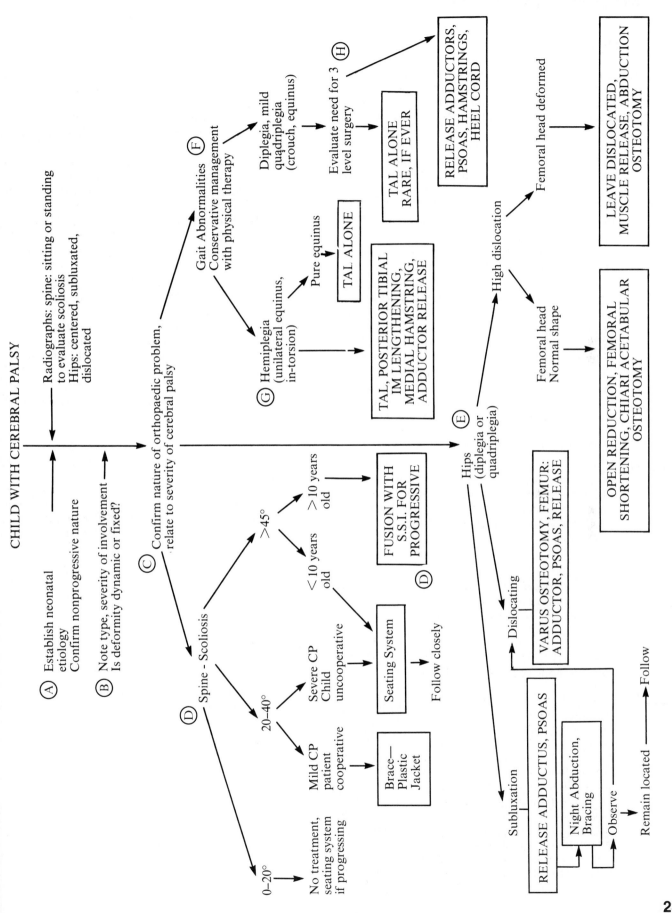

# CHILD WITH CEREBRAL PALSY

Radiographs: spine: sitting or standing
to evaluate scoliosis
Hips: centered, subluxated,
dislocated

(A) Establish neonatal
etiology
Confirm nonprogressive nature

(B) Note type, severity of involvement
Is deformity dynamic or fixed?

(C) Confirm nature of orthopaedic problem,
relate to severity of cerebral palsy

Gait Abnormalities
Conservative management
with physical therapy

(F) Diplegia, mild
quadriplegia
(crouch, equinus)

Evaluate need for 3
level surgery (H)

TAL ALONE
RARE, IF EVER

RELEASE ADDUCTORS,
PSOAS, HAMSTRINGS,
HEEL CORD

Femoral head deformed

LEAVE DISLOCATED,
MUSCLE RELEASE, ABDUCTION
OSTEOTOMY

(G) Hemiplegia
(unilateral equinus,
in-torsion)

Pure equinus

TAL ALONE

TAL, POSTERIOR TIBIAL
IM LENGTHENING,
MEDIAL HAMSTRING,
ADDUCTOR RELEASE

Femoral head
Normal shape

OPEN REDUCTION, FEMORAL
SHORTENING, CHIARI ACETABULAR
OSTEOTOMY

High dislocation

(E) Hips
(diplegia or
quadriplegia)

(D) Spine - Scoliosis

>45°

>10 years
old

<10 years
old

FUSION WITH
S.S.I. FOR
PROGRESSIVE (D)

20-40°

Severe CP
Child
uncooperative

Seating System

Follow closely

Mild CP
patient
cooperative

Brace—
Plastic
Jacket

0-20°

No treatment,
seating system
if progressing

Dislocating

VARUS OSTEOTOMY, FEMUR:
ADDUCTOR, PSOAS, RELEASE

Subluxation

RELEASE ADDUCTUS, PSOAS

Night Abduction,
Bracing

Observe

Remain located ——▶ Follow

235

# SPINA BIFIDA

## COMMENTS

A. This algorithm will provide a general outline of care, since specific details of treatment can be found elsewhere.[1,2] Determining the neurologic level (lowest functioning nerves) will help to establish the prognosis. Multidisciplinary care—including regular orthopaedic, urologic, neurosurgical, and orthotic attention—must be established. Proper shunting (and shunt maintenance) for hydrocephalus will be a greater determinant of adult function (intellectual capacity) than any orthopaedic treatment.

B. All children must have an IVP, cystogram, and regular urology follow-up because almost all spina bifinda patients have neurogenic bladders.

C. Early accurate establishment of neurologic level determines the degree of orthopaedic care that will be needed and allows you to better advise the parents about long-term prognosis. Isolated distal spastic muscle function (not controlled voluntarily) is common, and when present, makes early level determination more difficult. Another reason for early accurate documentation of the functional level is the establishment of a baseline, which allows early detection of functional deterioration if hydromyelia, tethered cord, or other problems develop.

D. The feet are partially or completely insensate and must be plantigrade to fit shoes and orthoses. Otherwise, skin ulcers will develop. Corrective casts, tendon releases or transfers, and later bony procedures may be needed to keep the feet braceable. Knees should be kept straight (and braceable) with casts, soft tissue release, or extension osteotomy.

E. Kyphosis occasionally occurs in thoracic level lesions and is present at birth. Bracing may protect the skin, but does little to affect the deformity. The indications for surgical correction are cosmetic concern and recurrent skin breakdown over the deformity. The surgery is difficult, but new methods have improved results.

F. Scoliosis is not usually present at birth, but develops because of congenital vertebral anomalies and/or muscle weakness. Curves that progress to 25° are braced (under-arm plastic orthosis). Curves over 45° are surgically corrected and fused when the child is 10 years of age or older. If the child is younger, bracing is often used in curves of over 40° in an attempt to gain trunk height prior to fusion. Anterior disc excision and grafting (± Dwyer) plus posterior segmental fusion (Luque) to the sacrum produces predictable results. Relentless scoliosis progression in a juvenile (3 to 9 years) should arouse suspicion of a tethered cord or hydromyelia, a common, treatable development in spina bifida.

G. The treatment of hip subluxation and dislocation in spina bifida is changing. Children with thoracic and upper lumbar levels do *not* benefit from having their hips maintained in the acetabulum. However, muscle releases are indicated (flexors, adductors, sometimes external rotators) to keep the limbs well aligned for weight bearing (Menelaus).[2] Patients with lower lumbar level *may* benefit from hip stabilization, which is achieved by femoral or femoral plus pelvic osteotomies.

H. Treatment of spina bifida in childhood emphasizes the ambulatory status, which improves socialization, self-image and bladder drainage. Thoracic and upper lumbar level patients change to wheelchair mobility by adolescence or the early teenage years. Some lower lumbar patients prefer ambulation in adult life; however, many find wheelchair mobility to be quicker and more practical. Parents should be aware of these patterns, and mobility (not necessarily walking) should be emphasized, particularly as the child becomes a teenager.

## REFERENCES

1. Drennan JC. *Orthopaedic Management of Neuromuscular Disorders*. Philadelphia: JB Lippincott, 1983.
2. Menelaus MB. *The Orthopaedic Management of Spina Bifida Cystica*. 2nd Ed. New York: Churchill-Livingstone, 1980.

# CHILD WITH SPINA BIFIDA

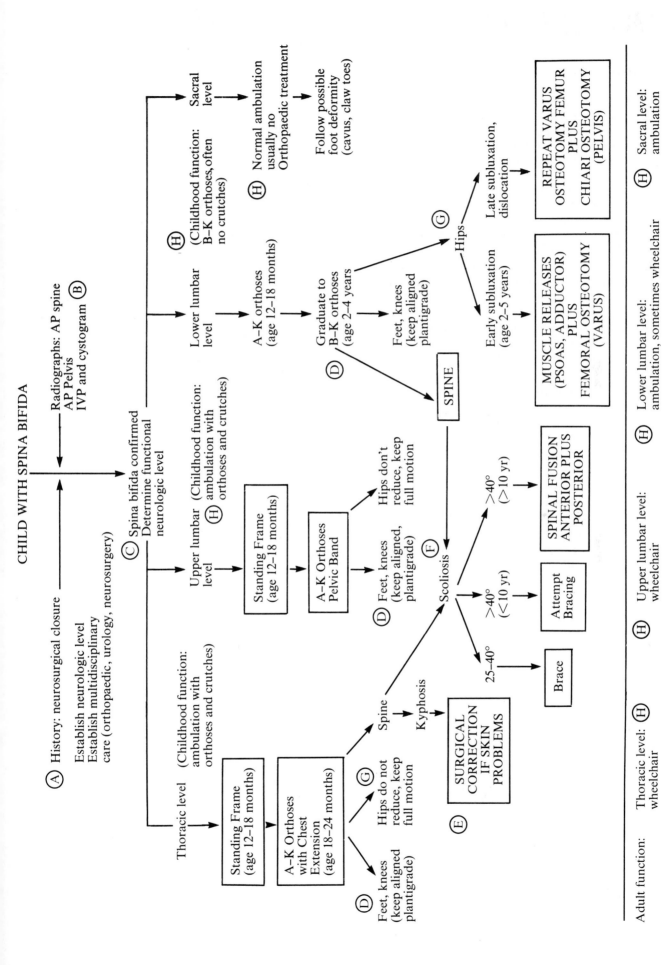

A. History: neurologic closure

Radiographs: AP spine
AP Pelvis
IVP and cystogram B.

Establish neurologic level
Establish multidisciplinary
care (orthopaedic, urology, neurosurgery)

C. Spina bifida confirmed
Determine functional
neurologic level

**Thoracic level** (Childhood function: ambulation with orthoses and crutches)

Standing Frame
(age 12–18 months)

A–K Orthoses
with Chest
Extension
(age 18–24 months)

D. Feet, knees
(keep aligned
plantigrade)

G. Hips do not
reduce, keep
full motion

Spine → Kyphosis

E. SURGICAL
CORRECTION
IF SKIN
PROBLEMS

**Upper lumbar level** (Childhood function:
H. ambulation with
orthoses and crutches)

Standing Frame
(age 12–18 months)

A–K Orthoses
Pelvic Band

Hips don't
reduce, keep
full motion

D. Feet, knees
(keep aligned,
plantigrade)

F. Scoliosis

25–40° → Brace

>40°
(<10 yr) → Attempt
Bracing

>40°
(>10 yr) → SPINAL FUSION
ANTERIOR PLUS
POSTERIOR

SPINE

**Lower lumbar
level**

A–K orthoses
(age 12–18 months)

Graduate to
B–K orthoses
(age 2–4 years)

D. Feet, knees
(keep aligned
plantigrade)

G. Hips

Late subluxation,
dislocation → REPEAT VARUS
OSTEOTOMY FEMUR
PLUS
CHIARI OSTEOTOMY
(PELVIS)

Early subluxation
(age 2–5 years) → MUSCLE RELEASES
(PSOAS, ADDUCTOR)
PLUS
FEMORAL OSTEOTOMY
(VARUS)

**Sacral
level**

H. (Childhood function:
B–K orthoses, often
no crutches)

H. Normal ambulation
usually no
Orthopaedic treatment

Follow possible
foot deformity
(cavus, claw toes)

Adult function:

Thoracic level: H.
wheelchair

Upper lumbar level: H.
wheelchair

Lower lumbar level: H.
ambulation, sometimes wheelchair

Sacral level: H.
ambulation

237

# MUSCLE DISEASE (FLOPPY INFANT)

## COMMENTS

A. This algorithm is meant to aid in establishing a diagnosis. Treatment schemes for children with muscle disease are available in several excellent texts and journals.[1,2,4,5] Remember that the floppy infant may have cerebral palsy. Carefully review the birth history for possible hypoxic episodes. Spasticity develops, along with myelination of the nerve fibers, as the child reaches the usual walking age. All floppy infants should have thyroid studies performed to rule out hypothyroidism.

B. Meryon's sign: when the child is picked up by the arms, he slips out of the examiner's grasp because of weak shoulder muscles.[2]

C. An experienced child neurologist should evaluate the floppy child whom you suspect of having muscle disease. An orthopaedist should have some knowledge of the subject; however, the neurologist will probably pursue the diagnosis.

D. Congenital myopathies include central core disease, nemaline myopathy, myotubular myopathy, and congenital fiber-type disproportion.

E. Electromyography (EMG) terminology: BSAP = brief duration, small amplitude muscle potentials.[1,3,4]

F. Muscle biopsy is usually performed on a muscle at the proximal end of the limb  biceps humerus or quadriceps femoris. Consult your neurologist, pathologist, or a text[3] concerning technique.

G. Infantile botulism has become more common in counter-culture groups who feed their infants honey and other organic products. Honey is often contaminated with *Clostridia botulinum*.

## REFERENCES

1. Brooke MH. *A Clinician's View of Neuromuscular Disease*. 2nd Ed. Baltimore: Williams & Williams, 1982.
2. Drennan JC. *Orthopaedic Management of Neuromuscular Disorders*. Philadelphia: JB Lippincott, 1983.
3. Dubowitz V, Brooke MH. *Muscle Biopsy: A Modern Approach*. London: WB Saunders, 1973.
4. Dubowitz V. *Muscle Disorders in Childhood*. Philadelphia: WB Saunders, 1978.
5. Shapiro F, et al. Orthopaedic management of childhood neuromuscular disease—Parts I, II, and III. J Bone Joint Surg. 1982;64A:785-789, 949-953, 1102-1107.

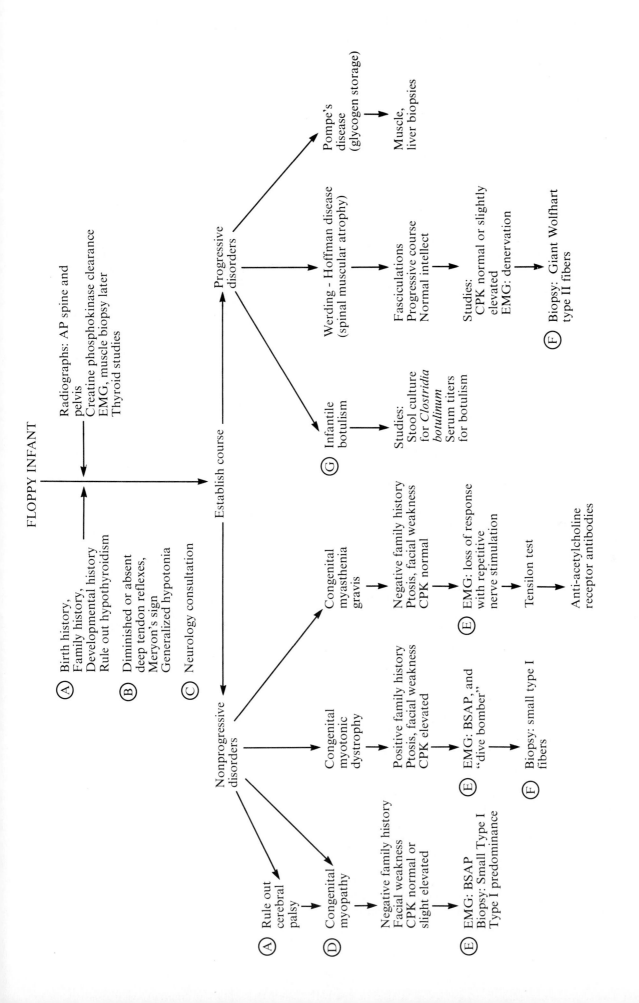

FLOPPY INFANT

Radiographs: AP spine and pelvis
Creatine phosphokinase clearance
EMG, muscle biopsy later
Thyroid studies

(A) Birth history,
Family history,
Developmental history
Rule out hypothyroidism

(B) Diminished or absent
deep tendon reflexes,
Meryon's sign
Generalized hypotonia

(C) Neurology consultation

Establish course

**Nonprogressive disorders**

(A) Rule out cerebral palsy

(D) Congenital myopathy

Negative family history
Facial weakness
CPK normal or slight elevated

(E) EMG: BSAP
Biopsy: Small Type I
Type I predominance

Congenital myotonic dystrophy

Positive family history
Ptosis, facial weakness
CPK elevated

(E) EMG: BSAP, and "dive bomber"

(F) Biopsy: small type I fibers

Congenital myasthenia gravis

Negative family history
Ptosis, facial weakness
CPK normal

(E) EMG: loss of response with repetitive nerve stimulation

Tensilon test

Anti-acetylcholine receptor antibodies

**Progressive disorders**

Infantile botulism

(G) Studies:
Stool culture for *Clostridia botulinum*
Serum titers for botulism

Werding - Hoffman disease (spinal muscular atrophy)

Fasciculations
Progressive course
Normal intellect

Studies:
CPK normal or slightly elevated
EMG: denervation

(F) Biopsy: Giant Wolfhart type II fibers

Pompe's disease (glycogen storage)

Muscle, liver biopsies

239

# SUSPECTED MUSCLE DISEASE (AGE 2–10 YEARS)

## COMMENTS

A. At the initial presentation, children with early weakness due to muscle disease are hard to distinguish from normal children. Delay in walking, clumsiness, and flatfeet are common. Meryon's sign suggests shoulder weakness (child slips through the examiner's hands when picked up by the arms). Gower's sign suggests proximal weakness in the lower limbs (child "climbs" his legs with his hands when attempting to rise from the seated position on the floor).

B. EMG (electromyography) terminology: BSAP = brief duration, small amplitude, muscle potentials.[1,3,4] Nerve conduction terms: lower extremities—normal = 40 to 50 meters/second; delayed = 20 to 30 meters/second (as seen in Charcot-Marie-Tooth disease).

C. Weakness patterns (distal, proximal, facial) help to initiate the differential diagnosis. Patients with distal weakness often have neuropathies (Charcot-Marie-Tooth). Proximal weakness suggests muscular disease (Duchenne muscular dystrophy). Facial weakness without distal limb weakness may suggest facioscapulohumeral muscular dystrophy or a myriad of miscellaneous disorders (congenital facioscapulohumeral dystrophy, congenital myotonic dystrophy, congenital myopathy, myasthenia gravis, acute organophosphate poisoning, and others.)

D. Charcot-Marie-Tooth disease is a common orthopaedic conditon that presents with cavus feet and distal weakness. Slowing of nerve conduction time in the lower extremities is diagnostic.[2,5,6] Progressive cavus foot deformity requires surgical correction, either with soft tissue procedures, including tendon transfers, or with bony procedures.[2]

E. Duchenne muscular dystrophy is transmitted as a sex-linked recessive trait; therefore, only boys are affected. Early signs include clumsiness, Gower's sign, and enlarged calves. Orthopaedic treatment includes muscle releases (tendo-Achilles release, tibialis posterior transfer, abduction-contracture release) followed by long-leg orthoses. After the heel cord is released, the very weak quadriceps will no longer be adequate; therefore, postoperative bracing is essential. Limb surgery will keep the child walking for several additonal years. Scoliotic spinal collapse is best treated by spinal fusion, with Luque SSI (Segmental Spinal Instrumentation) performed if the curve progresses to 30°. This method is extremely effective, but must be done before progressive decline in respiratory function becomes severe. Some centers do not advise spinal surgery because children with Duchenne muscular dystrophy all eventually die, no matter how they are treated. Spinal fusion clearly improves the quality of life, however.

F. Limb gridle and facioscapulohumeral muscular dystrophy can be distinquished by evaluating for facial weakness and deltoid weakness. Limb girdle patients have normal facial muscles, but weak deltoids. Facioscapulohumeral dystrophy patients have facial weakness and upper limb girdle weakness, but maintain deltoid strength. This characteristic is important because the scapulae can be surgically fused to the thorax (segmental wires plus bone graft—medial scapular border to ribs) with resulting improved upper extremity function.

G. Muscle biopsy is performed on a proximal limb muscle (biceps, humerus, quadriceps femoris).

## REFERENCES

1. Brooke MH. A Clinician's View of Neuromuscular Disease. 2nd Ed. Baltimore: Williams & Wilkins, 1982.
2. Drennan JC. *Orthopaedic Management of Neuromuscular Disorders*. Philadelphia: JB Lippincott, 1983.
3. Dubowitz V, Brooke MH. *Muscle Biopsy: A Modern Approach*. London: WB Saunders, 1973.
4. Dubowitz V. Muscle Disorders in Childhood. Philadelphia: W. B. Saunders Company, 1978.
5. Dyck PJ, et al. Lower motor and primary sensory neuron diseases with peroneal muscular atrophy. Arch Neurol. 1968:18:619.
6. Shapiro F, et al. Orthopaedic management of childhood neuromuscular disease. Parts I, II, III. J Bone Joint Surg. 1982:64A:785-789, 949-953, 1102-1107.

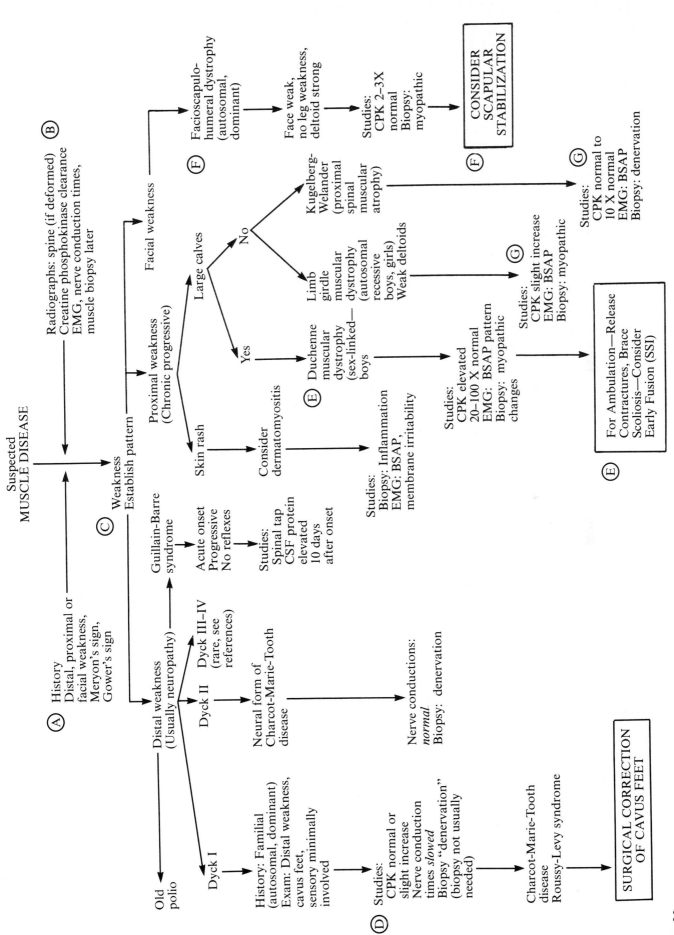

Suspected
MUSCLE DISEASE

(A) History
Distal, proximal or
facial weakness,
Meryon's sign,
Gower's sign

(B) Radiographs: spine (if deformed)
Creatine phosphokinase clearance
EMG, nerve conduction times,
muscle biopsy later

(C) Weakness
Establish pattern

Distal weakness
(Usually neuropathy)

Old
polio

Guillain-Barre
syndrome

Dyck I

Dyck II

Dyck III-IV
(rare, see
references)

Acute onset
Progressive
No reflexes

Studies:
Spinal tap
CSF protein
elevated
10 days
after onset

Neural form of
Charcot-Marie-Tooth
disease

(D) History: Familial
(autosomal, dominant)
Exam: Distal weakness,
cavus feet,
sensory minimally
involved

Studies:
CPK normal or
slight increase
Nerve conduction
times *slowed*
Biopsy "denervation"
(biopsy not usually
needed)

Nerve conductions:
*normal*
Biopsy: denervation

Charcot-Marie-Tooth
disease
Roussy-Levy syndrome

SURGICAL CORRECTION
OF CAVUS FEET

Proximal weakness
(Chronic progressive)

Facial weakness

(F) Facioscapulo-
humeral dystrophy
(autosomal,
dominant)

Face weak,
no leg weakness,
deltoid strong

Studies: CPK 2-3X
normal
Biopsy:
myopathic

(F) CONSIDER
SCAPULAR
STABILIZATION

Large calves

Skin rash

Consider
dermatomyositis

Studies:
Biopsy: Inflammation
EMG: BSAP,
membrane irritability

Yes

No

(E) Duchenne
muscular
dystrophy
(sex-linked—
boys)

Limb
girdle
muscular
dystrophy
(autosomal
recessive
boys, girls)
Weak deltoids

Kugelberg-
Welander
(proximal
spinal
muscular
atrophy)

Studies:
CPK elevated
20-100 X normal
EMG: BSAP pattern
Biopsy: myopathic
changes

(G) Studies:
CPK slight increase
EMG: BSAP
Biopsy: myopathic

(G) Studies:
CPK normal to
10 X normal
EMG: BSAP
Biopsy: denervation

(E) For Ambulation—Release
Contractures, Brace
Scoliosis—Consider
Early Fusion (SSI)

# DISTAL INTERPHALANGEAL JOINT INJURY

## COMMENTS

A. Avulsion of the insertion of either the flexor or extensor tendons may occur with or without a bony fragment. Specific tendon function should be tested and radiographs should be examined for the presence of a fragment either dorsally over the distal interphalangeal (DIP) joint or in the flexor sheath.

B. A nondisplaced fracture extending into the DIP joint should be splinted so that proximal interphalangeal motion is allowed.

C. A mallet fracture is one in which a large fragment of dorsal articular surface of the distal phalanx is attached to the extensor tendon. Frequently, this is rotated and tilted; the remainder of the phalanx may subluxate palmarly. Splinting alone will usually not control this fracture and open reduction with K–wire or internal fixation is indicated.

D. In general, displaced fractures involving the DIP joint result in minimal long term disability for a majority of patients. A single large fragment or split in the articular surface should be reduced and fixed where this is technically possible. A majority of fractures do not fit this pattern and do well if treated with splinting and early motion.

E. Dislocations of the DIP joint are likely to be open injuries. After appropriate debridement, irrigation and reduction, the integrity of the long flexor and extensor tendons should be ascertained. Delayed wound closure and splinting in stable position for 3 weeks usually results in a stable joint. A supplemental K-wire may be used for a very unstable injury.

## REFERENCE

1. Green DP, Rowland SA. Fractures and dislocations in the hand. In *Fractures* Rockwood CA, Green DP, eds. Philadelphia: Lippincott, 1975.

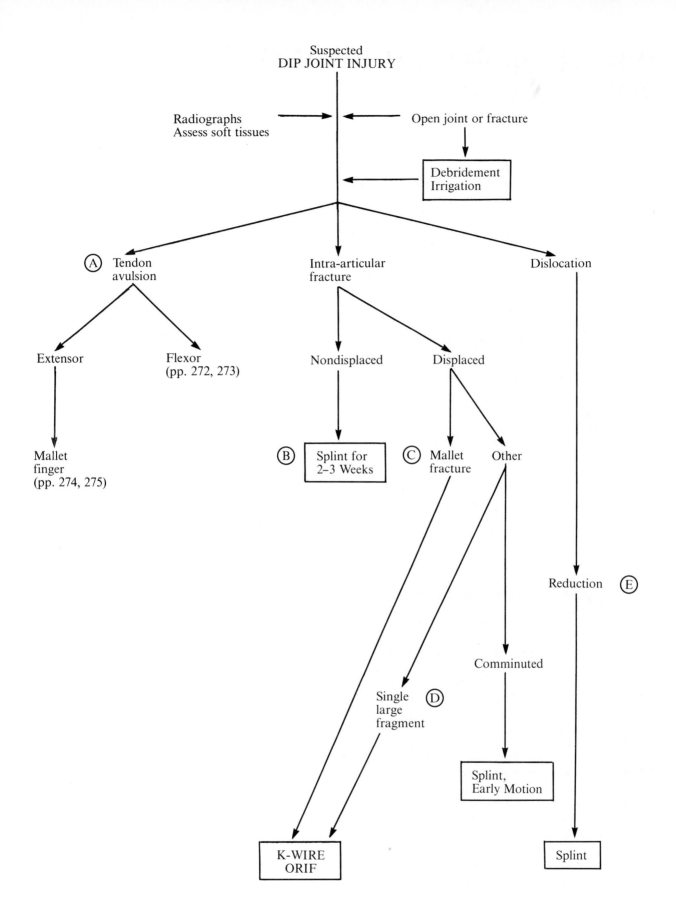

Suspected
**DIP JOINT INJURY**

Radiographs
Assess soft tissues

Open joint or fracture

Debridement
Irrigation

Ⓐ Tendon
avulsion

Intra-articular
fracture

Dislocation

Extensor

Flexor
(pp. 272, 273)

Mallet
finger
(pp. 274, 275)

Nondisplaced

Displaced

Ⓑ Splint for
2–3 Weeks

Ⓒ Mallet
fracture

Other

Reduction Ⓔ

Single
large
fragment Ⓓ

Comminuted

Splint,
Early Motion

K-WIRE
ORIF

Splint

# PROXIMAL INTERPHALANGEAL JOINT INJURY—I

## COMMENTS

A. A true lateral view is essential to detect dorsal subluxation; supplemental stress views or oblique radiographs may be needed.

B. Dislocations are often reduced "on the sidelines." A high index of suspicion is needed in order not to miss the diagnosis. Open dislocations are not uncommon; the principles of irrigation, debridement, and antibiotic coverage should be followed.

C. Volar or volar-lateral dislocation of the middle phalanx may cause the head of the proximal phalanx to buttonhole between the central slip and a lateral band of the extensor mechanism. If gentle manipulation fails to reduce the dislocation, open reduction and repair of the injured soft tissue should be performed.

D. Functional stability is tested by medial and lateral stress and active motion through the full range. Comparison with the normal side and radiographs taken at the extremes of motion are useful if stability is in doubt. Intermetacarpal block anesthesia is used when necessary, as digital block anesthesia is hazardous in view of swelling already present, and wrist block anesthesia interferes with normal motion by paralyzing the intrinsic musculature.

E. The PIP joint should be splinted in 10 to 20° more flexion than the position of instability for 14 to 21 days. A dorsal splint may be incorporated in a gauntlet cast to block extension while allowing active flexion. Hyperextension may be prevented during the second 3 weeks by taping small pieces of splint material over the dorsum of the proximal and middle phalanges so that they slightly overlap the PIP joint, or by using a molded or ready-made hyperextension block splint.

F. Central slip disruption may result in chronic boutonniere deformity. At no time should the PIP joint be allowed to assume a flexed position during the first 6 weeks of splinting. DIP motion should be encouraged. A "reverse-knuckle-bender" type of dynamic splint is useful in the second 6 weeks of treatment.

G. Repair of completely disrupted collateral ligaments is probably indicated in the index and small PIP joints. Nonoperative splint treatment usually results in satisfactory stability in the nonborder digits.

## REFERENCES

1. Burton RI, Eaton RG. Common hand injuries in the athlete. Ortho Clin N Am. 1973; 4:809–835.
2. Eaton RG. Joint injuries in the hand. Springfield, Il: Charles C Thomas, 1971.
3. McElfresh EC, Dobyns JH, O'Brien ET. Management of fracture-dislocation of the proximal interphalangeal joints by extension block splint. J Bone Joint Surg. 1972; 54A:1705–1717.
4. Wood GL, Burton RI. Avoiding pitfalls in the diagnosis of the acutely injured proximal interphalangeal joint. Clin Plast Surg. 1981;8:95–105.

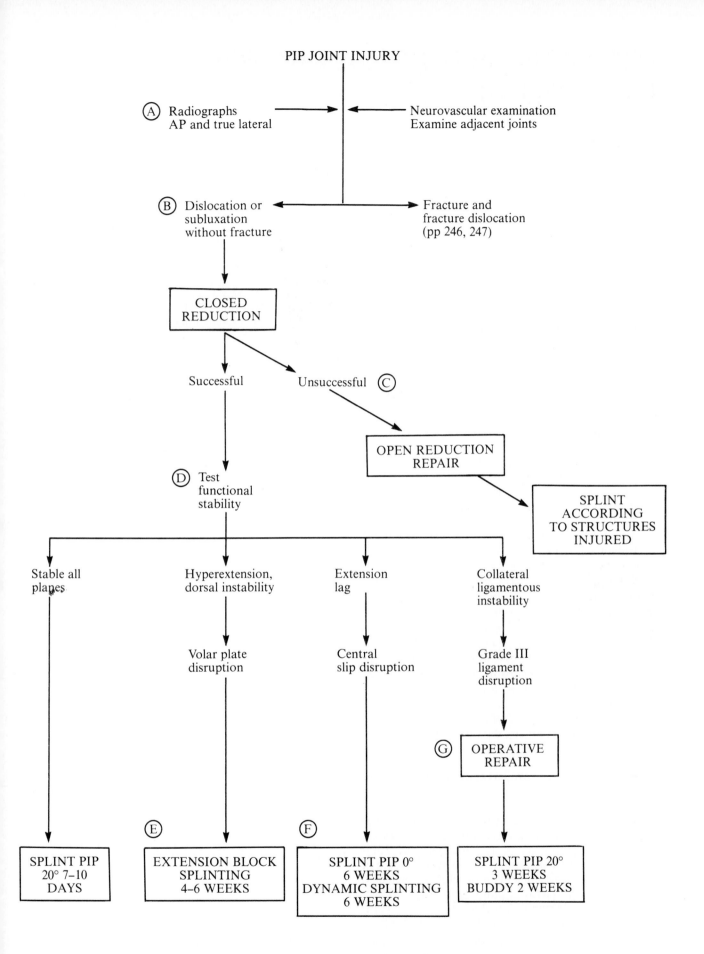

PIP JOINT INJURY

(A) Radiographs
AP and true lateral → ← Neurovascular examination
Examine adjacent joints

(B) Dislocation or
subluxation
without fracture ←→ Fracture and
fracture dislocation
(pp 246, 247)

CLOSED
REDUCTION

Successful    Unsuccessful (C)

OPEN REDUCTION
REPAIR

(D) Test
functional
stability

SPLINT
ACCORDING
TO STRUCTURES
INJURED

Stable all
planes

Hyperextension,
dorsal instability

Extension
lag

Collateral
ligamentous
instability

Volar plate
disruption

Central
slip disruption

Grade III
ligament
disruption

(G) OPERATIVE
REPAIR

SPLINT PIP
20° 7–10
DAYS

(E) EXTENSION BLOCK
SPLINTING
4–6 WEEKS

(F) SPLINT PIP 0°
6 WEEKS
DYNAMIC SPLINTING
6 WEEKS

SPLINT PIP 20°
3 WEEKS
BUDDY 2 WEEKS

# PROXIMAL INTERPHALANGEAL JOINT INJURY—II

## COMMENTS

A. A true lateral view is essential to detect dorsal subluxation. Supplemental stress views or oblique radiographs may be needed.

B. Fractures of the volar lip of the base of the middle phalanx are often associated with dorsal or hyperextension instability. The position at which subluxation occurs during active extension of the PIP joint should be noted. Intermetacarpal block anesthesia may be necessary.

C. Condylar shear or split condyle fractures are particularly unstable. Fractures extending into the volar recess at the junction of the proximal phalanx head and neck often result in osseous mechanical obstruction to flexion or significant scarring of the volar plate.

D. Extension block splinting[3] maintains congruity of the intact portion of the joint surface while allowing active motion in the stable range. A dorsal aluminum splint incorporated in a plaster gauntlet cast limits PIP extension to 10° to 15° short of the demonstrated position of subluxation. The degree of the extension block is decreased by 25% each week. Full extension is delayed for 6 to 12 weeks, depending on the amount of initial instability. A K-wire to transfix the joint for the initial 2 weeks may be useful in the more unstable fracture-dislocations.

E. When greater than 40% of the volar lip of the middle phalanx is involved, the collateral ligaments no longer insert onto the middle phalanx, but rather onto the volar fragment. Reduction is difficult to maintain and comminution is often more extensive than radiographically apparent.

F. Volar plate advancement arthroplasty, as described by Eaton[2] provides fibrocartilage resurfacing of the fracture defect and restoration of joint stability. This technique offers the greatest potential for recovery of joint function in the comminuted fractures. Alternately, dynamic skeletal traction by means of an outrigger on a plaster cast can be used to maintain length while holding the PIP joint reduced in 30° flexion. A few degrees of further active flexion should be encouraged while in traction. At 3 to 4 weeks, the traction can be removed and extension block splinting continued as described earlier. Joint function is usually limited following this form of treatment, although it is useful in selected patients. If reduction cannot be maintained or if interposed fragments preclude reduction, volar plate advancement arthroplasty is indicated.

G. Accurate reduction and stabilization by interfragmental compression, where technically possible, is the treatment of choice.

## REFERENCES

1. Burton RI, Eaton RG. Common hand injuries in the athlete. Orthop Clin N Am. 1973; 4:809–835.
2. Eaton RG. *Joint Injuries in the Hand.* Springfield, Il, Charles C Thomas, 1971.
3. McElfresh EC, Dobyns JH, O'Brien ET. Management of fracture-dislocation of the proximal interphalangeal joints by extension block splint. J Bone Joint Surg. 1972; 54A:1705–1717.
4. Woods GL, Burton RI. Avoiding pitfalls in the diagnosis of the acutely injured proximal interphalangeal joint. Clin Plast Surg. 1981; 8:95–105.

# PIP JOINT INJURY

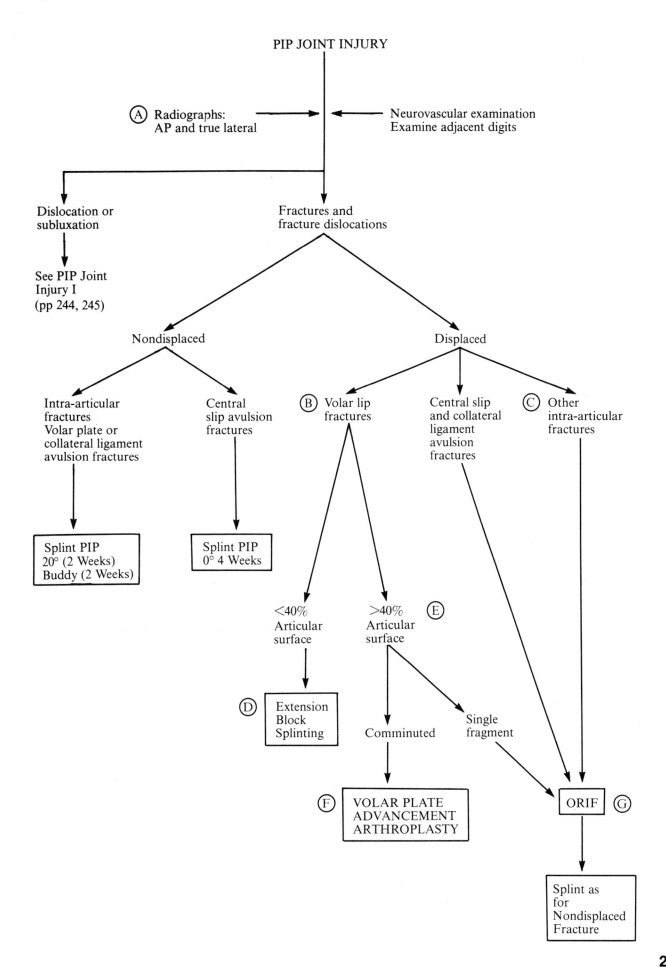

A Radiographs:
AP and true lateral

Neurovascular examination
Examine adjacent digits

Dislocation or
subluxation

See PIP Joint
Injury I
(pp 244, 245)

Fractures and
fracture dislocations

Nondisplaced

Displaced

Intra-articular
fractures
Volar plate or
collateral ligament
avulsion fractures

Central
slip avulsion
fractures

B Volar lip
fractures

Central slip
and collateral
ligament
avulsion
fractures

C Other
intra-articular
fractures

Splint PIP
20° (2 Weeks)
Buddy (2 Weeks)

Splint PIP
0° 4 Weeks

<40%
Articular
surface

>40%
Articular
surface

E

D Extension
Block
Splinting

Comminuted

Single
fragment

F VOLAR PLATE
ADVANCEMENT
ARTHROPLASTY

ORIF G

Splint as
for
Nondisplaced
Fracture

# PHALANGEAL FRACTURE

## COMMENTS

A. Open fractures are common. In all cases principles of debridement, irrigation, delayed wound closure and antibiotic coverage apply.

B. Intra-articular fractures and tendon avulsion injuries are covered in other algorithms (pp. 244–249, 272–275).

C. Nondisplaced fractures and impacted fractures which have no malalignment may be treated by buddy taping with or without an initial period of splinting.

D. Phalangeal fracture displacement is the result of both the mechanism of injury and the deforming forces of the tendons inserting in the digit. Rotational malalignment is of particular importance in the digits; it should be checked with the fingers in flexion, noting the plane of the nail plates and comparing with the opposite hand. Most displaced fractures can be reduced and held using external immobilization. Certain patterns are inherently unstable (e.g., oblique or spiral fractures of the proximal phalanx) and supplemental fixation is needed. Salter–Harris II fractures of the distal phalanx are common in the smashed finger in the child. Accurate reduction may require removal of a portion of the nail plate. These fractures are often open and require recognition and treatment as such. Subungual hematomas may occur with distal phalanx fractures. Evacuation of the hematoma by the "hot-paper-clip" method relieves pain, but theoretically converts a closed fracture into an open one. If the nail bed has been disrupted or irregularly lacerated, a better result will be obtained by removal of the nail plate and careful repair of the nail bed.

E. Markedly comminuted fractures or those with bone loss require skeletal traction to maintain length. Supplemental bone graft after soft tissue stabilization may be needed.

## REFERENCE

Green DP, Rowland SA. Fractures and dislocations in the hand. In, *Fractures*. Rockwood CA, Green DP, eds. Philadelphia, Lippincott, 1975.

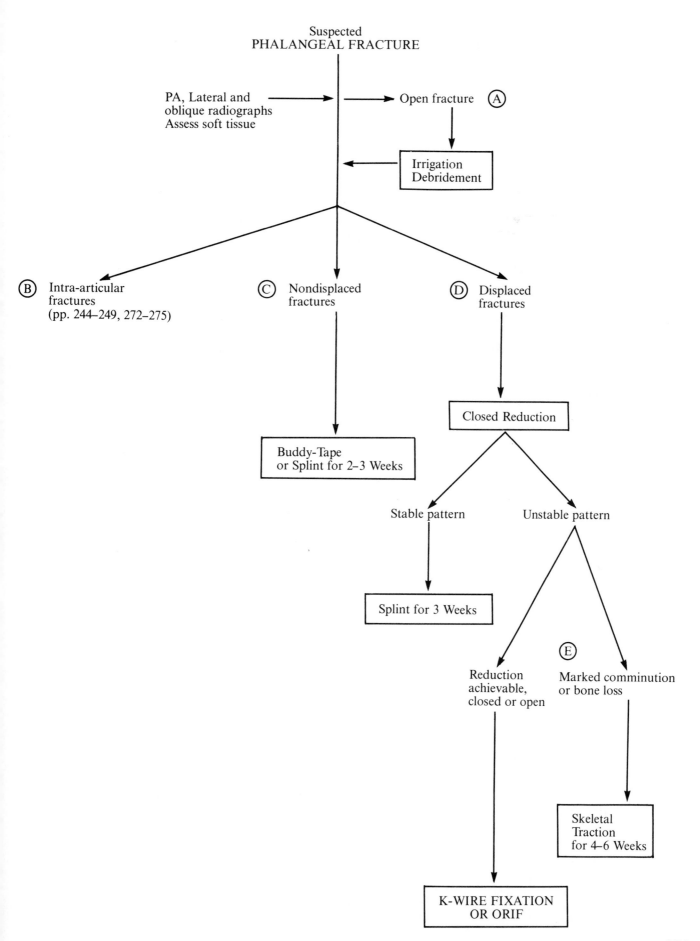

Suspected
PHALANGEAL FRACTURE

PA, Lateral and
oblique radiographs
Assess soft tissue → Open fracture (A)

Irrigation
Debridement

(B) Intra-articular
fractures
(pp. 244–249, 272–275)

(C) Nondisplaced
fractures

(D) Displaced
fractures

Buddy-Tape
or Splint for 2–3 Weeks

Closed Reduction

Stable pattern    Unstable pattern

Splint for 3 Weeks

Reduction
achievable,
closed or open

(E) Marked comminution
or bone loss

Skeletal
Traction
for 4–6 Weeks

K-WIRE FIXATION
OR ORIF

# CARPAL DISRUPTION I

## COMMENTS

A. The usual history is of a significant load applied to the wrist, more commonly in the dorsiflexed position. Special effort may be needed to identify these injuries in the comatose, restrained, or multiply injured patient.

B. Avulsion fractures or dorsal chip fractures can be treated by 4 to 6 weeks of immobilization after more serious injury has been excluded. Dislocations of the distal radioulnar joint should be reduced and immobilized for 6 weeks, with the forearm in supination for dorsal dislocations and in pronation for palmar dislocations. Open reduction with ligament reconstruction should be undertaken for the irreducible dislocation, usually due to delayed recognition, or for the symptomatic, recurrent subluxating distal radioulnar joint. An isolated ulnar styloid fracture implies an injury to the ulnocarpal ligament complex; the wrist should be immobilized for 5 to 6 weeks in slight ulnar deviation. Radial styloid fractures may be associated with major perilunate ligamentous injury, or may allow ulnar translocation of the carpus if reduction and stabilization are inadequate. Isolated fractures of other carpal bones, e.g., hook of hamate or pisiform, may require special radiographic views for identification. These usually heal with early and sufficient immobilization. Symptomatic nonunions may require excision of the offending fragments.

C. AP and true lateral radiographs are repeated after a minimum of 10 minutes of fingertrap distraction with the elbow flexed to 90° and 10 pounds of weight applied to the upper arm. Adequate anesthesia and relaxation are necessary.

D. Volar perilunate or dorsal lunate dislocations are extremely rare. The approach toward treatment follows the same principles as outlined.

E. Closed reduction is performed by continuing manual distraction, bringing the wrist into dorsiflexion and then into palmar flexion while stabilizing the lunate with the opposite thumb. This maneuver disengages the head of the capitate and repositions it into the cup of the lunate.

F. Careful and frequent radiographic inspection for instability must be carried out. Special attention should be paid to the capitolunate angle (CLA) and the scapholunate relationship on both the AP and lateral views.

G. Scaphoid fractures must be accurately reduced and pinned, and the capitolunate and lunatotriquetral articulations reduced. Whenever possible, pins should not cross the radiocarpal joint. Bone graft should be used early when it will enhance stability and bone apposition.

H. Avascular necrosis of the proximal scaphoid and lunate are not uncommon, but revascularization and union may occur. Late post-traumatic arthrosis is also common.

## REFERENCES

1. Dobyns JH, Linscheid RL, Chad EYS, Weber ER, Swanson GE. Traumatic instability of the wrist. AAOS Instructional Course Lecture, 1975; 24:182–199.
2. Green DP (Ed.). Carpal disruption. In *Operative Hand Surgery*. New York: Churchill-Livingstone, 1982.
3. Sebald JR, Dobyns JH, Linscheid RL. Natural history of collapse deformity of the wrist. Clin Orthop. 1974; 104:140–148.

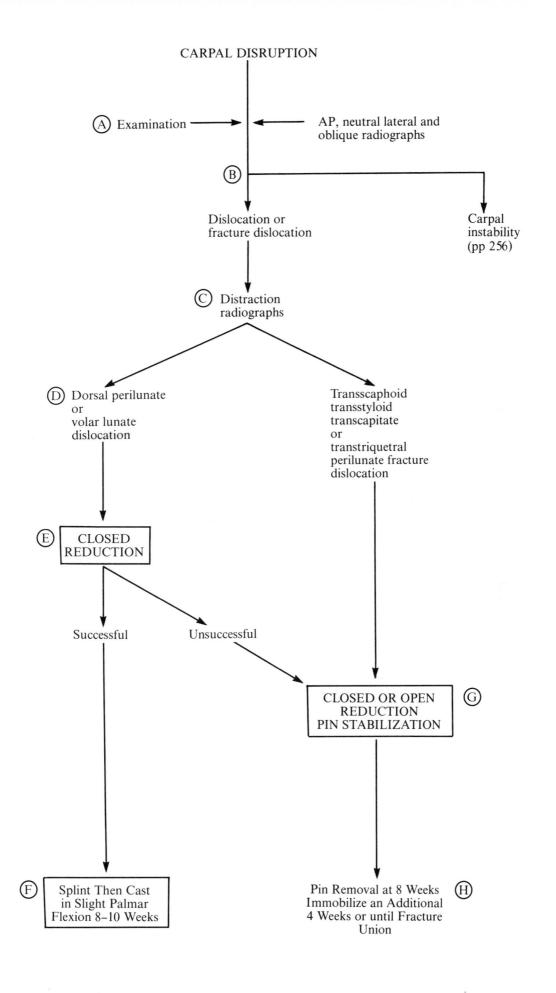

CARPAL DISRUPTION

Ⓐ Examination → ← AP, neutral lateral and oblique radiographs

Ⓑ

Dislocation or fracture dislocation

Carpal instability (pp 256)

Ⓒ Distraction radiographs

Ⓓ Dorsal perilunate or volar lunate dislocation

Transscaphoid transstyloid transcapitate or transtriquetral perilunate fracture dislocation

Ⓔ CLOSED REDUCTION

Successful     Unsuccessful

Ⓖ CLOSED OR OPEN REDUCTION PIN STABILIZATION

Ⓕ Splint Then Cast in Slight Palmar Flexion 8–10 Weeks

Ⓗ Pin Removal at 8 Weeks Immobilize an Additional 4 Weeks or until Fracture Union

# SCAPHOID FRACTURE

## COMMENTS

A. Tenderness in the anatomic snuffbox or over the scaphoid tubercle associated with a dorsiflexion injury of the wrist suggests scaphoid fracture. If the initial radiographs are negative, but the history and examination are suggestive, a well-molded short-arm thumb spica cast should be applied and radiographs re-evaluated at 10 to 14 days. If a fracture is present, early resorption at the fracture edges should make it apparent; if radiographs are normal and symptoms have abated, treatment has been appropriate for a Grade I or II ligament strain.

B. Median nerve deficit is unusual but, if present, should be treated by early exploration and decompression. K–wire fixation should be considered to augment fracture stability and facilitate soft tissue care.

C. Any displacement of a scaphoid fracture should initiate a systematic search for more extensive carpal disruption, ranging from mild DISI or VISI patterns to fracture dislocations. Assessment of radiocarpal and intercarpal relationships, particularly on radial and ulnar deviation, and clenched-fist radiographs will identify significant instability patterns (pp. 256, 257).

D. Reduction and immobilization are carried out in slight palmar flexion and radial deviation, namely, the reverse of the usual injury mechanism.

E. Fracture union is assessed by serial radiographs documenting bridging trabeculae in all planes. Tomography is useful in the more oblique patterns and following bone grafting procedures. Cooney reported that the single most significant factor in the development of nonunion was haste in discontinuing immobilization.[1]

F. The development of avascular necrosis does not preclude healing. With continuous, rigorous immobilization, revascularization and healing do occur. Serial radiographs should show no loss of reduction and progression of union. Pronation, supination, and metacarpophalangeal motion should be controlled during the first 6 weeks of treatment.

G. Smooth articular margins with apposition of the fracture fragments constitute acceptable reduction. Late degenerative changes correlate more with incongruity of the joint surfaces than with the development of avascular necrosis. Displacement can occur in the first 6 to 8 weeks of treatment and radiographic checks should be made at biweekly intervals for the first 2 months.

H. An anatomic reduction of a fracture dislocation or subluxation is tenuous at best. The decision whether to treat by closed measures alone or to implement percutaneous K–wire fixation, or to proceed to open reduction depends on the surgeon's assessment of the soft tissue injury and, hence, the instability present.

I. The need for bone graft is determined at the time of direct examination of the fracture. Cancellous or corticocancellous bone graft should be used without hesitation if it will enhance stability of the fixation or apposition of the fracture fragments.

J. Severely comminuted scaphoid fractures are most often associated with extensive carpal disruption and are highly unlikely to be isolated injuries. Restoration of inter- and radiocarpal relationships as well as external scaphoid dimensions by soft tissue repair and bone grafting should be achieved initially. Early silastic sca-

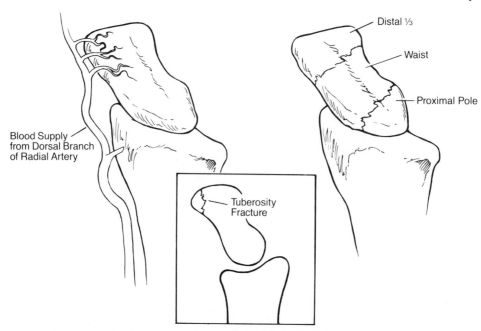

Blood Supply from Dorsal Branch of Radial Artery

Tuberosity Fracture

Distal ⅓

Waist

Proximal Pole

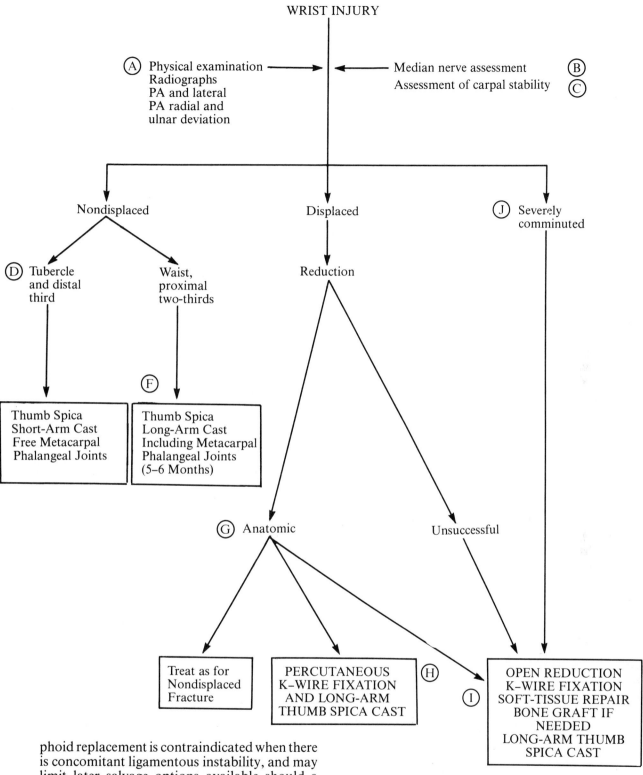

WRIST INJURY

(A) Physical examination
Radiographs
PA and lateral
PA radial and
ulnar deviation

(B) Median nerve assessment
(C) Assessment of carpal stability

Nondisplaced

Displaced

(J) Severely comminuted

(D) Tubercle and distal third

Waist, proximal two-thirds

Reduction

(F)

Thumb Spica
Short-Arm Cast
Free Metacarpal
Phalangeal Joints

Thumb Spica
Long-Arm Cast
Including Metacarpal
Phalangeal Joints
(5–6 Months)

(G) Anatomic

Unsuccessful

Treat as for
Nondisplaced
Fracture

PERCUTANEOUS
K–WIRE FIXATION
AND LONG-ARM
THUMB SPICA CAST

(H)

(I)

OPEN REDUCTION
K–WIRE FIXATION
SOFT-TISSUE REPAIR
BONE GRAFT IF
NEEDED
LONG-ARM THUMB
SPICA CAST

phoid replacement is contraindicated when there is concomitant ligamentous instability, and may limit later salvage options available should a painful, unstable wrist be the eventual outcome. After the initial 6 months of treatment, a more accurate assessment of residual instability, bone necrosis, and articular damage will be possible.

## REFERENCES

1. Cooney WP, Dobyns JH, Linscheid RL. Nonunion of the scaphoid; Analysis of the results from bone grafting. J Hand Surg. 1980; 5:343–354.

2. Gelberman RH. The vascularity of the scaphoid bone. J Hand Surg. 1980; 5:508–513.

3. Linscheid RL, Dobyns JH, Beabout JW, et al. Traumatic instability of the wrist. J Bone Joint Surg. 1972; 54A:1612–1632.

4. Mazet R, Hohl M. Fractures of the carpal navicular. J Bone Joint Surg. 1963; 45A:82–112.

5. Melone CP. Scaphoid fractures: concepts of management. Clin Plast Surg. 1981; 8:83–94.

6. Russe O. Fractures of the carpal navicular: diagnosis, nonoperative treatment and operative treatment. J Bone Joint Surg. 1960; 42A:759–768.

# PENETRATING INJURY

## COMMENTS

A. The examination for damage to underlying structures should be based on both the location of the injury and the posture of the hand at the time of injury.

B. Clean puncture wounds at digital flexor creases often gain entry into tendon sheaths. Early immobilization and antibiotics, especially in the diabetic, may forestall the development of serious infection.

C. Obtain details about the penetrating object, particularly if contaminated with animal or vegetable material or soil. In addition to clostridia, consider fungi, atypical mycobacteria and other unusual microorganisms in selecting antibiotics and dealing with resulting infections. Prophylaxis for hepatitis B may be indicated in health care workers.

D. Stabilization of fractures and local wound healing are the initial goals of treatment. Nerve and tendon grafts and other reconstructive procedures can be done under more favorable conditions. Retrieval of the missile is indicated if it lies within a synovial space, interferes with function, or otherwise causes symptoms.

E. Extensive damage results from high-velocity gunshot wounds and close range shotgun wounds. All nonviable tissue must be debrided while salvaging all structures of potential use in later reconstruction. Skeletal stabilization and control of infection must precede soft tissue coverage and reconstructive procedures.

F. High pressure injection injuries, often appearing innocuous at first, are associated with great morbidity and a high amputation rate. Solvents cause the greatest damage, followed by paints, grease, and other chemicals; water and air, the least. The extent of injury depends on the type and temperature of the injected substance, the pressure, and the site and direction of entry. Dissection along soft tissue planes and synovial spaces is common. Radiographs may show the extent of injection in lead-based paints, but are not helpful in other cases. Ischemia, chemical and foreign body inflammation, and infection contribute to the poor results. Thorough, early decompression, debridement and drainage, coupled with broad-spectrum intravenous antibiotics (e.g., cefalothin or penicillinase-resistant penicillin derivative plus an aminoglycoside) and high-dose steroids offer the best chance for salvage. Extensile exposure and removal of all foreign material are crucial in treating these wounds. A recommended course of steroids is hydrocortisone succinate, 100 mg IV, Q6 h. until swelling and erythema subsides, followed by prednisone, 25 mg PO b.i.d., and tapering unless signs and symptoms worsen.

G. Assessment of the amount of contamination and the pressure of the injected water must be made. If there is doubt as to the nature of the injected substance, early debridement is the safest course.

## REFERENCE

1. Schoo MJ, Scott FA, Boswick JA Jr. High-pressure injection injuries of the hand. J Trauma. 1980; 20:229–238.

PENETRATING INJURY

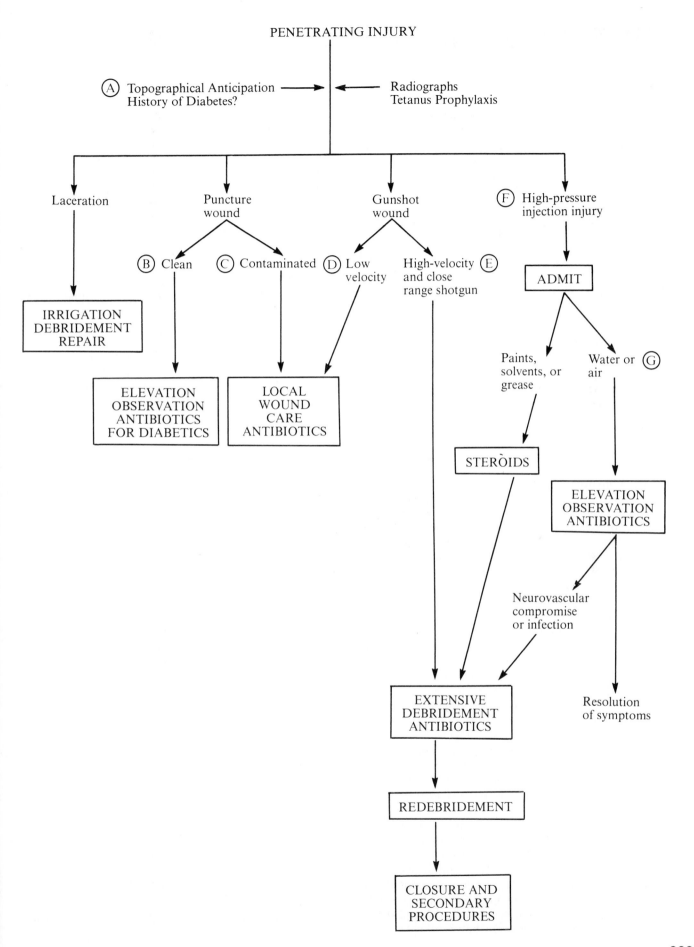

# BITE WOUNDS

## COMMENTS

A. A history should be obtained as to the exact nature and time of the incident, the species involved, allergies, and known sensitivities or exposure to horse serum or insect venom.

B. Exploration to the depths of the wound and debridement of contaminated tissue, followed by pressure irrigation to reduce the bacterial inoculum, is the mainstay of treatment of fresh bite wounds. Delayed primary closure is usually the safest course. Established infections should be treated as such.

C. Skunks, foxes, coyotes, raccoons, and bats—as well as unknown dogs or cats—should be considered rabid. Whenever possible, the animal should be captured for fluorescent antibody examination of its brain.

D. Guidelines for administration of rabies immune globulin and duck embryo vaccine are provided by the Public Health Service Advisory Committee.[6]

E. Each wound must be evaluated individually. Superficial wounds need not require antibiotic treatment. Any bite that penetrates a synovial or closed space or violates the superficial fascia constitutes a deep wound. Patients with deep bite wounds should be hospitalized for observation and administration of parenteral antibiotics for the first 48 to 72 hours of a 5–day course. Other bite wounds may be managed on an outpatient basis in the reliable patient. In deep human bite wounds patients should be hospitalized until "dismissal would not endanger the hand should they neglect follow-up".[5] When antibiotics are indicated, penicillin in high doses (8 to 12 million units per day) is the recommended drug for dog and cat bites (usual organism—*Pasturella multocida*). A combination of a pencillinase-resistant penicillin derivative or cephalosporin *and penicillin* is recommended for human bite wounds (frequent organism—*Eikenella corrodens* sensitive to penicillin, but resistant to the penicillinase-resistant derivatives and variably sensitive to the cephalosporins; human bites usually cause mixed infections).

F. Jellyfish, anemones, cone snails, echinoderms, and a variety of fish have mechanisms for introducing toxins. Specific antivenins either do not exist or are not readily available. Adverse human reactions range from the bothersome to the life-threatening.

G. Venomous snakes in the United States commonly include rattlesnakes, cotton-mouths, watermoccasins, massasaugas, copperheads, and coral snakes. Snake venom is a complex mixture of toxins, and when envenomation occurs, the snakebite should be considered a "multiple poisoning." Spreading necrosis, coagulopathy, peripheral vascular collapse, and neurotoxicity may occur simultaneously or in sequence, necessitating aggressive treatment.[7]

H. The bite of the brown recluse spider (*Loxosceles reclusa*) causes both systemic effects and local spreading necrosis. Early excision of the bite area speeds healing.

I. Specific antitoxins exist for rattlesnake bites (polyvalent antivenin, crotalidae) and for other snake venoms. The Oklahoma Poison Control Center, in cooperation with the Oklahoma City Zoo, publishes and maintains a National Anti-venin Index. Information on availability and location of antivenins can be obtained by calling their 24-hour telephone number: (405) 271-5454. Antitoxin exists for the black widow spider bite (Lyovac, Merck Sharp and Dohme), but not for the brown recluse spider. Systemic signs of serious envenomation require administration of specific antivenin. Steroids and antihistamines should be available to treat antivenin hypersensitivity reactions.

J. Wasps, bees, hornets, scorpions, and centipedes usually produce only local reaction, but anaphylactic reaction in sensitized persons may occur. Certain caterpillars and moths produce an intense dermatitis when handled. Meperidine hydrochloride and morphine sulfate potentiate the effect of scorpion venom and are contraindicated.[1]

K. Wound care as necessary and antibiotics are indicated in snake bites and marine animal envenomation. Supportive care includes preparation for volume and drug treatment of circulatory collapse, mechanical ventilatory support, treatment of anaphylaxis, and blood transfusion, should they be needed.

## REFERENCES

1. Beeson PB, McDermott W, Wyngaarden JP (eds). *Cecil Textbook of Medicine*. 15th Ed. Philadelphia: 1979.
2. Goldstein EJC, Miller TA, Citron DM, Finegold SM. Infections following clenched-fist injury: A new perspective. J Hand Surg. 1978; 3:455–457.
3. Huang TT, Lynch JB, Larson DL, Lewis SR. The use of excisional therapy in the management of snakebite. Ann Surg. 1974; 179:598–607.
4. McDonald I. Eikenella corrodens infections of the hand. Hand. 1979; 11:224–227.
5. Peeples E, Boswick JA Jr, Scott FA. Wounds of the hand contaminated by human or animal saliva. J Trauma. 1980; 20:383–389.

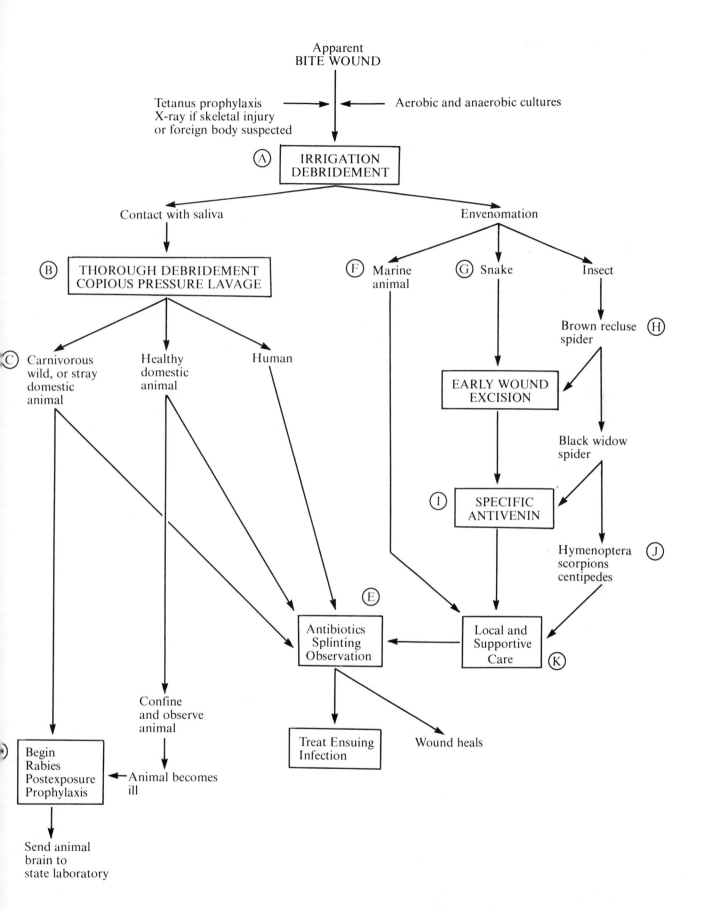

6. Rabies: Risk, Management, Prophylaxis and Immunization. Public Health Services Advisory Committee. Ann Int Med. 1977; 86:452–455.

7. Russell FF, Carlson RW, Wainschel J, Osborne AH. Snake venom poisoning in the United States. JAMA. 1975; 233:341–344.

# HAND INFECTION

## COMMENTS

A. Important points in the history of a patient with a hand infection include whether or not the patient is a diabetic (the organisms will likely be gram negative and multiple, and host defences are compromised[3]); exposure to the human mouth; and employment or recreational exposure to fresh or salt water, or plant or animal materials. Radiographs will help assess skeletal trauma or retained foreign material. Laboratory evaluation includes fasting serum glucose, WBC, and ESR. Gram stain and culture of infected material should be taken when possible.

B. Infectious gangrene is rare but requires immediate treatment. Gas in the soft tissues, rapid spread of tissue necrosis, and signs of systemic toxicity indicate life-threatening infection. Gram stain and culture of the exudate may reveal clostridial gram positive rods or the microaerophilic or anaerobic streptococci of Meleney's infection. Treatment consists of high doses of penicillin, decompression of tightly swollen areas, debridement of non-viable tissue, splinting, and careful frequent observation. Radical amputation may be necessary in relentlessly advancing infection.[2]

C. Early hand infections present with swelling, pain, cellulitis, but no localized purulence. At this stage the process can often be arrested and reversed by aggressive nonoperative measures. Gonococcal tenosynovitis, in particular, can often be treated without surgery. Septic arthritis requires open irrigation and debridement early in the course of the infection.

D. The infected hand should be splinted with the wrist in slight dorsiflexion, MCPs flexed to 70°, IPs extended, and the thumb maintained in palmar abduction. In addition, strict elevation, antibiotics, and close observation for 24 hours will enhance the patient's response to infection. Intermittent, nondependent soaks may be added for the infection expected to "point" (e.g., paronychia, pulpspace infection, or subcutaneous abscess). If the infection localizes, drainage is indicated. If the infection is resolving or no worse after 24 hours, continue with nonoperative care. The choice of antibiotics should consider both patient and infection factors. Most hand infections are due to *Stapholococcus aureus*; cellulitis is usually due to streptococcal species. Diabetic patients tend to have gram negative and mixed infecting organisms. Bite wound infections are often due to mixed anaerobic species (pp. 264, 265). Surgical drainage is indicated to decompress accumulated pus, clear infection from synovial space, or debride non-viable tissue.

E. In infections in which the body's response is adequate, (especially with *S. aureus*) purulence will become localized. Abscesses, paronychia, pulp space infections, deep space infections, purulent flexor tenosynovitis, and septic arthritis should be drained. Infected open wounds should be debrided, irrigated and dressed open early in the course of treatment.

F. Drainage incisions should be made so as to minimize tissue damage and avoid problematic scars.

G. *Herpes simplex* infection (herpetic whitlow) is most often seen in those who contact the human mouth (e.g., dental personnel). These painful, vesicular lesions should be treated with soaks, analgesics, and protection from autoinnoculation. Acyclovir* ointment may be beneficial in controlling symptoms and decreasing viral shedding in first-time infections.

H. Chronic infections result from nearly any organism, may present as soft tissue or skeletal neoplasms, and may be long standing and difficult to eradicate. Cutaneous infections such as *Candida* paronychia may best be treated with topical antimicrobial agents. Deep infections require debridement, and histologic and bacteriologic evaluation. Atypical mycobacterial infections have a predilection for the synovial spaces of the hand.[4] Chronic skeletal infection usually implies necrotic bone sequestra or lack of skeletal stability. Consultation with the infectious disease service is recommended in these cases.

*Acyclovir is not yet specifically recommended for this purpose.

## REFERENCES

1. Balcomb TV. Acute gonococcal flexortenosynovitis in a woman with asymptomatic gonorrhea: case report and literature review. J Hand Surg. 1982; 7:521–522.
2. Linscheid RL, Dobyns JH. Common and uncommon infections of the hand. Orthop Clin N Am. 1975; 6:1063–1104.
3. Mann RJ, Peacock JM. Hand infections in patients with diabetes mellitus. J Trauma. 1977; 17:376–380.
4. Sutker WL, Lankford L, Thomsett R. Granulomatous synovitis: the role of atypical mycobacteria. Rev Infect Dis. 1979; 1:729–735.

HAND INFECTION

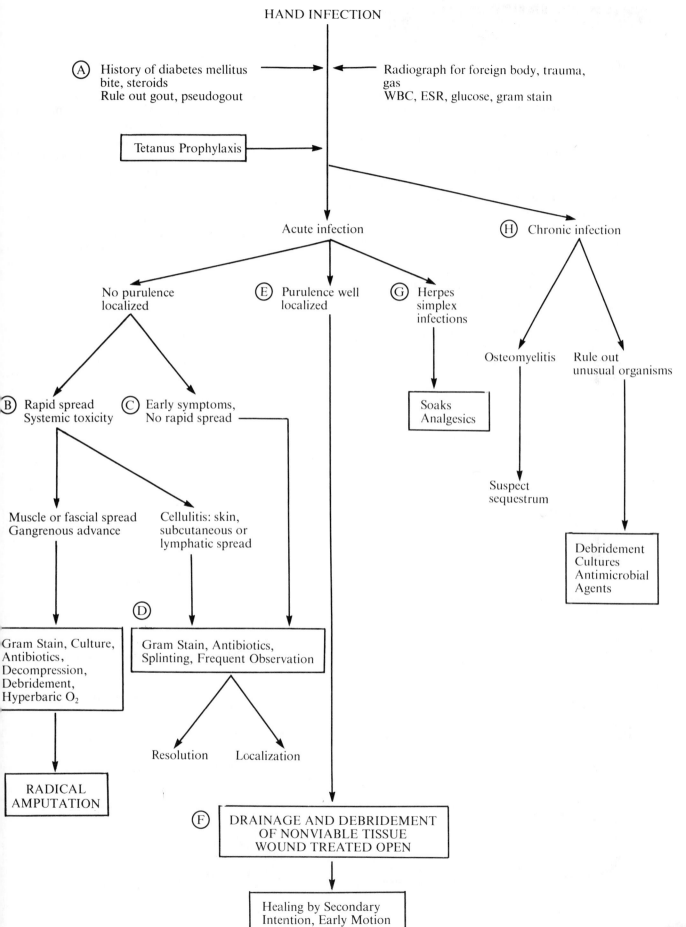

# FINGERTIP INJURY

## COMMENTS

A.  Fingertip injuries are those that involve the structures distal to the insertions of the flexor and extensor tendons on the distal phalanx. Primary suture of the wound under no tension is recommended when possible, but often the nature of the wound prevents this. A closed, healed, nonpainful wound, which functions as a part of the hand and is cosmetically acceptable, is the goal in treating these injuries. The initial examination should include information on tetanus immunization status, possibility of injury to the skeleton or foreign body retention, and the nature of contamination of the wound.

B.  In closed injuries, bleeding into a closed space may cause subungual hematoma or actual "compartment syndrome" of the pulp space. A simple subungual hematoma may be evacuated for pain relief. If there is an underlying fracture with nail bed disruption, it is preferable to remove the nail plate for appropriate debridement and repair of the nail bed.

C.  In children, the defatted skin of the severed part may be applied as a biological dressing with good results.

D.  Shortening with primary closure may be considered in the adult in a digit other than the thumb or digit adjacent to the thumb. Usually the patient prefers to preserve the remaining length of the injured digit.

E.  Where sensibility is crucial for function, the defect can be secondarily reconstructed by means of a neurovascular island pedicle flap.

## REFERENCES

1.  Atasoy E, Ioakimidis E, Kasden ML, Kutz JE, Kleinert HE. Reconstruction of the amputated fingertip with a triangular volar flap. A new surgical procedure. J Bone Joint Surg. 1970; 52A:921–926.
2.  Kutler W. A new method for fingertip amputation. JAMA. 1947; 133:29–30.
3.  Sandzen SC, Jr. Treating acute fingertip injuries. Am Fam Phys. 1972; 5:68–79.
4.  Sandzen SC, Jr. Management of acute fingertip injury in the child. The Hand, 1974; 6:190–196.

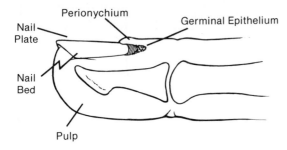

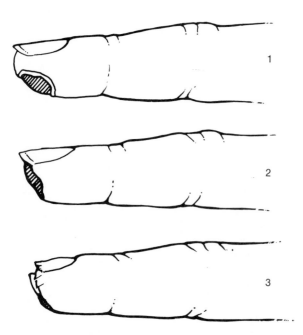

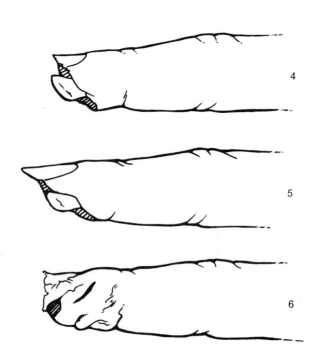

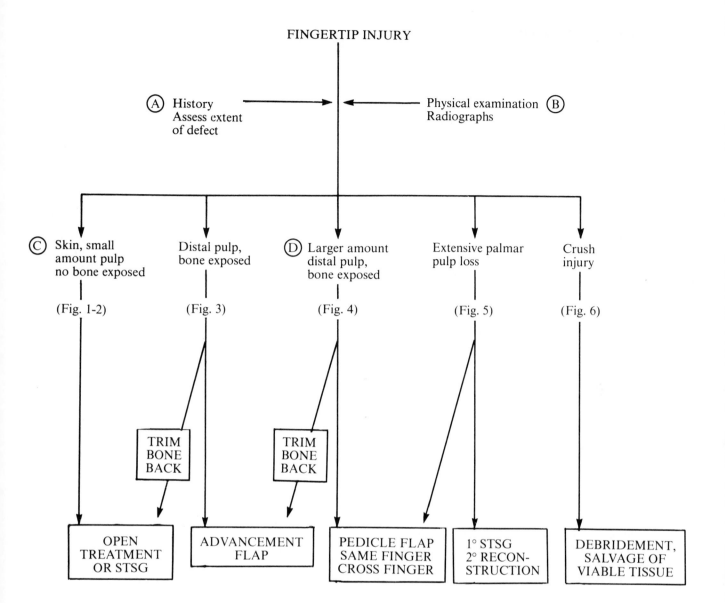

FINGERTIP INJURY

A History
Assess extent of defect

B Physical examination
Radiographs

C Skin, small amount pulp no bone exposed (Fig. 1-2)

Distal pulp, bone exposed (Fig. 3)

D Larger amount distal pulp, bone exposed (Fig. 4)

Extensive palmar pulp loss (Fig. 5)

Crush injury (Fig. 6)

TRIM BONE BACK

TRIM BONE BACK

OPEN TREATMENT OR STSG

ADVANCEMENT FLAP

PEDICLE FLAP SAME FINGER CROSS FINGER

1° STSG 2° RECON-STRUCTION

DEBRIDEMENT, SALVAGE OF VIABLE TISSUE

# AMPUTATION IN THE HAND

## COMMENTS

A. Age, medical condition (particularly diabetes or peripheral vascular disease), occupation, avocation, and hand dominance are important points in treating the amputation in the hand. Tetanus prophylaxis is mandatory. Initial treatment consists of irrigation of the wound and application of dressing. Bleeding is controlled by elevation and compressive dressings, never by blind clamping.

B. The goals of treatment are a clean, healed wound; stable, non-painful soft tissue with sensibility; preservation of functional length without joint contracture; and rapid return to function with minimum morbidity. In single digit amputations all efforts should be made to preserve the length of the thumb. Amputations distal to the IP joint of the thumb will function well if stable soft tissue and sensibility are secured. In amputations through a finger, it is important to preserve tendon insertions (i.e., the base of the distal phalanx and the proximal half of the middle phalanx) and to obtain closure with palmar skin when possible. In single finger amputations, a loose primary closure can usually be obtained by minimal shortening and reshaping of the phalanx into a tuft-like configuration similar to the distal phalanx. Amputations proximal to the superficialis insertion will lack PIP flexion and have only lumbrical action at the MCP joint, but will contribute to the breadth of the hand and to overall function. Single digit amputations proximal to the PIP joint are minimally functional and create a deficit in the palm. These can be considered for later ray deletion. Digital nerves should be shortened and placed where neuromas will not be caught in scar or be easily traumatized. Where it is necessary to preserve length (e.g., to preserve a tendon insertion, or in a multiple digit or thumb amputation) local or pedicle flaps or grafts can be used for coverage. Late reconstruction of the thumb is jeopardized by initial shortening of its length, or by local flap rearrangement. Wound closure with split thickness skin graft or distant pedicle flap is the primary goal.

C. Hand motion, desensitization and stump hardening should be started as soon as the wound heals.

D. In amputations through the thumb or multiple digits where the severed part is available and in good condition, the patient should be evaluated for possible reattachment. The parts must be cleanly severed or with minimal damage to the tissue edges. Avulsion injuries are usually not suitable for replantation in a finger but may be so in the thumb. Indications for replantation are somewhat broader in a child. The severed part should be kept clean and cold, wrapped loosely in gauze moistened with saline, placed in a clean plastic bag, and then placed on ice, *not on dry ice.* The patient must be evaluated for other injuries in the hand or elsewhere, systemic or local disease, and arteriosclerotic vessels. The patient's mental and emotional ability to cope with prolonged rehabilitation following replantation should be considered. A facility which has a microsurgical team available must be reachable within 12 hours of injury.

E. In amputations involving multiple digits or through the palm, any tissue which can be preserved may significantly contribute to the function of the hand. Flap coverage is indicated instead of shortening to obtain closure.

F. In treating complex hand injuries, principles of irrigation and debridement, skeletal stabilization, and initial open wound care apply. Potentially viable tissue should be preserved at the first debridement. A "second look" and redebridement at 48 hours will give a clearer picture of wound status.

## REFERENCES

1. Louis DS. Amputations. In, *Operative Hand Surgery.* Green DP, ed. New York: Churchill-Livingstone, 1982.
2. Milford L. The hand. In, *Campbell's Operative Orthopaedics.* Crenshaw AS, ed. St. Louis: CV Mosby, 1980.
3. Urbaniak JR. Replantation of amputated parts: technique, results, and indications. In, *AAOS. Symposium on Microsurgery: Practical Use in Orthopaedics.* St. Louis: CV Mosby, 1979.

# AMPUTATION IN THE HAND

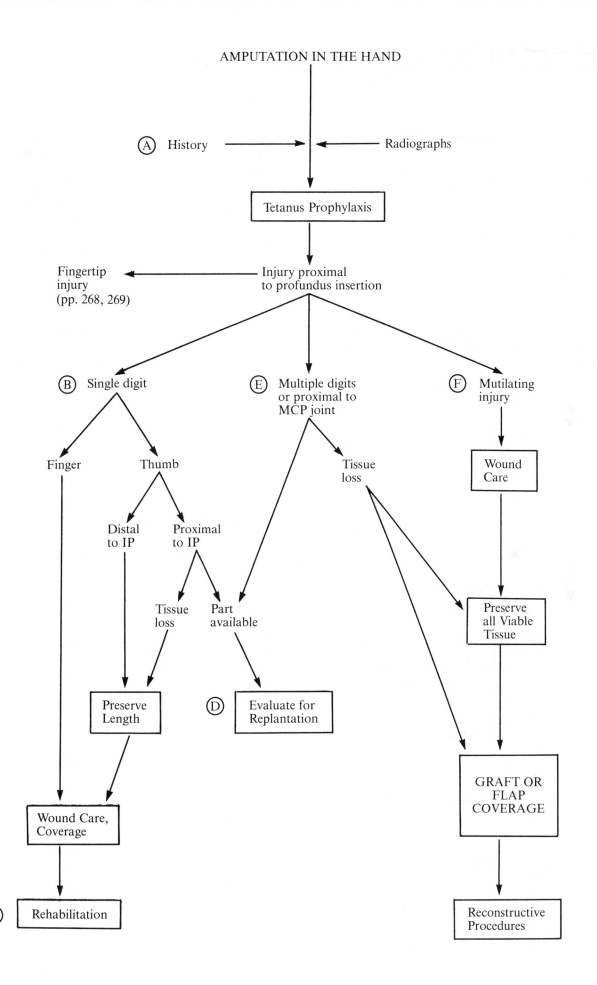

# FLEXOR TENDON INJURY

## COMMENTS

A. The anatomic proximity of the flexor mechanism to nerves in the forearm, wrist, and hand makes neurological examination crucial. Wound care including tetanus prophylaxis takes priority in management. Individual tendon function testing is needed to detect injury. A history of position of the hand and fingers at the time of injury will help localize the injury. Laceration of the sheath in zone II (see figure) suggests at least partial laceration of the tendons.

B. A tidy laceration is one in which skin edges are cleanly incised and contamination is minimal; the wound may be closed primarily without risk of infection. Primary or delayed (within 3 days to 3 weeks) primary repair in an end-to-end fashion is possible. Soft tissue coverage must be satisfactory, tendon bed and pulleys free from disruption and scar, and the tendon itself without gap in the substance. Tendons lacerated in zones III, IV, and V should be repaired where possible. In zone I the flexor digitorum profundus (FDP) may be repaired or advanced into bone if the advancement is less than 1 cm. Tendon lacerations within zone II are particularly hazardous. This fibro-osseous, synovial sheath known as "no man's land" bears an intimate and complex

relationship of tendons in a confined space. If conditions are favorable, (i.e., patient, wound, surgeon, equipment, and rehabilitation availability), the FDP and flexor digitorum superficialis (FDS) should be both repaired or the FDP may be repaired and the FDS excised. Partial tendon lacerations should be repaired. Meticulous repair, splinting, and experienced hand therapy are essential for satisfactory results. Flexor tendon surgery should not be undertaken by the inexperienced.

C. An untidy wound is one in which damage to the skin edges and soft tissue prevents safe primary closure. Any wound with significant contamination must be considered untidy, as must any wound that has gone 12 hours or more without attention.

D. If an untidy wound has been rendered tidy by adequate debridement, local care, and closure within 3 weeks of injury, and if end-to-end repair of the tendon is possible, surgical care is the same as for a tidy wound.

E. When direct repair of a tendon laceration is not possible within 3 weeks of injury, reconstructive procedures will likely be needed. Inadequate soft tissue coverage, inadequate tendon bed and lack of pulleys (especially in zone II), and gaps in the substance of the tendon demand attention prior to one-or two-stage tendon grafting.

Zone 1

Zone 2

Zone 3

Zone 4

Zone 5

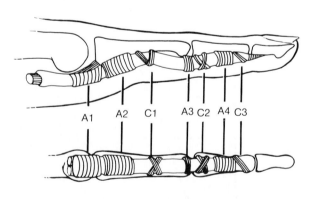

Zone I is distal to the superficialis insertion. Zone II is the area of the digital flexor sheath. Zone III is the palm distal to the carpal tunnel; Zone IV, the carpal tunnel and Zone V, the area proximal to the carpal tunnel. The pulley system in the digital flexor sheath consists of a number of discrete thickenings named "A" for annular and "C" for cruciform. The A2 and A4 are the most important of the pulleys to preserve.

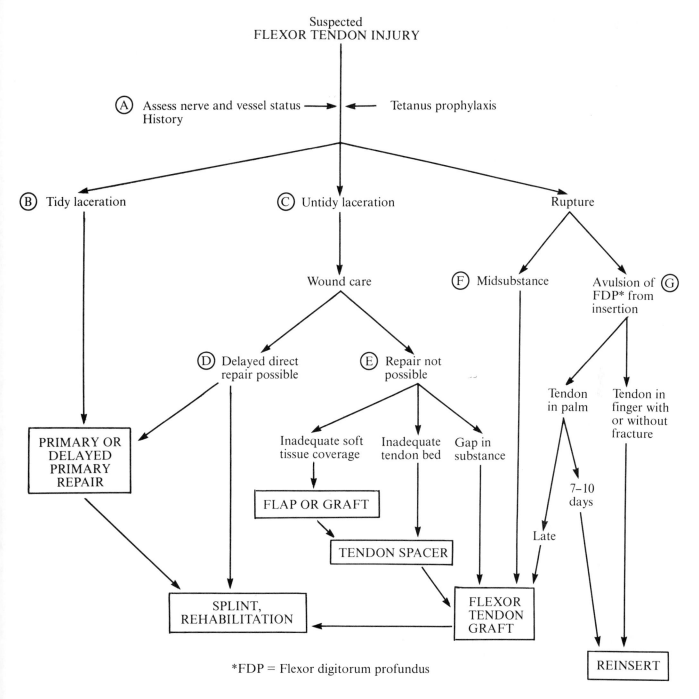

Suspected
FLEXOR TENDON INJURY

(A) Assess nerve and vessel status ——→ ←—— Tetanus prophylaxis
History

(B) Tidy laceration          (C) Untidy laceration                    Rupture

Wound care          (F) Midsubstance          Avulsion of (G)
FDP* from
insertion

(D) Delayed direct          (E) Repair not          Tendon          Tendon in
repair possible          possible          in palm          finger with
or without
fracture

PRIMARY OR          Inadequate soft          Inadequate          Gap in
DELAYED          tissue coverage          tendon bed          substance
PRIMARY
REPAIR          FLAP OR GRAFT                    7–10
days

TENDON SPACER          Late

SPLINT,          FLEXOR
REHABILITATION          TENDON
GRAFT          REINSERT

*FDP = Flexor digitorum profundus

F. Midsubstance ruptures of flexor tendons are unusual. Rheumatoid involvement of the tendon sheath or underlying joint, or fraying of the tendon over a bony prominence after fracture are the most common causes. Repair of the underlying condition should precede tendon reconstruction.

G. Avulsion of the FDP from its insertion on the distal phalanx is commonest in the ring finger. If the tendon has retracted into the palm through the decussation of the superficialis, all vincula will be ruptured. The tendon will rapidly become avascular, necrotic, and contracted. Advancement and reinsertion is recommended within 7 to 10 days of injury, but will be difficult and usually unsuccessful thereafter. Flexor tendon graft or

arthrodesis of the distal interphalangeal joint are options. If the tendon remains in the finger distal to the superficialis decussation, with or without a fragment of bone from the distal phalanx, reinsertion may be successful up to several months after injury.

## REFERENCES

1. Kleinert, HE, Kutz JE, Cohen MJ. Primary repair of zone II flexor tendon lacerations. In, *AAOS Symposium on Tendon Surgery in the Hand*. St. Louis: CV Mosby, 1975.
2. Leddy JP. Flexor tendons: acute injuries. In, *Operative hand Surgery*, Green DP, ed. New York: Churchill-Livingstone, 1982.

# EXTENSOR TENDON INJURIES

## COMMENTS

A.  A history of contact with the human mouth should be sought in any open wound on the extensor aspect of the hand. Injury to the underlying joint or skeletal structure should be investigated and treated appropriately.

B.  Distal to the wrist the excursion of extensor tendons is limited by the presence of junctura, and by the absence of extensive synovial sheaths. Retraction of tendon ends is less of a problem here than in flexor tendon lacerations. End-to-end repair should be undertaken if wound conditions are satisfactory, if there is no loss of tendon substance, and if soft tissue coverage can be obtained. A portion of retinaculum at the wrist may require excision to prevent adhesion of repaired tendon.

C.  Primary end-to-end repair is not possible where there has been loss of gliding soft tissue coverage or loss of tendon substance, especially over the dorsum of the hand and finger joints. Wound care, stabilization of underlying skeletal injury, and attainment of stable soft tissue coverage precede tendon reconstruction.

D.  The extensor mechanism in the finger comprises extrinsic and intrinsic components. If direct repair is not possible, reconstruction using locally recruited tissues or tendon graft to restore continuity and balance will be needed. Splinting should be with PIP and DIP in extension and MCP in approximately 20° to 30° of flexion.

E.  Function of a common extensor tendon with substance loss proximal to the MCP joint may be restored by suturing its distal end to an intact adjacent common extensor tendon in a balanced position, or by tendon transfer. When thumb extensor or abductor tendon, or multiple common extensor tendons, have defects, tendon grafts to bridge the defect or tendon transfer will be needed.

F.  Ruptures or avulsions of extensor tendons in mid substance are usually associated with rheumatoid synovitis or attenuation over a bony prominence. Correction of the predisposing condition should precede reconstruction of the tendon.

G.  Avulsion of the insertion of the extensor mechanism from the middle phalanx or distal phalanx can occur as an isolated one-plane injury or in conjunction with a dislocation. Assessment of joint stability and tendon function is crucial (pp. 242–247). Avulsion associated with a fracture fragment displaced more than 2 mm and/or rotated so that it does not reduce in extension, or one with articular surface disruption, should be treated by reattaching the frag-

ment. Rupture of the tendon insertion without associated fracture is often overlooked. Treatment by splinting is recommended for boutonniere and mallet tendon injuries seen even 3 to 6 months after injury.

H.  Ruptures of the transverse fibers of the extensor hood over the MCP joint allow the extensor tendon to sublux into the intermetacarpal valley, creating an extensor lag. Repair is indicated, using local tissue for reinforcement where needed.

I.  A boutonniere injury is splinted with the PIP joint in extension while allowing active and passive flexion of the DIP joint. PIP joint extension is increased by adjusting the splint as tolerated. When full passive PIP extension and full active DIP flexion is achieved, splinting can be changed to a dynamic "reverse knuckle bender" or boutonniere splint which will allow protected motion for an additional 3 to 6 weeks.

J.  Splinting of a mallet injury consists of maintaining the DIP joint in maximum tolerated extension while encouraging PIP motion. Mallet injuries should be splinted for a minimum of 6 weeks.

## REFERENCES

1.  Doyle JR. Extensor tendons: acute injuries. In, *Operative Hand Surgery*. Green DP, ed. New York: Churchill-Livingstone, 1982.
2.  Nalebuff EA. The recognition and treatment of tendon ruptures in the rheumatoid hand. *AAOS Symposium on Tendon Surgery in the Hand*. St. Louis: CV Mosby, 1975.

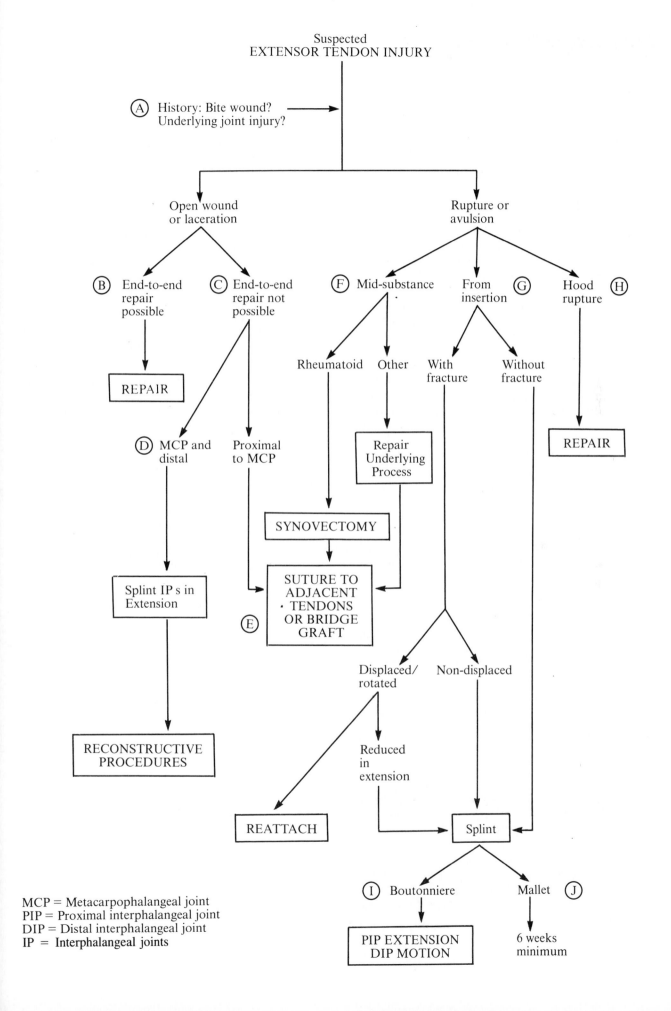

Suspected
EXTENSOR TENDON INJURY

(A) History: Bite wound?
Underlying joint injury?

Open wound or laceration

Rupture or avulsion

(B) End-to-end repair possible
(C) End-to-end repair not possible
(F) Mid-substance
From insertion
(G)
Hood rupture (H)

REPAIR

(D) MCP and distal
Proximal to MCP
Rheumatoid
Other
With fracture
Without fracture

Repair Underlying Process

REPAIR

SYNOVECTOMY

Splint IP s in Extension

(E) SUTURE TO ADJACENT TENDONS OR BRIDGE GRAFT

Displaced/ rotated
Non-displaced

RECONSTRUCTIVE PROCEDURES

Reduced in extension

REATTACH

Splint

(I) Boutonniere
Mallet (J)

PIP EXTENSION DIP MOTION

6 weeks minimum

MCP = Metacarpophalangeal joint
PIP = Proximal interphalangeal joint
DIP = Distal interphalangeal joint
IP  =  Interphalangeal joints

275

# THERMAL INJURY

## COMMENTS

A. Resuscitation of the patient as a whole takes priority. Other injuries and medical problems must be sought. Concomitant internal trauma, fractures, cardiac conduction abnormalities, and pulmonary difficulty may be present. The very young and the very old are at particular risk for complications. Tetanus prophylaxis is important in the care of any thermal injury.

B. Superficial second degree burns are treated by dressing with antibiotic-impregnated gauze and splinting of the burned part for 5 to 10 days, or by a program of active range of motion of the hand, dressed b i d only with silver sulfadiazine, and placed in a clean plastic bag. Pain control is excellent and motion is not lost. Oral penicillin for streptococcal coverage is indicated.

C. Electrical injury is usually more severe than initially appreciated. Electrical energy travels through soft tissue selectively. Nerves and vessels are more conductive than other tissues; electrical injury may occur at a distance from the point of contact. The patient should be monitored for cardiac arrythmias. Muscle damage may be extensive; nuclear medicine scanning techniques may elucidate the degree and location of myonecrosis.

D. Escharotomy is indicated in cases where distal perfusion is compromised due to circumferential tissue injury, edema, and constriction, and not where perfusion pressure is low due to inadequate resuscitation and hypovolemia. The arm, forearm, hand, and digits all may require decompression. Fascial release should be added in cases of deep burns and electrical injury. Interosseous release should not be neglected. Decompression of median and ulnar nerves following electrical injury is mandatory if sensory deficit is present or develops.

E. Early removal of eschar with preservation of dermal elements where possible, and removal of deep necrotic tissue as needed, is done to prevent extension of the depth of the wound due to secondary infection.

F. Where elements of dermis remain, biologic dressings or antibiotic impregnated dressings will allow healing of excised wounds without grafting; full-thickness burns require autogenous graft coverage, usually split-thickness grafts. Flap coverage may be necessary where later tendon reconstruction is planned, but this is often best done as a secondary procedure. Splinting and aggressive physical and occupational therapy are the mainstays of post-coverage treatment.

G. Frostbite involves ice crystal formation within living tissues resulting in direct injury to cells and in vascular impairment. Frozen tissue is relatively durable, but thawing and refreezing yield disastrous results. Care of frostbite should, therefore, not be initiated until comprehensive, ongoing treatment is available.

H. Rapid rewarming in a whirlpool or water bath at 40° to 44° C is the procedure of choice. Local skin care with topical antibacterial agents, non-occlusive dressings, and splinting should follow. Systemic antibiotics are given based on culture and sensitivity reports of infection should it develop. Other treatment modalities are still debated and include low molecular weight dextran infusions, steriods, and chemical or surgical sympathectomy.

I. As long as infection does not become an uncontrollable problem, it is wisest to allow tissue demarcation prior to debridement. When amputation is performed adequate soft tissue for closure should be allowed.

## REFERENCES

1. Evans EB. Orthopaedic measures in the treatment of severe burns. J Bone Joint Surg. 1966; 48A:643–669.
2. House JH, Fidler M. Frostbite of the hand. In, *Operative Hand Surgery*. Green DP, ed. New York: Churchill-Livingstone, 1982.
3. Salisbury RE and Dingeldein GP: The burned hand and upper extremity. In *Operative Hand Surgery*. Green DP, ed. New York: Churchill-Livingstone, 1982.

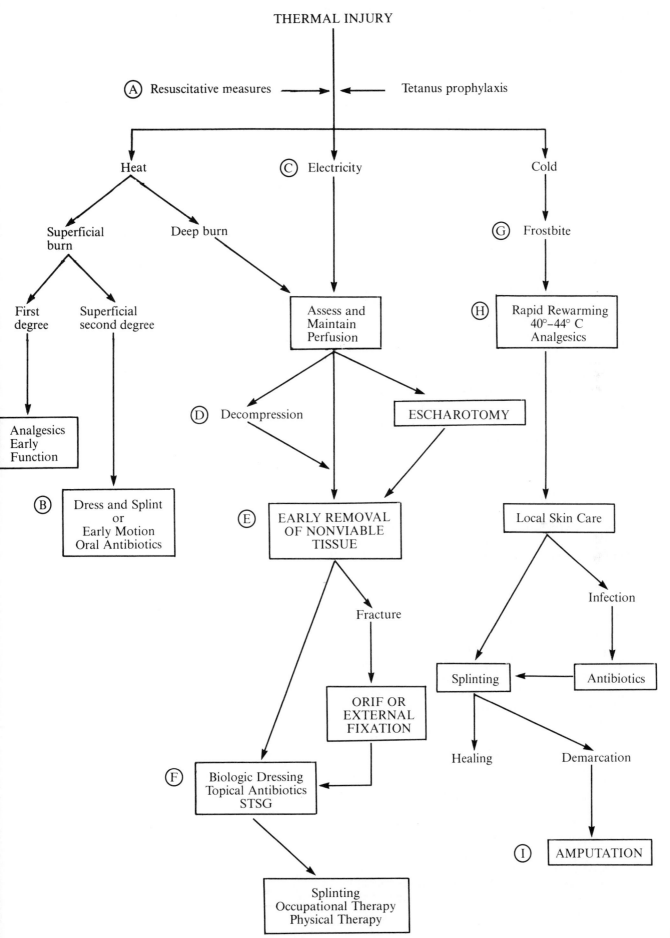

THERMAL INJURY

(A) Resuscitative measures ← → Tetanus prophylaxis

Heat  (C) Electricity  Cold

Superficial burn  Deep burn  (G) Frostbite

First degree  Superficial second degree

Assess and Maintain Perfusion

(H) Rapid Rewarming 40°–44° C Analgesics

Analgesics Early Function

(B) Dress and Splint or Early Motion Oral Antibiotics

(D) Decompression  ESCHAROTOMY

(E) EARLY REMOVAL OF NONVIABLE TISSUE

Local Skin Care

Fracture

Infection

Splinting ← Antibiotics

ORIF OR EXTERNAL FIXATION

Healing  Demarcation

(F) Biologic Dressing Topical Antibiotics STSG

Splinting Occupational Therapy Physical Therapy

(I) AMPUTATION

**277**

# SKELETAL TUMORS IN THE HAND

## COMMENTS

A.  The vast majority of skeletal tumors in the hand fall into one of several categories of benign lesions. It must be remembered that every type of skeletal lesion can occur in the hand and that a rational plan for diagnosis and treatment should be thought out prior to any surgical intervention. Certain lesions can be identified with relative certainty by their clinical and radiographic presentation. The exact nature of other lesions is less clear and, in these, open biopsy must be the initial surgical step. The final outcome may be compromised by surgical treatment designed without benefit of definitive diagnosis. Infection can usually be excluded from the differential diagnosis preoperatively. Material for culture should be obtained at the time of biopsy whenever doubt remains, and the potential for unusual organisms should not be overlooked. As clues to the identity and behavior of the lesion are usually obtained from radiographs, this algorithm proceeds from that starting point.

B.  Radiographic evidence of malignant behavior should initiate a preoperative evaluation of the extent of the disease. The prognosis for primary skeletal malignant tumors in the hand is better than for similar, more central lesions when appropriate treatment is rendered. In contrast, skeletal metastases in the hand are a grim prognostic feature, usually signifying hematogenous seeding of the primary lesion. Malignant degeneration of an enchondroma in Ollier's disease or Maffuci's syndrome is estimated at a risk of 1% or less for the individual lesion. The conversion will be heralded by the same indicators of malignancy seen with other lesions, namely, rapid growth and/or bony destruction.

C.  A suspected malignant lesion or one in which the diagnosis is unclear should undergo incisional biopsy prior to definitive treatment. The biopsy site must be planned so that any seeding of the tract can be completely eliminated at the time of ablative surgery. Surgical procedures for extremity tumor (or infection) should be performed under tourniquet control, but without Esmarch bandage exsanguination of the limb. There will be certain tumors in which the diagnosis of malignancy can be made at the time of biopsy, such as chondrosarcoma, whose malignancy correlates more closely with its clinical behavior than with its histology. In these cases the definitive surgical procedure can be performed immediately. However, in a majority of cases, the time needed to obtain a diagnosis based on permanent sections allows more thorough assessment of the tumor potential and better planning of the surgical treatment.

D.  Except for osteoid osteoma, a tumor is unlikely to involve cortex preferentially. In the absence of demonstrable lucent nidus (by tomography when indicated by history and plain radiographs), the material excised should be cultured for indolent infection and also sent for histologic examination. A fibrous cortical defect may occur in rare instances in the short tubular bones.

E.  Infection, eosinophilic granuloma, myeloma deposit, and brown tumor are examples of diagnoses in this category.

F.  Skeletal metastases in the hand constitute less than 1% of secondary deposits in bone.

## REFERENCE

1.  Dick HM. Bone tumors. In *Operative Hand Surgery*. Edited by Green DP. New York: Churchill Livingstone, 1982.

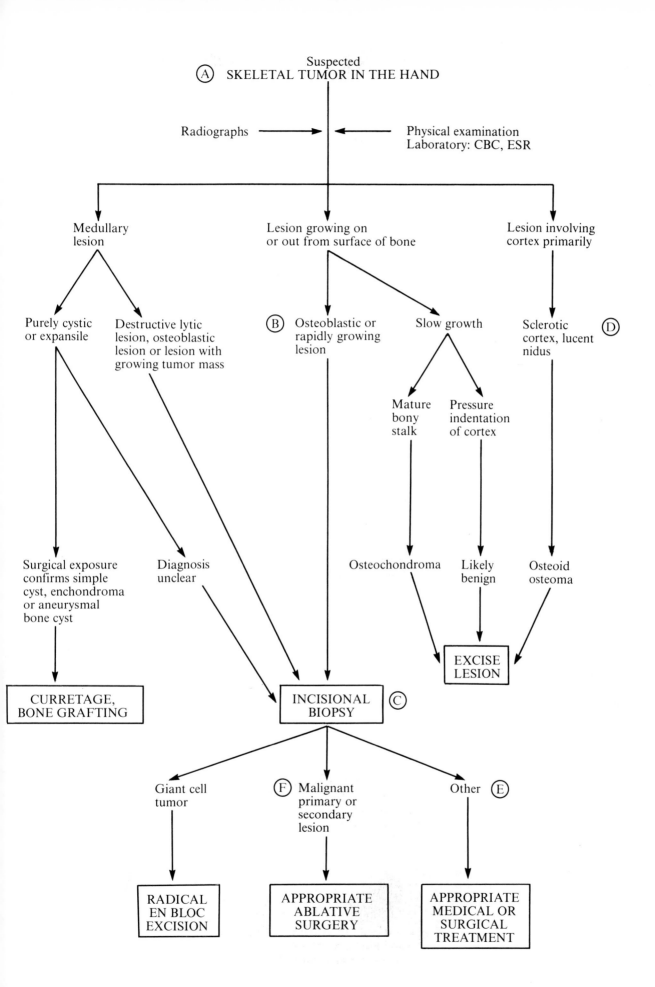

Suspected
(A) SKELETAL TUMOR IN THE HAND

Radiographs ⟶ ⟵ Physical examination
Laboratory: CBC, ESR

Medullary lesion

Lesion growing on or out from surface of bone

Lesion involving cortex primarily

Purely cystic or expansile

Destructive lytic lesion, osteoblastic lesion or lesion with growing tumor mass

(B) Osteoblastic or rapidly growing lesion

Slow growth

Sclerotic cortex, lucent nidus (D)

Mature bony stalk

Pressure indentation of cortex

Surgical exposure confirms simple cyst, enchondroma or aneurysmal bone cyst

Diagnosis unclear

Osteochondroma

Likely benign

Osteoid osteoma

EXCISE LESION

CURRETAGE, BONE GRAFTING

INCISIONAL BIOPSY (C)

Giant cell tumor

(F) Malignant primary or secondary lesion

Other (E)

RADICAL EN BLOC EXCISION

APPROPRIATE ABLATIVE SURGERY

APPROPRIATE MEDICAL OR SURGICAL TREATMENT

# SOFT TISSUE TUMORS IN THE HAND

## COMMENTS

A. In addition to a regional and general history and physical examination, specific information should be obtained regarding injury, penetration of the skin, fever, pain, drainage, cold intolerance, adenopathy, and vascular status. Skin testing or antibody titers may prove helpful in distinguishing an unusual infection from a neoplasm.

B. Most tumors can be determined to arise primarily from either the skin or deep soft tissue structures. However, eroding deep soft tissue tumors may present clinically as skin lesions and, conversely, invading skin tumors can involve deeper structures. Infection can occasionally mimic either a deep or superficial neoplasm, especially when the lesion is tender or there has been a history of penetrating trauma (e.g., pyogenic or foreign body granulomata).

C. Skin tumors may also arise in the subungual tissues. A nonhealing lesion, whether pigmented or not, arising in this site warrants biopsy. Surgical ablation of a subungual malignancy usually requires amputation.

D. Excisional biopsy with removal of a margin of normal skin is preferable to incisional biopsy. The width of the recommended margin varies with the suspected diagnosis. Incisional biopsy should be reserved for the very large lesion, that is, one in which extirpation of the tumor would require extensive surgery or amputation. The collaboration of an experienced pathologist is crucial.

E. Common benign skin lesions include juvenile warts, benign nevi, keratoacanthomata, and seborrheic keratoses, most of which are easily recognizeable and do not require removal. Any suspicious or premalignant lesion, such as actinic keratosis, should be excised with a margin of normal tissue. A patient's concern about a particular lesion is sufficient indication for treatment.

F. Deep soft tissue tumors in the hand are far more common than skeletal tumors. Certain lesions are common and easily identifiable by location, texture, and intraoperative inspection. Among these are ganglia, mucous cysts, epidermoid inclusion cysts, and giant cell tumors of tendon sheaths. Ganglia are by far the most common, comprising more than 50% of all deep soft tissue masses in the hand. Any neoplasm can occur in the hand and a plan for diagnosis and treatment must be available when the unfamiliar lesion is encountered. Dupuytren's nodules should not be excised.

G. Soft tissue calcification seen radiographically is usually associated with vascular malformation. Primary soft tissue cartilage tumors in the hand are, with rare exception, benign.

## REFERENCES

1. Angelides AC. Ganglions of the hand and wrist. In *Operative Hand Surgery*. Edited by Green DP. New York: Churchill Livingstone, 1982.
2. Fleegler EJ, McFarland GB. Soft tissue tumors. In *Operative Hand Surgery*. Edited by Green DP. New York: Churchill Livingstone, 1982.

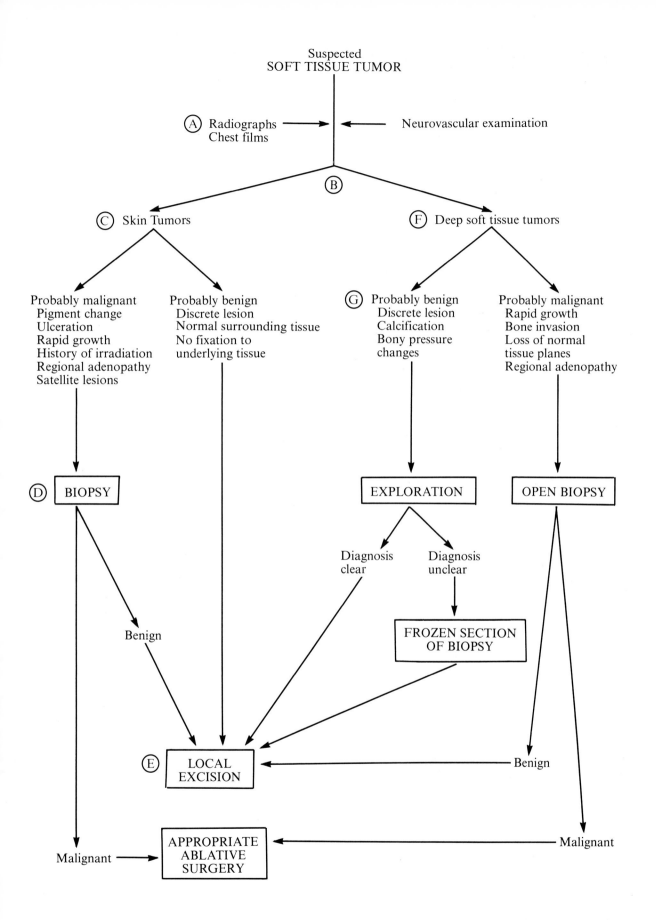

Suspected
SOFT TISSUE TUMOR

Ⓐ Radiographs
Chest films → ← Neurovascular examination

Ⓑ

Ⓒ Skin Tumors

Ⓕ Deep soft tissue tumors

Probably malignant
Pigment change
Ulceration
Rapid growth
History of irradiation
Regional adenopathy
Satellite lesions

Probably benign
Discrete lesion
Normal surrounding tissue
No fixation to
underlying tissue

Ⓖ Probably benign
Discrete lesion
Calcification
Bony pressure
changes

Probably malignant
Rapid growth
Bone invasion
Loss of normal
tissue planes
Regional adenopathy

Ⓓ BIOPSY

EXPLORATION

OPEN BIOPSY

Benign

Diagnosis
clear

Diagnosis
unclear

FROZEN SECTION
OF BIOPSY

Ⓔ LOCAL
EXCISION

Benign

Malignant

Malignant → APPROPRIATE
ABLATIVE
SURGERY

← Malignant

# STENOSING TENOSYNOVITIS

## COMMENTS

A. Stenosing tenosynovitis of the first dorsal extensor compartment at the wrist (de Quervain's disease), or of the extensor pollicis longus tendon, and trigger finger and thumb share a common anatomical feature of a tendon gliding within a rigidly enclosed synovial-lined space. The stenosing tenosynovitides occur most frequently in women and may be idiopathic or related to overuse. There is also a significant association with rheumatoid arthritis, degenerative joint disease, previous trauma, and metabolic conditions such as diabetes, hyperuricemia, hypothyroidism, and pregnancy, so that these diagnoses should be considered should symptoms persist. Treatment of a medical condition should precede any surgical release. In addition, septic tenosynovitis, particularly with a low virulence organism, including gonococcus, must be ruled out at the initial evaluation.

B. A trial of conservative nonoperative care with splinting, local steroid injection, and nonsteroidal anti-inflammatory agents should be given in cases of de Quervain's stenosing tenosynovitis and in trigger finger and trigger thumb. When the extensor pollicis longus tendon is involved, early decompression should be carried out because of the high rate of rupture of this tendon.

C. Trigger finger or thumb in an infant may resolve spontaneously by the age of three in 30% of cases noted at birth, and in 10% of cases noted later. Surgical release can be carried out anytime after the age of one year if spontaneous release does not occur.

D. Longstanding or recurrent trigger finger or a locked digit is best treated surgically.

E. Nonoperative treatment includes splinting, rest, nonsteroidal anti-inflammatory agents, and injection of a mixture of soluble steroid and local anesthetic into the tendon sheath, taking care not to inject into the tendon itself.

F. Surgical release of the constricting structures can be followed by early motion, provided the tendon is intact. Care should be taken to ensure complete release and not to disturb the tendon itself unless there is invading synovitis. Tenosynovectomy may be indicated in rheumatoid arthritis patients (see p. 289). Lister's tubercle should be smoothed to prevent further abrasion of the extensor pollicis longus tendon, and a retinacular pulley may need to be constructed for this tendon.

## REFERENCES

1. Fahey JJ, Bollinger JA. Trigger finger in adults and children. J Bone Joint Surg. 1954; 36A:1200–1218.
2. Medl WT. Tendonitis, tenosynovitis, "trigger finger" and Quervain's disease. Orthop Clin N Am. 1970; 1:375–382.

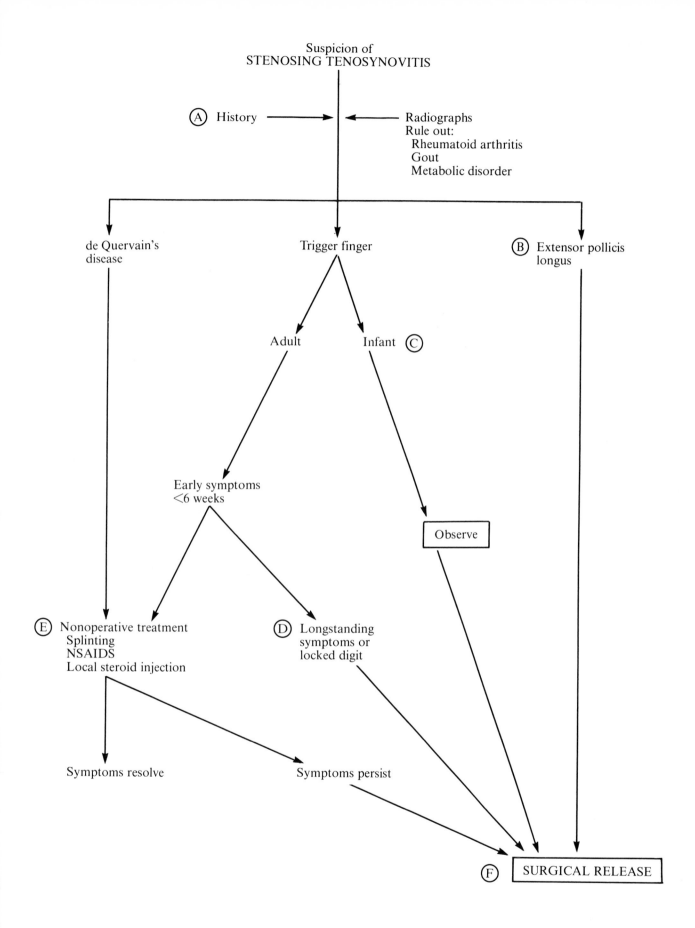

Suspicion of
STENOSING TENOSYNOVITIS

(A) History → ← Radiographs
Rule out:
Rheumatoid arthritis
Gout
Metabolic disorder

de Quervain's disease

Trigger finger

(B) Extensor pollicis longus

Adult

Infant (C)

Early symptoms <6 weeks

Observe

(E) Nonoperative treatment
Splinting
NSAIDS
Local steroid injection

(D) Longstanding symptoms or locked digit

Symptoms resolve

Symptoms persist

(F) SURGICAL RELEASE

# UPPER EXTREMITY NERVE COMPRESSION

## COMMENTS

A. Peripheral nerve compression lesions in the upper extremity are often difficult to localize. Many lesions are idiopathic but other types of pathology must be excluded in each. The patient's general medical condition, the possibility of trauma, the existence of any inflammatory condition, symptoms of generalized neuropathy, or possibility of tumor should be assessed. Symptoms may be nonspecific. Heaviness, weakness, aching, and pain, particularly after exertion of the extremity, are common complaints. Night pain, specific areas of sensory loss or specific motor weakness, are more discrete signs that may help to localize the level of compression.

B. Physical examination as well as careful examination of the limb in question should be made. A compressed nerve is irritable, and palpation or percussion in the injured area will elicit tenderness or paresthesias. The course of the nerve should be palpated for tenderness, masses, and provocation of symptoms. Maneuvers to increase pressure on the nerve (e.g., Phelan's test) may localize the lesion. Pulses should also be checked for concomitant vascular compression.

C. Radiographs may reveal certain bony and soft tissue abnormalities. A supracondylar process and ligament of Struthers occur in 1% of the population. Post-traumatic changes in the elbow or at the wrist may be the cause of nerve compression. A cervical rib may be associated with lower plexus lesions. Soft tissue contours should not be neglected in searching for causes of compression.

D. Electrodiagnostic studies may help confirm and localize a peripheral nerve compression lesion. Prolonged latency in conduction velocity suggests that damage to the myelin sheaths of the nerve fibers is sufficient to interfere with conduction. EMGs may be useful in primarily motor nerves to document either denervation or recovery. Lesions may coexist in a single nerve at more than one level; electrodiagnostic techniques may help to identify both lesions. Abnormal nerve conduction velocity or EMG is corroborative evidence of pathology; a normal study does not exclude a compression lesion.

E. Localization of the level of compression requires an understanding of the anatomy of the upper extremity and the sites of potential compression neuropathy. Careful, repeated examinations with provocative maneuvers are the key to a correct diagnosis. Anatomical variations such as Martin-Gruber connections should be kept in mind.

F. Once the probable location of compression is identified, other causes of nerve injury must be excluded (i.e., tumor, infection, inflammation, vascular malformation, congenital anomalies, trauma and degenerative changes). Correctable problems should be addressed.

G. Symptoms of nerve compression lesions represent a continuum of injury. By the time sensory loss and motor weakness are present, significant damage has occurred. Paralysis of muscles supplied by a pure motor nerve (e.g., anterior or posterior interosseous nerve) indicates long-standing pathology and a relatively poorer prognosis. In these lesions exploration and decompression should be undertaken at 6 weeks if motor function does not improve with conservative treatment. The risk of not treating a compression neuropathy is that ultimately the compression may result in a neuroma in continuity with no chance of spontaneous recovery.

## REFERENCES

1. DeLagi EF. Electrodiagnosis in peripheral nerve lesions. In, *Management of Peripheral Nerve Problems*. Omer GE, Spinner M, eds. Philadelphia: WB Saunders, 1980.
2. Spinner, M. Management of nerve compression lesions of the upper extremity. In, *Management of Peripheral Nerve Problems*. Omer GE, Spinner, M, eds. Philadelphia: WB Saunders, 1980.

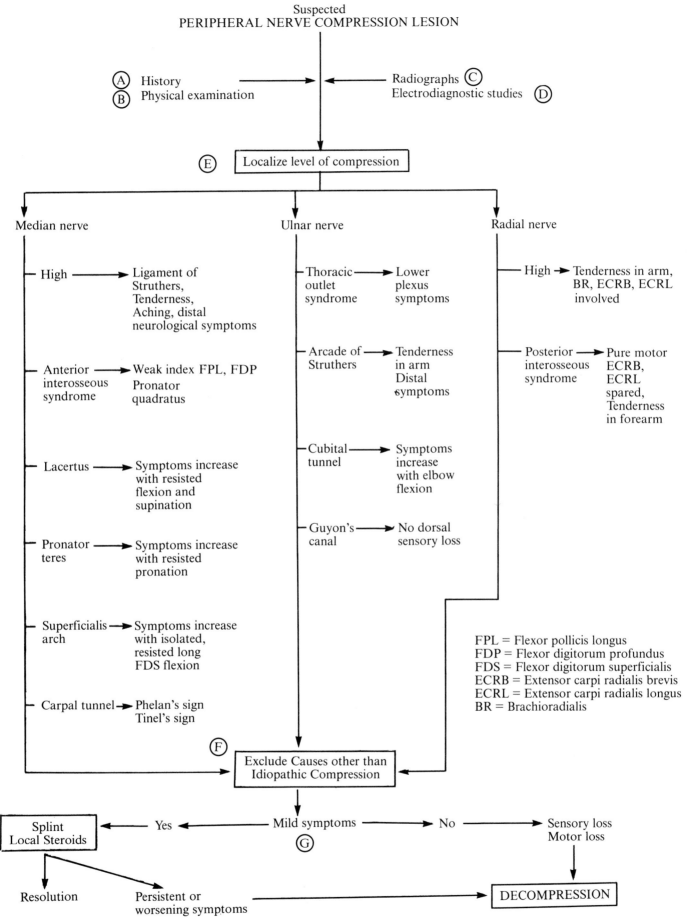

Suspected
PERIPHERAL NERVE COMPRESSION LESION

Ⓐ History
Ⓑ Physical examination
Radiographs Ⓒ
Electrodiagnostic studies Ⓓ

Ⓔ Localize level of compression

Median nerve

- High → Ligament of Struthers, Tenderness, Aching, distal neurological symptoms
- Anterior interosseous syndrome → Weak index FPL, FDP Pronator quadratus
- Lacertus → Symptoms increase with resisted flexion and supination
- Pronator teres → Symptoms increase with resisted pronation
- Superficialis arch → Symptoms increase with isolated, resisted long FDS flexion
- Carpal tunnel → Phelan's sign Tinel's sign

Ulnar nerve

- Thoracic outlet syndrome → Lower plexus symptoms
- Arcade of Struthers → Tenderness in arm Distal symptoms
- Cubital tunnel → Symptoms increase with elbow flexion
- Guyon's canal → No dorsal sensory loss

Radial nerve

- High → Tenderness in arm, BR, ECRB, ECRL involved
- Posterior interosseous syndrome → Pure motor ECRB, ECRL spared, Tenderness in forearm

FPL = Flexor pollicis longus
FDP = Flexor digitorum profundus
FDS = Flexor digitorum superficialis
ECRB = Extensor carpi radialis brevis
ECRL = Extensor carpi radialis longus
BR = Brachioradialis

Ⓕ Exclude Causes other than Idiopathic Compression

Splint
Local Steroids ← Yes ← Mild symptoms → No → Sensory loss Motor loss
Ⓖ

Resolution    Persistent or worsening symptoms → DECOMPRESSION

# BRACHIAL PLEXUS INJURY

## COMMENTS

A. Brachial plexus injuries (BPI) range from mild compression lesions to insoluble avulsion of nerve roots. Most BPI are partial and have some potential for recovery, although the time course may be prolonged. The prognosis for a closed BPI is related to the amount of energy dissipated by the soft tissues of the neck. Compression lesions have the best prognosis; traction lesions, the worst. The most common mechanism of traction injury is the motorcycle accident in which the helmeted head is distracted from the unprotected shoulder. Details of speed, position of the body at the time of impact, and associated injuries are important.

B. After initial stabilization of the patient, examination is directed toward identifying vascular injury, cervical spinal cord injury, and skeletal injury (clavicle, shoulder, first rib, and C-spine).

C. At the time of exploration for vascular repair, repair of a clean laceration of a plexus structure is optimal if patient, surgeon, and surgical team and facilities are ideal. Nothing is to be gained by attempting primary repair of a traction injury.

D. In closed injuries the most important aspect of BPI care is the repeated, detailed documentation of the neurologic status of the extremity. Only with time does the nature and extent of the injury become apparent. Splinting should be accomplished early, especially with the upper plexus injuries, to support the shoulder and elbow and allow positioning of the hand. An exercise program to maintain supple joints is also important. Detailed examination and special diagnostic studies may help to separate a lesion in continuity, which will recover, from a ruptured structure or avulsed nerve root. These studies include: myelography (4 weeks if root avulsion is suspected), nerve conduction studies and EMG (after 8 weeks), histamine tests and sensory evoked potentials.

E. Good prognostic signs indicate a postganglionic lesion and include: absence of a Horner's sign, presence of a clavicle or shoulder injury (energy dissipated by bone), abnormal nerve conduction, normal myelogram, negative flare reaction on histamine test, and proximal muscle sparing. Spotty sparing of distal function or early spotty recovery are particularly favorable signs.

F. Poor prognostic signs include: a persistent Horner's sign, long tract signs, first rib or transverse process fracture, persistent burning pain, meningoceles on myelography, normal nerve conduction studies in the presence of paralysis and anesthesia, flare reaction on histamine testing, and fibrillation potentials in posterior spinal muscles. All indicate a preganglionic location of the lesion.

G. Grafting of brachial plexus postganglionic ruptures is being carried out in selected patients in specialized centers.

H. Reconstructive surgery such as tendon transfers or arthrodeses, may provide functional improvement in carefully selected patients. Orthotic or prosthetic fitting may be indicated in others.

## REFERENCES

1. Leffert RD. Lesions of the brachial plexus, including thoracic outlet syndrome. Chapter 12 in AAOS Instructional Course Lectures. Vol 26. St. Louis, CV Mosby Co., 1977.
2. Narakas A. Surgical treatment of traction injuries of the brachial plexus. Clin Orthop Rel Res. 1978; 133:71–90.
3. Wynn-Parry CB. *Rehabilitation of the Hand.* London: Butterworths, 1981.

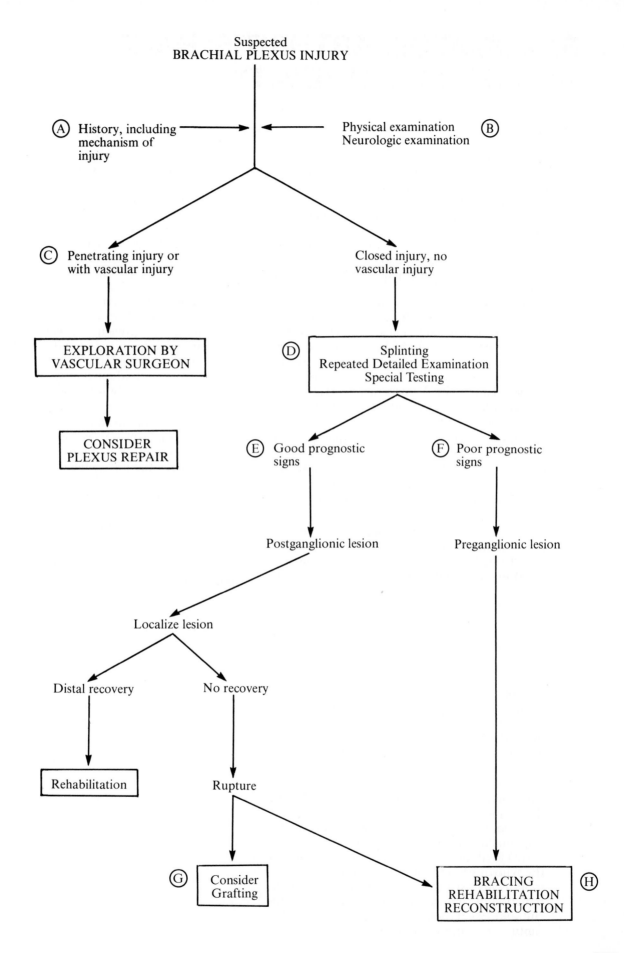

Suspected
**BRACHIAL PLEXUS INJURY**

Ⓐ History, including
mechanism of
injury

Ⓑ Physical examination
Neurologic examination

Ⓒ Penetrating injury or
with vascular injury

Closed injury, no
vascular injury

**EXPLORATION BY
VASCULAR SURGEON**

Ⓓ Splinting
Repeated Detailed Examination
Special Testing

**CONSIDER
PLEXUS REPAIR**

Ⓔ Good prognostic
signs

Ⓕ Poor prognostic
signs

Postganglionic lesion

Preganglionic lesion

Localize lesion

Distal recovery

No recovery

Rehabilitation

Rupture

Ⓖ Consider
Grafting

Ⓗ **BRACING
REHABILITATION
RECONSTRUCTION**

# RHEUMATOID ARTHRITIS: HAND AND UPPER EXTREMITY

## COMMENTS

A. Rheumatoid arthritis (RA) involves many tissues and requires a multidisciplinary approach to management; medical management has become the mainstay of treatment. Routine examination of the hands and upper extremities is necessary to detect early evidence of tendon and joint involvement and to prevent the functional loss which is the sequela of articular cartilage and supporting tissue destruction. Other clinical entities that mimic RA are erosive osteoarthritis, gout, pseudogout, and chronic infection. Juvenile chronic arthritis (JCA) may produce the same deformities and clinical problems as RA. Specific attention should be directed toward recognizing tendon rupture, nerve compression, and bacterial infections in patients with compromised immunity. Disease in the cervical spine may produce symptoms in the upper extremity and needs to be ruled out.

B. A hand therapist or occupational therapist will be able to assist the patient with activities of daily living. The patient needs instruction in avoiding situations which place excessive stress on joints and weakened supporting structures.

C. Signs and symptoms of flexor tenosynovitis include pain, stiffness, swelling, crepitus, triggering, and fullness along the digital flexor sheath. Bowstringing of the tendon may result from destruction or attenuation of the pulley system within the sheath. Carpal tunnel syndrome is common. Injection of the tenosynovium or tendon sheath, with a soluble or depot steroid preparation may preclude the need for surgical debridement. Tenosynovectomy is indicated by evidence of nerve compression; by persistent synovitis unresponsive to local steroids and medical management for a period of 4 months; by evidence of rupture. The flexor tendon most likely to rupture is the flexor pollicis longus because of the acute course the tendon takes around the scaphoid and trapezium on its way into the thumb.

D. Tenosynovitis involving the extensor tendons over the dorsum of the wrist requires splinting during medical management. The risk of rupture of tendons is high, particularly with concomitant synovitis of the distal radioulnar joint or radiocarpal joint, or with bony collapse deformity. If the synovitis has not improved or resolved by 4 months, tenosynovectomy is indicated. Reconstruction of ruptured tendons is far more difficult and less rewarding than prevention of the ruptures by early synovectomy.

E. Rheumatoid synovitis will destroy articular cartilage and surrounding supporting tissue. This synovitis may cause nerve compression lesions, especially at the elbow (posterior interosseous nerve). Progressive deformity of unstable joints is the result of normal and abnormal forces crossing the joint. The potential for swan-neck deformity, boutonniere deformity, and various collapse patterns must be recognized early and appropriate splinting initiated. In the case of rheumatoid synovitis of the metacarpophalangeal joints, these joints should be splinted in extension to prevent excessive laxity of the collateral ligaments. The wrist should be maintained in neutral and the interphalangeal joints in extension. Maintenance of the thumb web space, and the thumb in palmar abduction is also important.

F. If medical therapy does not control the synovitis, and if the articular cartilage is not yet eroded, synovectomy may control local disease. Postoperative therapy is demanding, but if carried out by a motivated patient, the results can be rewarding. In most situations, damage to the articular surfaces is already significant and the selection of reconstructive procedures is less clear.

## REFERENCE

1. Flatt AE. *Care of the Arthritic Hand*. St. Louis: CV Mosby, 1983.

RHEUMATOID ARTHRITIS

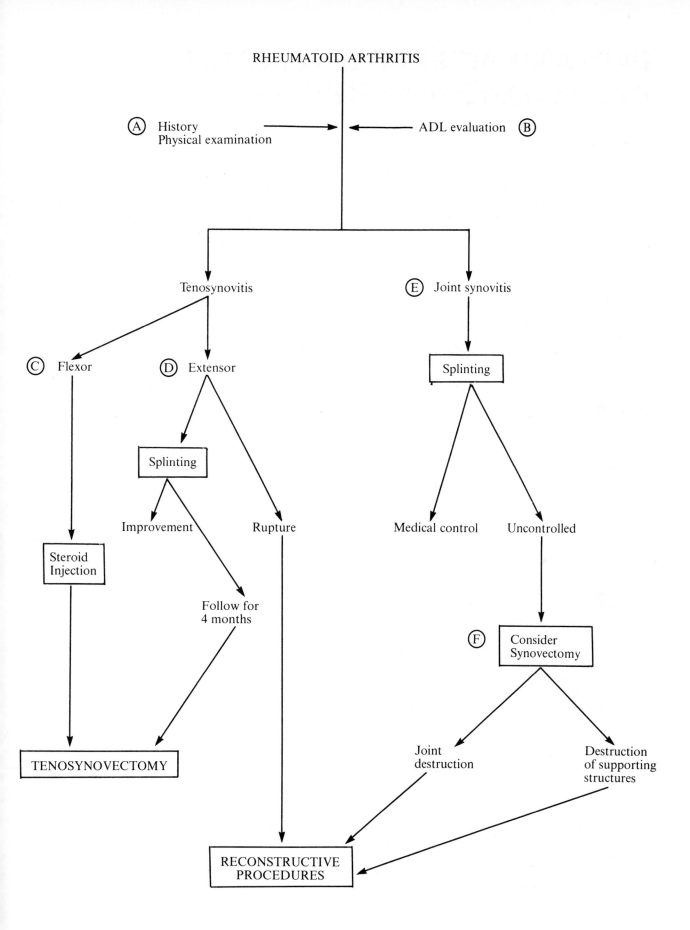

ⒶHistory
Physical examination

ⒷADL evaluation

Tenosynovitis

ⒺJoint synovitis

ⒸFlexor

ⒹExtensor

Splinting

Splinting

Improvement

Rupture

Medical control

Uncontrolled

Steroid
Injection

Follow for
4 months

ⒻConsider
Synovectomy

TENOSYNOVECTOMY

Joint
destruction

Destruction
of supporting
structures

RECONSTRUCTIVE
PROCEDURES

ADL = activities of daily living

# PAIN AND ALTERED SENSATION IN THE HAND AND FOREARM

## INTRODUCTION

The differential diagnosis of pain in the hand and forearm is one of the most difficult in medicine. By no means is this algorithm meant to be comprehensive, but rather to point out some of the common and uncommon diagnoses, and to demonstrate the wide variety of etiologies producing altered sensation.

Sensations are described, at best, inexactly. Often overlap of sensations, such as numbness in combination with aching pain in the case of a compression neuropathy, makes categorization and differential diagnosis based on the nature of the sensory abnormality very arbitrary. No attempt is made here to separate etiologies based on the nature of the altered sensation.

## COMMENTS

In addition to obtaining a complete and accurate history about the nature of the symptoms, inquiry should be made regarding previous trauma, similar complaints in other family members, status of general health, nutritional status, recent weight loss, symptoms of visceral malignancy, exposure to industrial toxins or solvents, exposure to heavy metals, current medications especially chemotherapeutic agents, relationship of symptoms to cold exposure and exertion, and associated cardiac symptoms.

The examination of the upper extremity should test all sensory modalities, particularly position and vibration sense. Note should be made of the presence or absence of sweating, trophic skin changes, atrophy, skin or nail lesions, and muscle strength and reflexes. Ataxia and astereognosis should also be looked for. Examination of the neck and cervical spine is frequently indicated and examination of the lower extremities is often helpful.

Many conditions can be readily diagnosed by a classic presentation, such as a carpal tunnel syndrome or a subungual glomus tumor (the former being far more common than the latter), but other diagnoses are more obscure. Clinical judgment must guide the selection of laboratory and diagnostic procedures. A CBC and sedimentation rate, and SMA 12 profile to check serum glucose, uric acid, creatinine, and liver functions along with a chest radiograph are a useful start. EMGs and nerve conduction velocities are helpful, but should not supplant careful physical examination. Metrizamide myelography often can define nerve root or cord pathology.

Pain and altered sensation in the hand and upper extremity arise from an array of disorders whose accurate diagnosis and treatment involve many medical and surgical specialties. Early consultation best serves the interest of the patient when the diagnosis is elusive or when the suspected diagnosis is out of the realm of one's expert treatment. The "trial of vitamins and physical therapy" approach without a diagnosis has no place in the treatment of these disorders.

## REFERENCES

Beeson PB, McDermott W, Wyngaarden JP (eds). Cecil Textbook of Medicine. 15th Ed. Philadelphia: WB Saunders, 1979.

Omer G E. Management of the painful extremity. Curr Pract Orthop Surg. 1977; 8:86–98.

Spengler D, Kirsch MM, Kaufer H. Orthopaedic aspects and early diagnosis of superior sulcus tumor of lung (Pancoast). J Bone Joint Surg. 1973; 55:1645–1650.

# PAIN AND ALTERED SENSATION IN THE HAND AND FOREARM

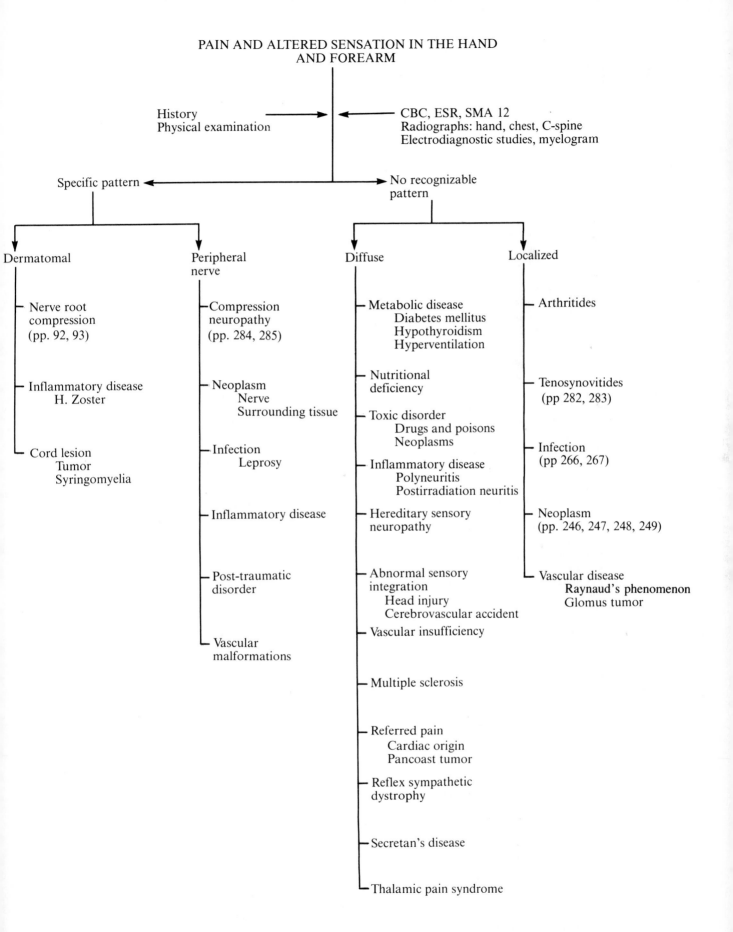

History
Physical examination

CBC, ESR, SMA 12
Radiographs: hand, chest, C-spine
Electrodiagnostic studies, myelogram

Specific pattern

No recognizable pattern

## Dermatomal

- Nerve root compression (pp. 92, 93)

- Inflammatory disease
  H. Zoster

- Cord lesion
  Tumor
  Syringomyelia

## Peripheral nerve

- Compression neuropathy (pp. 284, 285)

- Neoplasm
  Nerve
  Surrounding tissue

- Infection
  Leprosy

- Inflammatory disease

- Post-traumatic disorder

- Vascular malformations

## Diffuse

- Metabolic disease
  Diabetes mellitus
  Hypothyroidism
  Hyperventilation

- Nutritional deficiency

- Toxic disorder
  Drugs and poisons
  Neoplasms

- Inflammatory disease
  Polyneuritis
  Postirradiation neuritis

- Hereditary sensory neuropathy

- Abnormal sensory integration
  Head injury
  Cerebrovascular accident

- Vascular insufficiency

- Multiple sclerosis

- Referred pain
  Cardiac origin
  Pancoast tumor

- Reflex sympathetic dystrophy

- Secretan's disease

- Thalamic pain syndrome

## Localized

- Arthritides

- Tenosynovitides (pp 282, 283)

- Infection (pp 266, 267)

- Neoplasm (pp. 246, 247, 248, 249)

- Vascular disease
  **Raynaud's phenomenon**
  Glomus tumor

# INDEX